RACIAL AND ETHNIC DISPARITIES IN HEALTH AND HEALTH CARE

RACIAL AND ETHNIC DISPARITIES IN HEALTH AND HEALTH CARE

ELENE V. METROSA
EDITOR

Nova Science Publishers, Inc.
New York

Library of Congress Cataloging-in-Publication Data
Racial and ethnic disparities in health and healthcare / Elene V. Metrosa (editor).
    p. ; cm.
Includes bibliographical references and index.
ISBN 1-60021-268-9
1. Health services accessibility. 2. Discrimination in medical care. 3. Minorities--Medical care.
I. Metrosa, Elene V.
[DNLM: 1. Health Services Accessibility--United States. 2. Health Status--United States. 3. Ethnic Groups--United States. 4. Minority Groups--United States. 5. Socioeconomic Factors--United States. WA 300 R121 2006]
RA418.3.U6R33   2006
362.1089--dc22   2006017213

Published by Nova Science Publishers, Inc. ✥ *New York*

CONTENTS

69391439

PREFACE

It is generally conceded that there are significant disparities in health and health care based on a person's racial and ethnic background. Infant mortality rates for black babies remain nearly two-and-one-half times higher than for whites. The life expectancy for black men and women remains at nearly one decade fewer years of life compared with their white counterparts. Rates of death attributable to heart disease, stroke, prostate and breast cancer remain much higher in black populations. Diabetes disease rates are more than 30 percent higher among Native Americans and Hispanics than among whites. Minorities remain grossly under-represented in the health professions workforce relative to their proportions in the population. In addition, despite a large and growing body of scientific evidence, many patients and providers remain unaware that racial and ethnic health care disparities are a problem and perceptions about health care inequalities vary between minorities and whites. closing the disparity gap. This new book presents new research focusing on these disparities.

Numerous studies have examined racial and ethnic disparities in the treatment of pain. Although some research shows no difference in analgesic care for patients of various racial and ethnic backgrounds, the majority of studies in this area suggest that minorities are more likely than White patients to be undertreated for pain. Chapter 1 provides a comprehensive review of the literature related to racial/ethnic disparities in pain treatment, summarizing the results of published research, discussing discrepancies among studies, and outlining the mechanisms hypothesized to underlie disparities in analgesic care. In addition, this chapter describes an original study designed to examine racial and ethnic disparities in the pain outcomes of elderly home health care recipients. A large, nationally representative sample of home health care episodes was used to examine pain outcomes for White, Black, and Hispanic home health care recipients age 65 and older. Racial/ethnic differences in two outcome measures were assessed: (1) improvement in the frequency of pain and (2) hospitalization for the treatment of uncontrolled pain. Holding demographic characteristics and baseline health status constant, no racial/ethnic differences in the rate at which patients were hospitalized for the treatment of uncontrolled pain were identified. Although Hispanic and White patients did not differ in the rate of improvement in pain frequency, Whites were found to have a significantly lower rate of improvement than Black patients after controlling for potentially confounding factors (58.6% vs. 60.3%, respectively). Although statistically significant, however, this small difference is unlikely to be clinically meaningful and is hypothesized to be related to the greater severity of pain among White patients, in comparison with Black patients, at the start or resumption of care. The unique characteristics of home health care that may serve to diminish the likelihood of racial and ethnic differences in pain management are discussed.

Limited research has been done to examine emergency department (ED) admissions as a percentage all hospital admissions and to assess the trends in ED utilization over time. The objective of chapter 2 is to examine relationships between ED utilization, race, insurance status and access to care. To identify priority conditions upon which to explore implications for access and quality improvement efforts. Cross-sectional data of over 19 million patients hospitalized in the 1995-2001 National Inpatient Sample were weighted to reflect national totals. Percent and likelihood of ED admission among all hospital admission in general and as related to race, insurance status, specific clinical conditions, length of stay, and mortality rates. Percentages of hospital admissions through the ED has progressively increased over time; specifically as related to 16 clinical conditions, mostly chronic. Decreased utilization has been noted for diseases that have been focal points of improvement efforts (e.g., heart failure, acute myocardial infarction, asthma, and cerebral occlusion) while other conditions have shown increased utilization. Disparities of constant magnitude were noted with respect to race and most categories of insurance status. Disparities of increasing magnitude were observed with respect to the uninsured. While trends regarding mortality and length of stay have shown improvements, disparities persisted, especially with respect to the uninsured. Access to care was a significant etiologic factor with areas having higher provider to population ratios showing reduced ED utilization. Quality improvement efforts need to promote evidence based approaches to chronic conditions where increased ED utilization has been demonstrated including diabetes mellitus and affective psychosis. Access to care by promoting optimal provider to population ratios needs to be prioritized as a cost effective, quality improvement measure. Access to care for uninsured populations should be improved by expansion of availability of insurance benefits.

American ethnic minorities, particularly those of African and Hispanic descent have a greater risk of developing hypertension and type 2 diabetes compared to American Whites. Despite the consistency of the epidemiologic evidence of the racial/ethnic variation for these diseases, relatively little is known with confidence about the causes of the non-White dilemma. The objective of chapter 3 is to determine how much of the relative difference in the rates of hypertension and type 2 diabetes between high-risk Blacks and Hispanics and low-risk Whites is attributable to their differences in obesity. Data (n=5531) from the 1999-2002 U.S. National Health and Nutrition Examination Surveys were utilized for this analysis. Gender-specific proportions of White to non-White differences in odds of hypertension and diabetes that were due to their relative differences in the prevalence of obesity were estimated using relative attributable risk derived from multiple logistic regression modeling. Statistical adjustment was made for age, education, alcohol intake, education, and physical activity. 50.2% and 30.6% of differences in odds of hypertension between White men and Black men and between White men and Hispanic men, respectively, are attributable to their differences in rates of obesity. The analogous values for diabetes were 70.7% and 57.4% for Black men and Hispanic men. Also, 30.6 % and 13.4% of differences in odds of hypertension between White women and Black women and between White women and Hispanic women, respectively, are associated with their differences in rates of obesity. The analogous values for diabetes are 62.2% and 83.7% for Black women and Hispanic women when compared with White women. The magnitude of racial/ethnic differences in hypertension and diabetes due to their differences in obesity provides an encouraging reason to continue to implement public health obesity prevention programs in the United States' minority groups. Aggressive programs to reduce obesity and increase physical activity in Blacks and Hispanics may prove useful in reducing racial/ethnic disparities in hypertension and diabetes.

The genetic constituents of all human races are exceedingly similar, and racial diversity only accounts for less than 5 % of the overall genetic variations within our entire species. Nevertheless, this subtle difference is associated with an apparent asymmetry in health-related problems across the races. Chapter 4 focuses on the biological basis for the racial disparities in health and diseases, which will be interpreted from an evolutionary perspective. Firstly, the uneven distribution of genetic diseases among different ethnic groups can be attributed to some chance events in human history. This is illustrated by the aggregation of certain uncommon mutations in Ashkenazi Jews. Conversely, racially or geographically circumscribed diseases may merely reflect the pathogenic influences from environmental or cultural factors, rather than genuine race-specific biological differences. The examples used are haemorrhagic stroke in East Asians, megaloblastic anaemia in South Asians, kuru, and Japanese encephalitis. To enhance survival in the natural environment, our ancestors evolved adaptive mechanisms against the various environmental threats through natural selection. Therefore, the genetic compositions of different population groups may be modified by the specific selection pressures within their habitats. Relevant examples include the "anti-AIDS gene" *CCR5-Δ32* and the population pattern of pharmacogenetic polymorphisms. However, besides promoting successes in survival and reproduction, adaptive traits may be associated with tradeoffs that can result in human diseases. Moreover, relaxation of selection pressures upon urbanization can produce discordance between our biological makeup and the modern lifestyle. Such maladaptations are manifested as the so-called "diseases of civilization" or "afflictions of affluence". This is illustrated by the propensity for hypertension in African Americans and ethnic differences in susceptibility to diabetes mellitus.

The purpose of chapter 5 was to examine racial differences in the risk and protective factors for the initiation and maintenance of cigarette smoking during varying developmental periods from childhood through late adolescence. We used data from a sample of 503 males who were first recruited in the first grade and followed annually for 14 years. Trajectory analyses identified three trajectory groups for African Americans and whites: nonsmokers, light smokers, and regular smokers. The following domains of risk and protective factors were included in the analyses: individual [hyperactivity/impulsivity/attention problem (HIA), depression, attitudes toward substance use, school performance, delinquency frequency, and religiosity], family (parental smoking and relationship with parents), peer (peer delinquency), and environmental [socioeconomic status (SES) and neighborhood quality]. First analyses were conducted separately by race to determine which factors represented risk and which represented protection. Then hierarchical logistic regression analyses were conducted to determine how these factors differentiated among the three trajectory groups and whether race interacted with these factors. Many of the variables were both risk and protective factors across different developmental periods. School performance and religiosity were only significantly related to smoking for African Americans and SES was only related for whites. For both races HIA, depression, delinquency, and peer delinquency were significantly related to smoking. In the multivariate analyses, race, SES, and delinquency were related to smoking at younger ages and delinquent peers was related to smoking at all ages. Only four interactions with race were significant for smoking. Good school performance was protective for African Americans at ages 7-9, but not whites. Having many delinquent peers was a stronger risk factor for African Americans at ages 13-16, but having many at ages 17-19 was a risk factor only for whites. Being low in delinquency was a stronger protective factor for whites at ages 13-16. Depression was related to regular smoking only for African Americans and attitudes toward substance use, parental smoking, and neighborhood quality were related only for whites. For both races HIA, school performance, delinquency, and peer delinquency were related to regular smoking. In the multivariate analyses, being African American protected against regular smoking at all ages. Only one interaction was significant; low depression was a protective factor for African American but not white regular smoking. Overall, the fact that there were few significant interactions of risk and protective factors with race suggests that the same factors can be targeted for both whites and African Americans in cigarette prevention programs.

Racial and ethnic disparities in American health and healthcare are becoming increasingly apparent and are garnering a growing body of research attention (e.g., La Viest, 2005). These disparities are particularly problematic regarding mental health service delivery to multicultural populations (Snowden and Yamada, 2005; U.S. Department of Health and Human Services, 2001). Chapter 6 explores a variety of key parameters associated with the Multicultural Assessment Intervention Process (MAIP) model proposed by Dana (1993, 1998, 2000) and Dana, Aragon, and Kramer, (2002). This model provides a mental health agency and its practitioners with the necessary conceptual scaffolding and theoretical clarity to address service delivery disparities by positing that mental health consumers are best served when factors such as (1) consumer-provider ethnic/racial match, (2) consumer acculturation status and/or ethnic/racial identity, and (3) provider cultural competence are assessed and factored into the treatment process and clinical outcome. Toward this end, a sample of 123 university counseling center consumers was measured on the 4 previous independent variables (i.e., ethnic/racial match, acculturation status, ethnic identity, and staff cultural competence). Five clinical outcome dependent measures were assessed including Global Assessment of Function (GAF) pre and post treatment differences, and 4 subscales of the Brief Psychiatric Rating Scale (BPRS): Thinking Disturbance, Withdrawal/Retardation, Hostile-Suspicious, and Anxious-Depression, all of which served as dependent variables. A 2 x 2 x 2 x 2 factorial between-subjects multivariate analysis of covariance (MANCOVA) indicated a statistically significant multivariate interaction effect between Ethnic Match x Client Acculturation x Client Ethnic Identity for the BPRS-thinking disturbance measure. Implications for the MAIP model with this college student population are discussed.

The continuing racial and ethnic diversification of the youth population in the United States necessitates greater understanding of issues related to the delivery of appropriate youth mental health services. There is a dire need for greater research in this area, and recent studies have begun to form a strong foundation of knowledge regarding mental health service delivery for various racial and ethnic groups. Chapter 7 will review the empirical literature on racial and ethnic disparities in mental health care use, treatment retention, and outcomes for youth across a variety of service types (e.g., inpatient services, outpatient services, school-based services, clinical trials). Barriers that may explain racial and ethnic disparities in mental health care will be reviewed, and a model illustrating the influence of barriers in creating and sustaining disparities in the mental health treatment process will be introduced. Recent public policy documents highlighting the nation's priority upon addressing racial/ethnic disparities in mental health care for youth will be identified, and recommendations for future directions in research and clinical practice will be discussed.

Chapter 8 provides a brief overview of the devastating impact of drug abuse on many poor and/or minority American families. While all groups experience drug abuse and its negative consequences, research has classified individuals into broad groups that include Native Americans (which include American Indians and Alaska Natives), Hispanics, and African Americans. Within each broad minority grouping, fall many distinct ethnic populations; however for research purposes these groups are placed into these broad categories. Research has found that the adverse health consequences related to drug abuse and the associated violence are experienced disproportionately by members of minority groups. In this paper, drug abuse among the poor and specific minority groups will be examined with the following statements in mind:

- The relatively greater threat of drug use and its consequences for poor and minority adults and youth
- The reduced likelihood of drug abuse treatment and the inferior medical treatment of the poor and minority populations
- The greater risk of drug-related HIV/AIDS infection in these populations
- The developmental complexities observed among children residing in poor and/or minority families and their connections to drug abuse

In: Racial and Ethnic Disparities in Health and Health Care   ISBN 1-60021-268-9
Editor: Elene V. Metrosa, pp. 1-39   © 2006 Nova Science Publishers, Inc.

Chapter 1

THE EFFECT OF RACE AND ETHNICITY ON PAIN OUTCOMES AMONG ELDERLY HOME HEALTH CARE RECIPIENTS

*Angela G. Brega**

Division of Health Care Policy and Research, Department of Medicine,
University of Colorado at Denver and Health Sciences Center, Aurora, CO

ABSTRACT

Numerous studies have examined racial and ethnic disparities in the treatment of pain. Although some research shows no difference in analgesic care for patients of various racial and ethnic backgrounds, the majority of studies in this area suggest that minorities are more likely than White patients to be undertreated for pain. This chapter provides a comprehensive review of the literature related to racial/ethnic disparities in pain treatment, summarizing the results of published research, discussing discrepancies among studies, and outlining the mechanisms hypothesized to underlie disparities in analgesic care. In addition, this chapter describes an original study designed to examine racial and ethnic disparities in the pain outcomes of elderly home health care recipients. A large, nationally representative sample of home health care episodes was used to examine pain outcomes for White, Black, and Hispanic home health care recipients age 65 and older. Racial/ethnic differences in two outcome measures were assessed: (1) improvement in the frequency of pain and (2) hospitalization for the treatment of uncontrolled pain. Holding demographic characteristics and baseline health status constant, no racial/ethnic differences in the rate at which patients were hospitalized for the treatment of uncontrolled pain were identified. Although Hispanic and White patients did not differ in the rate of improvement in pain frequency, Whites were found to have a significantly lower rate of improvement than Black patients after controlling for potentially confounding factors (58.6% vs. 60.3%, respectively). Although statistically significant, however, this small difference is unlikely to be clinically meaningful and is hypothesized to be related to the greater severity of pain among White patients, in comparison with Black patients, at the start or resumption of care. The unique characteristics of home

* Phone: 303-724-2445; Fax: 303-724-2530; E-Mail: angela.brega@uchsc.edu

health care that may serve to diminish the likelihood of racial and ethnic differences in pain management are discussed.

INTRODUCTION

Despite the availability of powerful analgesic medications and practice guidelines designed to optimize pain control (e.g., Stjernsward, 1988; U.S. Department of Health and Human Services, 1992), undertreatment of pain is a common problem (e.g., Desbiens et al., 1996; Green, Wheeler, LaPorte, Marchant, and Guerrero, 2002; Selbst and Clark, 1990; Von Roenn, Cleeland, Gonin, Hatfield, and Pandya, 1993). Some research suggests that patients of minority racial or ethnic backgrounds may be particularly likely to experience inadequate pain management, a condition referred to as "oligoanalgesia" (e.g., Bernabei et al., 1998; Cleeland et al., 1994; Todd, Samaroo, and Hoffman, 1993). This chapter provides a comprehensive review of the literature related to racial and ethnic disparities in pain management. The results of published studies are summarized, discrepancies are discussed, and the mechanisms hypothesized to underlie disparities in analgesic treatment are outlined. (Throughout this chapter, the term "White" denotes patients of non-Hispanic White origin, "Black" refers to those of Black or African American descent, and "Hispanic" refers to anyone identified as Hispanic or Latino.)

In addition to synthesizing the literature, this chapter describes an original study examining racial/ethnic differences in the pain outcomes of elderly home health care recipients. Although disparities in the physical, functional, and psychiatric outcomes of home care services have been reported (Brega, Goodrich, Powell, and Grigsby, 2005; Peng, Navaie-Waliser, and Feldman, 2003), the relationship between patient race/ethnicity and pain outcomes has not been addressed. This study makes an important contribution to the literature by examining pain outcomes in a health care setting in which (1) racial and ethnic disparities in pain management have not been studied, (2) the patient population is largely elderly, a group found to be at high risk for undertreatment of pain (e.g., Bernabei et al., 1998; Cleeland et al., 1994), and (3) the nature of the interaction between care provider and patient is quite different from settings in which disparities in pain management have been reported.

LITERATURE REVIEW

The medical literature contains approximately two dozen papers examining the relationship between patient race/ethnicity and the treatment of pain. Although previous reviews of this research have emphasized studies demonstrating racial/ethnic differences in analgesic treatment (Bonham, 2001; Green et al., 2003; Meghani, 2005; Tait and Chibnall, 2005; Smedley, Stith, and Nelson, 2003; Sullivan and Eagel, 2005; Todd, 2001), a number of investigations have provided no evidence of such disparities. Papers reporting both positive and negative findings are summarized below.

Studies Showing Racial/Ethnic Disparities in Pain Management

A number of papers reporting racial and ethnic disparities in the management of pain have been published in the medical literature. These studies have assessed analgesic treatment in a variety of health care settings: (1) the emergency department (ED), (2) inpatient settings, (3) specialty cancer practices, and (4) primary care settings. The underlying medical conditions targeted in these studies also vary considerably and include fractures, post-operative care, childbirth, cancer, and chronic pain.

Management of Pain in the Emergency Department

Many of the studies that have examined racial and ethnic disparities in the treatment of pain have focused on care provided in the ED. Of these studies, several have shown differences in the way minority patients are treated in comparison with their White counterparts. In two well-known studies, Todd and his colleagues found disparities in the treatment of pain for patients presenting with long bone fractures. In a retrospective chart review conducted at the University of California at Los Angeles Emergency Medicine Center, Todd, Samaroo, and Hoffman (1993) examined the prescription of analgesics to Hispanic and White patients. The investigators found that Hispanic patients presenting with long bone fractures were twice as likely as Whites to receive no analgesic medications. In fact, after controlling for patient characteristics (sex, language, insurance), physician characteristics (ethnicity, sex, specialty), severity of injury (need for admission, open fracture, need for reduction), and potential for ethanol intoxication (time of presentation, occupational injury, mechanism of injury), Hispanic ethnicity was the strongest predictor of the receipt of no analgesic medication.

To ensure that their findings did not simply reflect isolated, institution-specific ethnic differences in the management of pain, Todd, Deaton, D'Adamo, and Goe (2000) conducted a second study examining racial differences in the treatment of pain at an urban ED in Atlanta, Georgia. In this retrospective chart review of patients presenting with isolated long bone fractures, the investigators found that Black patients were significantly less likely than White patients to receive analgesics in the ED (57% vs. 74%, respectively). Although complaints of pain were recorded in the medical records of Black and White patients with equal frequency, the risk of receiving no analgesic medications was 66% higher for Blacks than Whites after controlling for time since injury, total time in the ED, shift of presentation, need for reduction, and payer status. The investigators did not find racial differences in the receipt of parenteral medications or in the receipt of narcotics.

In 2002, Hostetler, Auinger, and Szilagyi examined racial/ethnic differences in the receipt of parenteral analgesic and sedative (PAS) in ED settings. The investigators examined disparities using six years of data collected as part of the National Hospital Ambulatory Medical Care Survey, a large nationally representative sample of hospital encounters. Examining pediatric and adult ED visits related to orthopedic injuries and wounds, the authors found Black race to be a significant risk factor for not receiving PAS. Black children covered by Medicaid appeared to be at particular risk for undertreatment of pain in the ED.

A second study using data from the National Hospital Ambulatory Medical Care Survey also found evidence for disparities in the treatment of pain in the ED. Tamayo-Sarver, Hinze, Cydulka, and Baker (2003b) investigated racial and ethnic disparities in ED analgesic care for 67,487 patients presenting with long bone fractures, migraine, or back pain. All analyses controlled for patient age and sex, insurance coverage, diagnoses, severity of injury, visit characteristics (e.g., discharge status), and hospital characteristics (e.g., urban versus rural). Although there were no racial or ethnic differences in the probability of receiving analgesics of any kind, Black patients were less likely than Whites to receive opioids for migraine or back pain (there were no racial or ethnic differences for patients presenting with long bone fractures). Hispanics did not differ from Whites in the receipt of opioids, although the investigators acknowledged that the small sample of Hispanics may have impeded the finding of significant results.

Management of Pain in the Inpatient Setting

Most studies of analgesic care in the inpatient setting have focused on post-operative pain. Several such studies have demonstrated racial and ethnic disparities in treatment. In 1981, Streltzer and Wade examined pain management in two hospitals located in Honolulu. Controlling for age, sex, pre-operative condition, time under anesthesia, number of post-operative hospital days, hospital, ward, and surgeon race, the authors found evidence for disparities in analgesic dose. Although the post-operative orders were quite similar for all patients, White and Hawaiian patients received significantly larger doses of parenteral narcotics during the first five post-operative days than did Japanese, Chinese, and Filipino patients. The investigators found that nurses often administered lower doses of medication than were ordered. Streltzer and Wade (1981) speculated that patients of Asian descent may have been more stoic about the severity of their pain and that the nursing staff may therefore have been particularly successful at limiting narcotic doses for this group of patients.

In 1994, McDonald obtained similar results in a study of pain treatment following appendectomy. The study's author retrospectively reviewed the medical charts of 180 patients from three teaching hospitals in New England. Although there were no racial/ethnic differences in the initial post-operative narcotic dose, differences in total post-operative narcotic dose were identified. Controlling for patient sex as well as the hospital in which care was provided, McDonald found that White patients received significantly larger doses of narcotics over the entire post-operative period than did minorities (a single comparison group combining Black, Hispanic, and Asian patients).

Ng and colleagues conducted two studies of the management of post-operative pain. Ng, Dimsdale, Shragg, and Deutsch (1996b) conducted retrospective reviews of the medical charts of 250 patients hospitalized for open reduction and internal fixation following limb fracture. Focusing on the initial post-operative period (the first seven days following surgery), the average dose of narcotics per day was computed for each patient. The investigators reported that White patients received a significantly higher narcotic dose per day than did Hispanic patients. Hispanics received approximately 60% of the dose that White patients received. Although Whites received a larger average daily dose of narcotics than did Blacks, this difference was not significant. (As the Black sample included in the study was quite small [36], the investigators may not have had enough statistical power to identify differences involving this group.)

To tease apart the effects of patient pain-related behavior and provider perception of pain, Ng and his colleagues sought to study the treatment of pain in a context in which patient-provider interaction is minimized. Ng, Dimsdale, Rollnik, and Shapiro (1996a) reported a study examining the relationship between race/ethnicity and pain management in a sample of 454 patients receiving patient-controlled analgesia (PCA) for post-operative pain. Although there were no significant racial/ethnic differences in the level of pain reported, nor in the amount of narcotics self-administered, there were significant differences in the narcotic doses prescribed to patients of different racial and ethnic groups. Controlling for age, patient gender, pre-operative use of narcotics, site of pain, and insurance status, doctors prescribed a significantly larger dose of narcotics for White than Hispanic patients and for Black than Hispanic and Asian patients. Although doctors prescribed a slightly higher dose of narcotics for Black than White patients, this difference was not significant.

Research also has suggested the presence of disparities in the treatment of pain associated with childbirth. Obst, Nauenberg, and Buck (2001) examined records for 121,351 births in New York with the goal of determining the influence of insurance coverage on the provision of epidural analgesia. Although insurance coverage was a significant predictor of the receipt of epidural pain medication, patient race influenced the use of epidural analgesia as well. Controlling for educational attainment, facility characteristics, and insurance coverage, Black women were significantly less likely than White women to receive epidural pain medication.

In 2004, Atherton, Feeg, and El-Adham explored the influence of race, ethnicity, and insurance coverage on the provision of epidural analgesia during childbirth. The investigators examined Medical Expenditure Panel Survey data for a nationally representative sample of 1,003 women with normal singleton deliveries. Controlling for age, pregnancy complications, and insurance type, the authors found that Hispanic women were twice as likely as Whites to go without epidural pain medication.

Management of Cancer Pain

The inadequate management of pain related to cancer has been widely reported in the literature (e.g., Bernabei et al., 1998; Cleeland et al., 1994). Some research has shown minority cancer patients to be at particular risk for oligoanalgesia. In two well-known studies, Cleeland and his colleagues examined the treatment of pain among cancer patients seen in outpatient settings. In 1994, Cleeland et al. assessed the severity and impact of pain for 1,308 cancer patients receiving treatment from cancer subspecialists in one of 54 health care settings affiliated with the Eastern Cooperative Oncology Group (ECOG). Controlling for potentially confounding factors, the investigators found that patients seen at centers that primarily treated minority populations (generally, of Black and Hispanic descent) were three times more likely to receive inadequate treatment for pain than were patients seen at centers primarily treating White patients. The authors also found older patients to be at greater risk of inadequate analgesic treatment.

In 1997, Cleeland, Gonin, Baez, Loehrer, and Pandya further examined disparities in the treatment of cancer pain across racial/ethnic groups. The investigators compared analgesic care in a sample of 281 minority patients (primarily Blacks and Hispanics) to the treatment received by the primarily White sample from the prior study conducted by Cleeland and his colleagues (i.e., patients treated in clinical settings primarily serving White patients; Cleeland et al., 1994). Controlling for confounding variables, the investigators reported that minority patients experiencing pain were less likely than patients in the primarily White sample to receive guideline-appropriate analgesic treatment.

In 1998, Bernabei and his colleagues examined the management of cancer pain among nursing home residents. Controlling for patient gender, cognitive status, communication skills, and severity of disease (terminal condition, bedridden, number of diagnoses, use of other medications), White patients in daily pain were significantly more likely than similar

Blacks to receive analgesic medication. Blacks had a 63% increased probability of receiving no medications for the treatment of pain. Although the pattern of results was similar when comparing Asian and Hispanic patients to their White counterparts, these differences were not statistically significant (perhaps due to the small sizes of these minority samples). The investigators also found that age predicted the receipt of analgesic medications. Among those in daily pain, older residents were less likely than their younger counterparts to receive any form of analgesia.

Management of Pain in the Primary Care Setting

The majority of studies examining racial and ethnic disparities in the treatment of pain have focused on treatment in the ED, inpatient settings, or cancer specialty clinics. Little research is available on disparities in the treatment of pain in the primary care setting. In 2005, Chen et al. examined pain treatment received by 397 chronic pain patients seen in the primary care clinics of 12 academic medical centers. Analyses controlled for age, patient sex, pain severity and duration, comorbid conditions, disability status, type of insurance, hours worked per week, annual income, years of schooling, and physician status (resident or attending). Although Blacks had significantly higher pain scores than did Whites, they were significantly less likely to receive opioids, particularly the more powerful and longer-acting varieties. The investigators found no differences in the use of nonopioid medications, physical therapy, or referral to pain specialist services.

Studies Showing No Evidence of Racial/Ethnic Disparities in Pain Management

Although many studies have shown disparities in pain treatment, a number of investigators have reported no racial or ethnic differences in the management of pain. Studies showing no relationship between race/ethnicity and analgesia have focused on the treatment of pain in the ED or have used experimental methods rather than assessing pain management in real clinical settings.

Management of Pain in the Emergency Department

Several studies have shown no racial or ethnic differences in the treatment of pain in the ED. Like the previously summarized studies conducted by Todd et al. (1993, 2000), four studies showing no evidence of disparities examined the management of pain in ED patients presenting with fractures. Fuentes, Kohn, and Neighbor (2002) studied racial and ethnic differences in the receipt of any analgesic medications and parenteral analgesics. The investigators reviewed the charts of 323 patients admitted to the San Francisco General Hospital ED. Controlling for the need for reduction, size of the bone fractured, and patient sex, race/ethnicity was not a significant predictor of the receipt of pain medication. The proportion of patients receiving analgesics and parenteral analgesics was equivalent for Whites and minorities (Blacks and Hispanics combined).

Karpman, Del Mar, and Bay (1997) studied pain treatment in the general and pediatric EDs at Maricopa Medical Center in Phoenix, AZ. The investigators examined the medical records of 84 adults presenting with isolated long bone fractures and 63 children with isolated closed distal radius and/or ulna fractures. Controlling for the need for reduction, Hispanic and White adults did not differ significantly in the probability of receiving analgesic medications or in the dose of medication received. No significant differences in receipt or dose of analgesics were found in the pediatric sample either. Although work conducted by Cleeland and his colleagues (1994, 1997) suggests otherwise, the investigators speculated that institutions serving a large population of minorities, such as Maricopa Medical Center, may be less likely to undertreat pain in these patients. The authors acknowledged, however, that sample size was a limitation of their study.

Two studies of pain management in children presenting with fractures in the ED also showed no racial or ethnic differences. Friedland and Kulick (1994) examined the trauma registry records of 99 children treated at a single pediatric ED for fractures of the pelvis, long bones, ankle, wrist, or clavicle. Although the authors noted a fairly low rate of analgesic use in their sample, which is consistent with other research suggesting that children may be undertreated for pain (e.g., Karpman et al., 1997; Petrack, Christopher, and Kriwinsky, 1997; Selbst and Clark, 1990), no racial differences were found in the probability of receiving analgesic medications in the ED.

Using data from the National Hospital Ambulatory Medical Care Survey, Yen, Kim, Stremski, and Gorelick (2003) examined racial and ethnic differences in the use of analgesia in the ED for a nationally-representative sample of 1,030 children treated for long bone fractures. Controlling for age, insurance type, hospital ownership, geographic region, survey year, and metropolitan status, the investigators found no racial or ethnic differences in the receipt of analgesics or in the receipt of opioid analgesics. Regional differences in analgesic use were identified, however. The authors suggest that earlier studies showing evidence of racial and ethnic disparities in the management of pain in the ED have reflected inequities isolated to single institutions and that these disparities are not present at the national level. It is noteworthy, however, that the findings of this study are not corroborated by two previously summarized studies that used the same national data set to examine racial and ethnic differences in the treatment of pain in the ED (Hostetler et al., 2002; Tamayo-Sarver et al., 2003b).

A prospective study of analgesic treatment provided to adult patients in the ED at Albany Medical Center Hospital showed no racial or ethnic differences in the management of pain. Bartfield, Salluzzo, Raccio-Robak, Funk, and Verdile (1997) examined the administration of analgesic medications to 91 adults presenting with non-traumatic low back pain. Analyses controlled for age, insurance coverage, and patient gender. Although the proportion of minorities who received analgesics appeared to be quite a bit smaller than the proportion of White patients receiving treatment for pain (28% versus 44%, respectively), race/ethnicity was not a statistically significant predictor of pain management. The authors acknowledge that the small sample size (59 White and 32 minority patients) may have reduced statistical power.

Experimental Studies of Pain Management

Three studies have used experimental designs to examine racial and ethnic disparities in the treatment of pain. In 2001, Weisse, Sorum, Sanders, and Syat assessed racial differences in the pain management decisions of 111 primary care physicians in the Northeastern United States. Physicians participating in the study reviewed three hypothetical patient vignettes, for which race (Black or White) and gender were varied. For two vignettes, one describing a patient with kidney stones and the other describing a patient with a back injury, pain was the primary complaint. A third vignette focused on a patient with sinusitis and served to disguise the objective of the study. Controlling for physician age and years in practice as well as patient gender, patient race, and physician race (and the interactions of these three variables), the investigators found no overall effect of race on the total dose of hydrocodone prescribed for the kidney stone or back injury vignettes.

Racial differences in treatment did appear when physician gender was considered (Weisse et al., 2001). In reviewing the vignette of the hypothetical patient suffering from kidney stone pain, female doctors prescribed larger doses of opioids to Black than White patients, whereas male physicians prescribed larger doses to Whites than Blacks. Because the physician sample in this study was evenly split by gender (55% male, 45% female), this interaction between patient race and physician gender eliminated any overall effect of patient race on pain management decisions. The investigators noted that, if these racial differences in the way male and female physicians treated patient pain could be generalized beyond this study, it might explain the appearance of racial disparities in pain treatment reported in studies including a larger proportion of male physicians (which is likely to be most studies).

In an attempt to replicate their findings related to the influence of physician gender on pain management decisions, Weisse, Sorum, and Dominguez (2003) repeated their study with a sample 712 practicing internists. Again, no overall effect of race was identified. In this study, physician gender did not appear to interact with patient race as it had in the authors' previous work (Weisse et al., 2001). This result suggests that the gender make-up of the physician sample is unlikely to contribute to the finding of disparities in other studies. There was a significant interaction between patient race and gender, however. In the kidney stone scenario, doctors prescribed significantly lower initial doses of hydrocodone for Black women than for White women, and significantly higher doses for Black men in comparison to White men.

In a third experimental study, Tamayo-Sarver et al. (2003a) examined the influence of patient race and socially desirable characteristics (i.e., high status occupation, socioeconomic status [SES], relationship with a primary care physician) on physician pain management decisions. A sample of 2,872 practicing emergency physicians made diagnostic and treatment recommendations for three hypothetical patients suffering from pain (ankle fracture, migraine, back pain). The race of the hypothetical patients was varied (Black, White, Hispanic) and socially desirable information was randomly included or not included in each vignette. Controlling for variables reflecting socially desirable information, the interaction of these terms with patient race/ethnicity, and position of the vignette within the survey, the investigators found no main effect of patient race/ethnicity. The inclusion of socially desirable information, however, did somewhat increase the rate at which opioids were prescribed.

Discrepancies in Research Findings

Many studies examining the relationship between race/ethnicity and analgesic care have provided evidence of disparities in the provision of pain medication. Other studies, however, have found no differences in pain management for patients of different racial and ethnic backgrounds. Although research providing evidence of disparities has addressed a wide range of treatment settings and conditions, research showing no relationship between patient race/ethnicity and analgesic care appears to be restricted to experimental paradigms and studies focusing on analgesic treatment provided in the ED. Possible explanations for the discrepancies in research results in these areas are discussed below.

Experimental Studies of Pain Management

As indicated previously, experimental studies of racial and ethnic disparities in pain treatment have not found a direct effect of patient race/ethnicity on the pain management decisions of physicians. (Note that Weisse et al. [2001] did find racial differences in doctors' analgesic decisions that depended on physician gender. This result was not replicated in a follow-up study, however.) In each of the three experimental studies summarized, practicing physicians reviewed hypothetical patient vignettes (for which the assignment of patient race was experimentally manipulated) and indicated their preferred treatment approach. Using this experimental paradigm, the investigators had a number of important advantages, including control over the mechanism, type, and severity of injury; patient reporting of pain and language barriers; physician communication style; patient preferences for or concerns about treatment; and patient characteristics, such as age, insurance coverage, SES, and physical appearance.

This experimental approach, however, may have disadvantages as well. Although the investigators attempted to heighten study participants' awareness of the race/ethnicity of the hypothetical patients (e.g., racially/ethnically identifiable names, photographs showing skin tone), it may be that physicians participating in these studies were not as aware of the race/ethnicity of the hypothetical patients as they would be of the race/ethnicity of a real patient during an actual clinical encounter. Further, although these studies used cover stories to disguise the research objective, it is conceivable that physician participants suspected the true purpose of the study and were motivated to respond in socially desirable ways.

Importantly, by employing an experimental design, the investigators removed some of the key factors hypothesized to underlie disparities in pain management. Many researchers have suggested that the interaction between physician and patient may be the critical determinant of differences in care (e.g., Bonham, 2001; Green et al., 2003; Tait and Chibnall, 2005). For example, there is some evidence that communication is less effective when the social distance between parties is greater (Tamayo-Sarver et al., 2003b), that physicians may be less comfortable interacting with minorities than Whites (Gregory, Wells, and Leake, 1987), that minorities experience less participatory interactions with physicians than do White patients (Cooper-Patrick et al., 1999), and that physicians perceive more involved patients in a positive light (Sleath, Rotor, Chewning, and Svarstad, 1999). In these experimental studies, the participating physicians had no interaction with the patients about which they were making treatment decisions. As a result, in addition to controlling numerous factors that had the potential to confound the relationship between patient race/ethnicity and analgesic care, the investigators necessarily controlled factors that may be at the root of that relationship. By eliminating any interaction between patient and physician, the investigators removed an important potential contributor to racial/ethnic disparities in pain management. Therefore, although these studies are very intriguing, they may not depict the true nature of a clinical encounter closely enough to call findings of racial/ethnic disparities in pain management in natural clinical settings into question.

Management of Pain in the Emergency Department

Research examining racial/ethnic differences in the management of pain in the ED has resulted in inconsistent findings. Although studies in this area share some important methodological similarities (e.g., similar dependent variables and underlying medical conditions), some have demonstrated racial and/or ethnic differences in ED analgesic treatment (Hostetler et al., 2002; Tamayo-Sarver et al., 2003b; Todd et al., 1993, 2000), whereas others have shown no effect of patient race/ethnicity on pain management (Bartfield et al., 1997; Friedland and Kulick, 1994; Fuentes et al., 2002; Karpman et al., 1997; Yen et al., 2003).

It is unclear why the results of these studies should be at odds. Some investigators have suggested that the publication of the studies conducted by Todd and his colleagues (1993, 2000) may have drawn attention to inequities in the treatment of pain in the ED, and in so doing, resulted in more egalitarian pain management practices (Fuentes et al., 2002; Tamayo-Sarver et al., 2003b). However, there does not appear to be a pattern of older studies showing disparities and more recent studies reporting negative findings. Indeed, three of the four studies providing evidence of racial/ethnic disparities in ED pain treatment were conducted since 2000 (Hostetler et al., 2002; Tamayo-Sarver et al., 2003b; Todd et al., 2000).

Some investigators have hypothesized that disparities in the treatment of pain in the ED may only be present in single-facility studies, indicating isolated problems with the treatment received by minorities (Tamayo-Sarver et al., 2003b; Yen et al., 2003). Two of the four studies finding disparities in ED pain management, however, were conducted using large, national samples (Hostetler et al., 2002; Tamayo-Sarver et al., 2003b). Of the five studies reporting no racial/ethnic differences in the treatment of pain in the ED, only the study conducted by Yen and colleagues utilized a national sample.

In 1997, Karpman et al. suggested that inconsistencies in research findings may be related to the demographics of the patient population typically treated by a facility. Having not found ethnic differences in the treatment of pain at their facility, which treats a large number of Hispanic patients, the authors speculated that providers at facilities with a large population of minority patients may be more sensitive to the analgesic needs of these patients. Although one might expect greater contact with minority patients to lead to better communication between patients and providers, and thus better treatment of pain, other research suggests that cancer patients treated at facilities with a large population of minority patients actually receive less adequate pain relief (Cleeland et al., 1994).

Fuentes et al. (2002) suggested that differences in injury severity may contribute to discrepancies in the research findings related to pain management in the ED. The investigators noted that their patient sample, in which no disparities were found, had a higher rate of open fractures, reduction, and hospital admission than did the samples examined by Todd and his colleagues (1993, 2000), whose work has provided evidence of racial and ethnic differences in the treatment of pain. The investigators speculated that patient race/ethnicity may be less likely to influence providers' analgesic decisions when the severity of the injury and the accompanying pain are more obvious to providers.

Some research has, indeed, suggested that patient race may influence the analgesic decisions of providers largely when objective evidence of patient pain is not available. Tamayo-Sarver et al. (2003b) found racial disparities in pain management only when the patient's medical condition was one for which objective evidence of pain cannot be obtained. Black patients were significantly less likely than White patients to receive opioid analgesics when presenting with back pain or migraine, but were equally likely to receive opioids for the treatment of pain associated with long bone fracture. (As discussed previously, however, a number of studies have found disparities for patients suffering fracture-related pain.)

Differences in analytic methods also may contribute to research discrepancies in this area. Although the studies examined similar dependent variables (e.g., receipt of analgesics, opioids, parenteral medications), the approach to controlling for potentially confounding variables varied widely across studies. For example, in some studies multiple variables were used to control for the severity of the patient's injury (e.g., Todd et al., 1993). In other studies, control of injury severity was less extensive or even absent (e.g., Karpman et al., 1997; Todd et al., 2000; Yen et al., 2003). Importantly, although there is strong evidence that patient SES accounts for some portion of racial/ethnic disparities in health care (e.g., Smedley et al. 2003), few studies of disparities in the treatment of pain have included direct measures of patient SES. Whereas the study by Chen et al. (2005) included direct measures of patient SES, most studies control only for patient insurance coverage, which can serve as a rough proxy for patient SES as well as access to care.

Another methodologic difference that may contribute to inconsistencies in the findings of ED pain management studies relates to the age of the study subjects. Of studies addressing analgesic treatment in the ED, some examine pediatric populations, whereas others focus on adult ED patients. Interestingly, only one of four studies showing disparities in ED pain management included pediatric patients (Hostetler et al., 2002), whereas three of the five studies showing no effect of patient race/ethnicity focused on the treatment of pain in children (Friedland and Kulick, 1994; Karpman et al., 1997; Yen et al., 2003). Although there is evidence that children often are undertreated for pain (Friedland and Kulick, 1994; Hostetler et al., 2002; Karpman et al., 1997; Petrack et al., 1997; Selbst and Clark, 1990), it is unclear why racial/ethnic disparities in pain treatment would be less prevalent in this population. Perhaps the factors that underlie analgesic disparities in adults do not operate similarly in the treatment of children.

Mechanisms Underlying Disparities in Pain Management

Investigators have proposed a number of mechanisms that may underlie racial and ethnic disparities in the treatment of pain. To clarify the possible stages at which disparities may occur, Todd (2001) outlined the four steps involved in the process of managing patient pain. The patient must perceive pain (step 1) and communicate his/her discomfort to a care provider (step 2). The care provider must assess the patient's pain, making judgments about the validity and severity of the complaint (step 3) and decide whether and how to treat the patient's symptoms (step 4). Constructs associated with each step in this process, as well as patient and provider characteristics that may influence each step, have been discussed as possible contributors to racial and ethnic disparities in pain management.

Perception and Expression of Pain

In order for a health care provider to prescribe adequate treatment for pain, the patient must experience pain and make the provider aware of it. A number of researchers have examined the possibility that individuals of different racial/ethnic backgrounds may differ in their perception and expression of pain. In 1990, Zatzick and Dimsdale reviewed the literature related to cultural differences in the perception of laboratory-induced pain, concluding that there was no definitive evidence of cultural differences in the ability to discriminate pain.

Other research suggests that the way a patient experiences and expresses pain varies by race/ethnicity (e.g., Tait and Chibnall, 2005; Wolff, 1985; Zborowski, 1969). Although some investigators have found no racial/ethnic differences (e.g., Jordan, Lumley, and Leisen, 1998; Pfefferbaum, Adams, and Aceves, 1990; Thomason et al., 1998; Tait and Chibnall, 2001), a number of studies have shown lower pain tolerance or higher reported pain intensity among Blacks and Hispanics in comparison with Whites (e.g., Bates, Edwards, and Anderson, 1993; Edwards, Doleys, Fillingim, and Lowery, 2001; McCracken, Matthews, Tang, and Cuba, 2001; Weisenberg, Kreindler, Schachat, and Werboff, 1975; Woodrow, Friedman, Siegelaub, and Collen, 1972). Investigators have noted that, in some of the studies in this area, the group differences reported are fairly small (Tait and Chibnall, 2005) and that within-group differences often are more prominent than those seen between groups (Todd, 2001).

Although research suggests that racial and ethnic differences in the tolerance and reaction to pain do exist, there is evidence that these differences are not the primary cause of disparities in the treatment of pain. One might expect that the lower pain tolerance often reported among minorities would result in more aggressive pain treatment. Many studies focusing on the prescription of analgesic medications show precisely the opposite effect, however. Further, the expression of pain does not precisely predict analgesic treatment. Todd et al. (2000) found undertreatment of pain in minorities despite the fact that minority subjects did not differ from Whites in the level of pain reported. Less aggressive analgesic treatment for minority patients has been identified even when the minority sample has pain scores reflecting more severe pain than the White sample (Chen et al., 2005).

Physician Assessment of Pain

Many researchers have suggested that health care providers' judgments about the severity of patient pain may be an important cause of racial and ethnic disparities in analgesic treatment. There is growing evidence that provider assessment of pain often does not correspond well with patient assessment of pain. In 1997, Chibnall, Tait, and Ross used medical vignettes depicting hypothetical patients suffering from low back pain to examine the degree of agreement between patient and provider judgments of pain intensity. Medical students overestimated the severity of pain when pain intensity (as reported by the patient) was low and underestimated the severity of pain when pain intensity was high. These results are corroborated by studies of pain assessment among internists (Tait and Chibnall, 1997); primary care nurses, residents, and oncology fellows (Grossman, Sheidler, Swedeen, Mucenski, and Piantadosi, 1991); and registered nurses (Zalon, 1993). In 1993, Von Roenn et al. reported that 76% of cancer specialists responding to a survey about pain management identified inadequate pain assessment as the predominant barrier to the successful management of cancer pain.

Many investigators have hypothesized that providers may be less adept at interpreting the pain cues and expressions of patients from racial or ethnic groups other than their own (e.g., Todd et al., 1993; Todd, 2001). Few studies examining racial/ethnic differences in physician assessment of pain have been conducted, however, and their results do not lend clear support to this hypothesis. In 2000, Anderson et al. examined the correspondence between patient and physician assessment of pain associated with cancer. The investigators found that physicians underestimated the severity of pain in 64% of Hispanic and 74% of

Black patients. Because White patients were not included in the study sample, however, it is unclear whether patient-physician agreement was influenced by patient race/ethnicity. Pain experienced by White patients might have been similarly discounted.

In 1994, Cleeland et al. found that patients treated at ECOG cancer centers primarily serving minorities were less likely to receive adequate analgesia than did patients treated in other centers. Given that the discrepancy between patients' and physicians' judgments of pain severity was a strong predictor of the adequacy of care, this study may suggest that doctors' ratings of pain severity were more divergent from those of minority than White patients. However, patient-level race/ethnicity data were not collected and thus the investigators were unable to test this hypothesis explicitly.

In a follow-up study, Cleeland et al. (1997) found that minority patients were less likely than patients from facilities treating primarily White patients to receive adequate pain management and more likely to have the severity of their pain underestimated by their physicians. Although these findings suggest that physician-patient discordance in pain judgments may mediate the relationship between patient race/ethnicity and analgesic treatment, this hypothesis was not tested directly, as race/ethnicity data were not available for the "nonminority" sample.

In the only direct test of racial/ethnic disparities in physician pain assessment identified in the literature, Todd, Lee, and Hoffman (1994) found no evidence that physicians are less capable of assessing the pain of minority patients. In that study, physicians underestimated pain to an equal degree in White and Hispanic patients. Thus, although some studies suggest the possibility of disparities in the adequacy of physicians' ability to assess pain, it appears that pain assessment may not be the key mechanism underlying disparities in pain management.

Provider Decision to Treat Pain

In making the decision to prescribe analgesic medications, a physician must not only estimate the severity of the patient's pain, but also must assess the likelihood that analgesics will be taken as intended (Cleeland et al., 1997; Tamayo-Sarver et al., 2003a). Some research suggests that physicians may have less confidence that prescribed medications will be used appropriately by minority patients. For example, there is evidence that providers believe Black and Hispanic patients to be less compliant with medical treatment than White patients (Gregory et al., 1987; Van Ryn and Burke, 2000). The expectation of noncompliance may limit physicians' willingness to prescribe analgesics, particularly medications such as opioids, which are prone to abuse. Other research has shown that patients' socially desirable characteristics, such as having a regular relationship with a primary care provider, enhance the likelihood that physicians will prescribe opioids for the treatment of pain (Tamayo-Sarver et al., 2003a). Knowing that a patient has a regular source of care may increase a provider's confidence that medications will be taken correctly. As minorities are less likely to have a regular source of health care (Collins, Hall, and Neuhaus, 1999), physicians may be more reluctant to prescribe strong analgesics to members of minority groups.

Many investigators have suggested that negative attitudes in general toward minorities may contribute to racial/ethnic differences in care (e.g., Chen et al., 2005; Tamayo-Sarver et al., 2003a, 2003b; Todd, 2001). For example, racial/ethnic stereotypes may cause physicians to be more likely to suspect minority patients of drug seeking (Tamayo-Sarver et al., 2003a). As mentioned previously, patient sociodemographic characteristics may be particularly likely to inform physician decision making when the underlying medical condition does not allow objective assessment (Tamayo-Sarver et al., 2003b). Although there is evidence that physicians hold more negative attitudes regarding Black than White patients (e.g., lower intelligence, higher potential for risky behavior), and feel less affiliation toward them (Van Ryn and Burke, 2000), no studies have directly tested the role that racial stereotypes and prejudice may play in racial/ethnic disparities in the management of pain.

Characteristics of the Patient

A variety of patient characteristics have been hypothesized to influence disparities in analgesic care, including (1) language barriers, (2) SES and access to care, and (3) beliefs, expectations, and preferences related to pain and its management. These factors have the potential to exert effects on patient expression of pain as well as physician pain assessment and decision to treat.

The language spoken by the patient is frequently hypothesized to influence disparities in analgesic treatment. However, although language barriers between patient and physician are likely to hinder the patient's ability to express his/her discomfort and the physician's ability to accurately interpret and assess the patient's pain, it appears that they are not the underlying determinant of ethnic disparities in care. Todd et al. (1993) found clear evidence of ethnic disparities in the receipt of analgesics among patients treated in the ED for long bone fractures, despite including primary language as a covariate. Further, if language barriers were to be the key mechanism underlying disparities, it would be difficult to explain why Black patients are frequently shown to receive inadequate pain control and sometimes to experience more substantial undertreatment of pain than do Hispanic patients. Bernabei et al. (1998) found no differences in the rate at which analgesics were provided to White and Hispanic nursing home residents suffering from cancer-related pain. Blacks, however, were significantly less likely than their White counterparts to receive pain medications. Tamayo-Sarver et al. (2003b) found a similar pattern of results in a national sample of ED encounters.

Patient SES and access to care also have the potential to influence disparities in pain management. As mentioned previously, most studies examining racial/ethnic disparities in analgesic care have included only limited control over the effects of SES, using insurance status as a proxy for SES as well as access to care (e.g., Atherton et al., 2004; Ng et al., 1996a; Obst et al., 2001; Tamayo-Sarver et al., 2003b; Todd et al., 1993, 2000). One of the studies reviewed involved more thorough measurement of SES. Chen et al. (2005) controlled for several aspects of SES, including annual income, years of schooling, and hours worked per week, in addition to insurance status. Despite the investigators' conscientious attempt to account for the influence of SES, racial disparities in the receipt of opioids remained.

This same study also provided some evidence that general access to care does not explain the effect of race/ethnicity on analgesic care (Chen et al., 2005). Although there were racial differences in the receipt of opioids, the investigators did not find differences in the other treatments provided to patients of different racial backgrounds. Although insurance status should affect all treatments, Blacks were as likely as Whites to receive nonopioid medications, as well as specialty referral and physical therapy.

One aspect of access to care that has received some attention in the pain management literature regards the availability of medications from local pharmacies. In 2000, Morrison, Wallenstein, Natale, Senzel, and Huang found that pharmacies in predominantly minority neighborhoods were substantially less likely than those in primarily White neighborhoods to have adequate supplies of opioid medications. Some have speculated that differences in the treatment decisions of physicians may reflect an understanding of the more limited access to opioid medications that minority patients may have (Tamayo-Sarver et al., 2003b).

Patients' beliefs, expectations, and preferences related to pain treatment also are hypothesized to influence disparities in analgesic care. Some investigators have found that minorities are often concerned about addiction and possible side effects of pain medication (Anderson et al., 2000; Cleeland et al., 1997). Other research suggests that patients from minority backgrounds may consider pain to be an expected part of illness or may be reluctant to report pain (Anderson et al., 2002; Green et al., 2003; Juarez, Ferrell, and Borneman, 1998, 1999). Although investigators have speculated that minority patients may have lower expectations for the effectiveness of pain-relieving medications and thus may be less likely to seek out or accept pain medication, there is evidence that Hispanic and White ED patients have equally high expectations for pain relief (Lee, Burelbach, and Fosnocht, 2001), suggesting that patient expectations are not the underlying cause of disparities in treatment. Although preferences for and concerns about the use of pain medications may contribute to racial/ethnic differences in pain treatment, this hypothesis has not been tested directly.

Characteristics of the Health Care Provider

Researchers have speculated that the demographic and psychological characteristics of health care providers may influence decision making regarding analgesic treatment. However, some studies have found that provider race/ethnicity (Streltzer and Wade, 1981; Todd et al., 1993) and training (Chen et al., 2005; Todd et al. 1993; Weisse et al., 2003) do not explain differences in pain management decisions. Although early work by Weisse and her colleagues (2001) suggested that physician gender may play a critical role in explaining disparities in pain management, these findings were not replicated in a follow-up study (Weisse et al., 2003).

Synthesis of the Literature

It is clear that not all research examining racial/ethnic differences in pain management provides evidence for a relationship between race/ethnicity and analgesic care. However, the majority of studies conducted to date suggest the presence of disparities in pain treatment. The body of literature reporting racial/ethnic differences in the prescription and use of analgesics includes more than a dozen studies covering a wide range of treatment settings (ED, inpatient, cancer specialty practices, primary care) and causes of pain (fractures, wounds, migraine, back pain, post-operative pain, childbirth, cancer, chronic pain). Studies showing no relationship between race/ethnicity and analgesic care in clinical settings are relatively few and appear to be restricted to the examination of pain control in the ED. Although three experimental studies have shown no main effect of patient race/ethnicity on pain management, it is unclear how well these studies reflect the decision-making processes employed in real clinical encounters with patients of various cultural backgrounds.

Although many factors have been hypothesized to influence the relationship between race/ethnicity and pain management, no single factor or set of factors has emerged to fully explain disparities in pain management. It is likely that characteristics of the patient (e.g., SES), physician characteristics (e.g., pain assessment skills), and injury factors (e.g., availability of objective medical evidence) interact to produce differences in the treatment of patients of various racial/ethnic groups. Most of the mechanisms hypothesized to underlie these effects have yet to be tested directly. For example, no studies have directly examined the role that patient preferences or physician racial attitudes may play in mediating the relationship between patient race/ethnicity and analgesic treatment.

Home health care for the elderly represents a segment of the U.S. health care system in which the presence of racial/ethnic disparities in the treatment of pain has not been studied. Because of the unique style of care delivery in home care, the examination of pain management in this setting provides an important complement to research already conducted in this area. Some of the factors hypothesized to underlie racial/ethnic disparities in analgesic care have the potential to be less influential in home care than they are in ED, inpatient, outpatient, and primary care settings. Although patient perception of pain is likely to be similar in the home and in other settings, the patient's expression of pain as well as the provider's assessment of and decision to treat pain may be quite different. Home care recipients generally see their providers numerous times over the span of weeks or months. Repeated interactions may enhance the quality of patient-provider communication, perhaps contributing to more effective patient communication regarding the experience of pain and more accurate provider assessment of pain. Further, the possible involvement of multiple care providers in treating the patient and the strong likelihood that the patient's family members will be involved in the provision and/or facilitation of care may enhance the chances that accurate information about the patient's need for pain relief will be communicated. Characteristics of the patients cared for by Medicare-certified home health care agencies also may alleviate concerns that doctors in other settings may have about their patients. For example, providers caring for elderly home care recipients may be less likely to suspect drug seeking and may be more comfortable coordinating pain treatment knowing that they (and family members) will continue to oversee the patient's care for some time.

Pain Outcomes in Home Health Care

Medicare home health care services have become an increasingly important component of the medical system for elderly Americans. Between 1989 and 1996, Medicare home health care expenditures rose from $2.5 to $16.8 billion (U.S. General Accounting Office, 1998). Increases in the use of these services can be traced to a variety of causes (Brega et al., 2002), the most significant being the implementation of the Prospective Payment System (PPS) for hospitals in 1983. The hospital PPS resulted in reduced durations for Medicare-funded hospital stays (Beebe et al., 1985; Feder et al., 1987; Health Care Financing Administration, 1986; Stern and Epstein, 1985) and dramatic increases in the percentages of Medicare inpatients discharged to skilled nursing facilities or home health agencies (Liu and Manton, 1988; Neu and Harrison, 1988). As inpatient lengths of stay decreased, the case mix of Medicare patients receiving post-acute care increased in complexity and severity (Shaughnessy and Kramer, 1990). As a result, the Medicare home health benefit has become an important safety net for elderly beneficiaries.

Given the important role that home care plays in maintaining elderly beneficiaries safely in the community, evidence of racial and ethnic disparities in the utilization and outcomes of in-home services is of concern. Numerous studies have examined racial and ethnic differences in the use of home care by the elderly. These studies have yielded disparate results. Several studies have shown that elderly Whites utilize more services than non-Whites (Chadiha, Proctor, Morrow-Howell, Darkwa, and Dore, 1995; Greene and Monahan, 1984; Jenkins and Laditka, 2003; Kemper, 1992; Miller, McFall, and Campbell, 1994; Mui and Burnette, 1994; Wallace, Levy-Storms, and Ferguson, 1995). Other studies suggest the reverse relationship, finding that minorities are more likely than Whites to receive formal home health care services (Bass and Noelker, 1987; Jackson et al., 2002; Mauser and Miller, 1994; Morrow-Howell, Chadiha, Proctor, Hourd-Bryant, and Dore, 1996; Schore, 1994). Other researchers have found no relationship between race/ethnicity and the utilization of home health care after important covariates are controlled (Baxter, Bryant, Scarbro, and Shetterly, 2001; Cagney and Agree, 1999; Dunlop, Manheim, Song, and Chang, 2002; Miller et al., 1996; Mindel, Wright, and Starrett, 1986; Netzer et al., 1997; Norgard and Rodgers, 1997; Peng, Navaie-Waliser, and Feldman, 2003; Wallace, Levy-Storms, Kington, and Andersen, 1998; White-Means and Rubin, 2004). Only two studies have examined racial and ethnic differences in the outcomes of home care for the elderly, each of which suggests that White patients obtain greater benefit from Medicare home health services than do minorities (Brega, Goodrich, Powell, and Grigsby, 2005; Peng et al., 2003). No known research has examined disparities in the effectiveness of home-based pain management.

Pain management in home health care is unique in comparison with the other health care settings in which disparities in pain treatment have been studied. The management of pain in home care rests heavily on the regular assessment of patient pain by home care nurses and therapists. At the time of each comprehensive assessment (e.g., start/resumption of care, every 60-day recertification visit, discharge), the home care provider assesses the presence, severity, and frequency of the patient's pain and completes a review of all patient medications. If pain is a significant problem for a patient, the provider generally will assess pain at each home care visit, which may occur multiple times per week. With the goal of controlling patient pain, the care provider may take a number of clinical actions. He/she is likely to address both pharmacologic approaches to controlling pain (e.g., prescription and over-the-counter medications, addressing concerns that may discourage appropriate use of analgesics) as well as non-pharmacologic treatments (e.g., the use of heat or cold, massage therapy, relaxation therapy, ultrasound, biofeedback). Any changes to the plan of care that are recommended to address patient pain must be approved by the physician who referred the patient to home care. Therefore, although the home care provider is responsible for ensuring that pain is adequately treated, he/she is not the ultimate decision maker with regard to the patient's treatment plan.

The objective of the current study was to assess the relationship between patient race/ethnicity and pain outcomes among elderly recipients of home health care services. Although there is little research examining the treatment of pain among the elderly (Green et al., 2003), some studies have found elderly individuals to be undertreated at a higher rate than younger individuals (Bernabei et al., 1998; Cleeland et al., 1994). Given the important role that home health care plays in the medical treatment of older Americans, it is important to examine the equity of pain outcomes in this setting.

METHODS

Sources of Study Data

The Centers for Medicare and Medicaid Services (CMS) requires that Medicare-certified home health agencies collect and submit Outcome Assessment and Information Set (OASIS) data for all Medicare patients and all Medicaid patients receiving skilled nursing or therapy services. (With the exception of agencies required by state law to meet the Medicare Conditions of Participation, home health agencies that are not Medicare-certified are not required to collect OASIS data.) The OASIS data set is used to collect information about patient demographics, living situation, and caregiver availability, as well as functional, physiologic, and cognitive/behavioral status. Agencies are required to collect these data at the start of care or resumption of care after an inpatient stay, at each 60-day recertification visit, and at the time of discharge, transfer to an inpatient facility, or death. OASIS data are collected by skilled home health care providers. In the majority of cases, registered nurses conduct required patient assessments and complete the OASIS data set. In a small percentage of cases (cases requiring only therapy services [e.g., physical therapy] and no skilled nursing care), therapists may complete the OASIS.

OASIS data from 2001 were obtained from the University of Colorado Outcome Reporting and Enhancement (CORE) Research Partnership, a non-profit public service venture that was based at the University of Colorado at Denver and Health Sciences Center. The CORE Research Partnership, which was in operation from mid-1999 to the end of 2005, analyzed OASIS data submitted by participating home health care agencies and provided agencies with graphical reports showing how their patients' case mix and outcomes compared with a reference sample composed of patients from all other participating agencies. These reports were used by agencies to monitor and enhance the quality of care they provided.

Because OASIS contains only limited information regarding patient financial status, data from the 2004 Area Resource File (ARF) were used to enhance the estimation of patient SES. The ARF data file, which is maintained by Quality Resource Systems, Inc., provides extensive information about the nation's health care system as well as basic demographic, economic, and environmental information. All data are derived from existing data sources and are aggregated to the county level. ARF data reflecting the 2001 per capita income in each patient's county of residence were used as part of this study.

In order to merge ARF data with OASIS data, it was necessary to identify the county of residence of each patient included in the OASIS data file. Although OASIS contains a patient's zip code, it does not identify his/her county of residence. Therefore, a third data set was used to allow a crosswalk between the ARF and the OASIS. Using a year 2000 version of ZIPList, a publicly available zip code database developed by ZipInfo.com, the Federal Information Processing Standards (FIPS) code associated with the zip code for each OASIS record was identified. The FIPS code reflects a patient's county of residence and was used to merge county-level income data from the ARF with the OASIS data.

Study Sample

Racial and ethnic differences in pain outcomes were examined using a sample of OASIS episodes that had been submitted to the CORE Research Partnership by participating agencies. An episode of care reflects a patient's complete case from the time of admission (or readmission following an inpatient stay) to the time of discharge. (Some patients are discharged and readmitted to home care repeatedly, and thus may have multiple episodes of care.) To ensure that study findings would not be confounded by changes in the system of payment for Medicare home health services and would be reflective of the current home health care environment, only data from calendar year 2001 were analyzed (the first full year that the Prospective Payment System for home care was in effect).

Because the agencies that participated in the CORE Research Partnership were self-selected (i.e., not all certified home health agencies participated in CORE) and were not geographically representative of the national population of home health agencies, a sample of patient episodes was drawn from the CORE data set. The sampling procedure ensured that the percentage of episodes in the sample from each of the ten CMS geographic regions matched the percentage of episodes that occurred in each region according to national data (e.g., the percentage of episodes in the study analysis file that originated in New England was equivalent to the percentage of all OASIS episodes that occurred in this region [7.23%]). Within each region, a random sample of patient episodes was selected. In all, 590 agencies located in 48 states contributed data to the final sample.

To be included in the final analysis sample, patients were required to meet three inclusion/exclusion criteria. First, only episodes for patients age 65 years or older were included in the final sample. Second, all episodes for patients who were nonresponsive (e.g., vegetative) at the start/resumption of care were eliminated because of the limited likelihood of clinical improvement. Third, because the dependent variables could not be computed for episodes that ended in death, only patients who were discharged or transferred to an inpatient facility at the conclusion of their home health episodes were included in the analyses.

After the inclusion/exclusion criteria were implemented, the resulting analysis file – referred to as the Hospitalization Sample – included a total of 144,178 home care episodes. Of these, 123,430 were for non-Hispanic White patients, 14,100 were for Black patients, and 4,391 were for Hispanic patients. The remaining 2,257 episodes, which were for patients of other or unknown race/ethnicity, were excluded from all analyses. Analyses of utilization of inpatient hospital care for the treatment of pain during the home care episode were conducted using the Hospitalization Sample.

A second sample was created for the purpose of examining improvement in the frequency of pain over the course of the episode of care. The Pain Frequency Sample included all episodes from the Hospitalization Sample that ended in discharge. Episodes ending in transfer to an inpatient facility were excluded as only minimal health status data are collected at the time of transfer, making the computation of outcomes related to pain frequency impossible. The total sample size for the Pain Frequency Sample was 105,160 episodes, of which 90,924 were for White patients, 9,277 were for Black patients, and 3,247 were for Hispanic patients. Of the episodes in this sample, 1,712 were for patients of other or unknown racial/ethnic backgrounds. These data were not included in the study analyses. Preliminary descriptive analyses as well as analyses related to improvement in pain frequency were conducted using the Pain Frequency Sample.

Dependent Variables

Analyses examined the effect of patient race and ethnicity on two outcome measures related to pain: (1) improvement in pain frequency and (2) hospitalization for uncontrolled pain. Improvement in pain frequency was a dichotomous variable (yes=1, no=0) indicating whether or not a patient improved over the course of his or her episode of care in the frequency with which pain interfered with his/her activity or movement. This measure was based on data collected for OASIS item M0420 (Frequency of Pain) at the start or resumption of care and again at discharge. Because they cannot show improvement, patients rated as having no pain at the start or resumption of care were excluded from analyses related to pain frequency outcomes.

Hospitalization for uncontrolled pain was a dichotomous variable (yes=1, no=0) indicating whether or not a patient's home care episode ended because the patient was admitted to the hospital specifically for the treatment of uncontrolled pain. This variable was based on option 14 of OASIS item M0895 (Reason for Hospitalization). Analyses related to this outcome included all patients, rather than just those patients whose episodes ended in hospitalization.

Key Independent Variables

Separate analyses compared the pain outcomes of White home health care recipients to those of Blacks and Hispanics. Race and ethnicity were measured using OASIS data item M0140 (Race/Ethnicity). This item is answered based on patient self-report and has been shown to have excellent interrater reliability (kappa = 1.0 and 100% agreement; Hittle et al., 2003). In categorizing patients by race/ethnicity, non-Hispanic White patients were identified as those individuals who chose only the "White" response option on the OASIS Race/Ethnicity data item. Blacks were identified as those patients who chose only the "Black or African-American" option. Patients who chose the "Hispanic or Latino" option, regardless of what other options also had been selected, were identified as Hispanic.

Covariates

Risk-adjusted analyses examining pain outcomes controlled for 22 variables expected to influence a patient's likelihood of improvement in pain frequency and hospitalization for the treatment of uncontrolled pain. With one exception, all covariates were based on OASIS data and reflected information about patient characteristics and health status collected at the start or resumption of care visit. Three demographic variables were included in the risk-adjusted analyses (i.e., age, sex [female=1, male=0], and per capita income). As mentioned previously, the financial status of patients was estimated using 2001 per capita income information from the ARF data set. Although these data are aggregated to the county level, they provide a degree of control over patient SES that would not be possible using OASIS data alone. Previous research has established the value of aggregated socioeconomic indicators in the measurement of patient SES (e.g., Bach, Guadagnoli, Schrag, Schussler, and Warren, 2002).

Two OASIS-based variables provided information about insurance coverage, which has the potential to influence the types and amounts of care that are available to a patient. A dichotomous variable indicating whether Medicare was a payer for the patient's home health services (yes=1, no=0) was included in all risk-adjusted analyses. A parallel variable indicating whether Medicaid was a payer for home health services (yes=1, no=0) also was included. In addition to controlling for access to services, this latter variable provided some degree of control over patient SES.

The existing literature on racial and ethnic disparities in analgesic treatment does not address the role that a patient's support network may play in determining the approach to pain management (Todd et al., 1993). Because of the important role family members and friends often play in providing informal health-related assistance to elderly home care recipients, the patient's support network may be particularly influential in facilitating appropriate pain treatment in home care. For this reason, an OASIS-based variable measuring the frequency of assistance provided by the patient's primary informal caregiver was included in risk-adjusted analyses (0-6 scale, with larger values reflecting more frequent assistance). Informal caregivers who provide more frequent assistance may be more likely to be involved in the facilitation of home health care services and may be more aware of the patient's experience of pain, perhaps informing the plan of care with regard to pain treatment.

Seven OASIS variables were included to reflect the complexity of patients' medical conditions. The number of acute medical conditions and the number of chronic medical conditions were included in all risk-adjusted analyses. These variables, as well as the variable reflecting frequency of caregiver assistance, were computed according to the analytic specifications used for the case mix reports provided by CMS to Medicare-certified home health care agencies (CMS, 2005). In addition, analyses controlled for a dichotomous variable indicating whether the patient was discharged from a hospital within 14 days prior to the start/resumption of home care (yes=1, no=0). Three prognosis variables also were included in risk-adjusted analyses. One dichotomous variable (yes=1, no=0) indicated whether the patient was rated by the home care provider conducting the start/resumption of care visit as having a good rehabilitative prognosis (i.e., marked improvement in functional status expected over the course of the episode of care). A second dichotomous variable (yes=1, no=0) indicated whether the patient was rated as having a good/fair overall prognosis for recovering from the current episode of illness (i.e., partial to full recovery expected). A third prognosis variable, referred to as "Terminal Condition," indicated whether the patient was rated by the care provider as having a life expectancy of six months or less (yes=1, no=0). Finally, a dichotomous variable indicating the length of the home care episode was included in all risk-adjusted regression models (greater than 31 days=1, less than or equal to 31 days=0).

Four specific diagnoses often associated with significant pain also were controlled in the risk-adjusted analyses. Dichotomous variables (yes=1, no=0) indicated whether or not a patient had a diagnosis reflecting a (1) neoplasm, (2) digestive system disease, (3) musculoskeletal system disease, or (4) fracture were included in risk-adjusted analyses. These variables were computed based on International Classification of Diseases, Ninth Revision (ICD-9) codes representing the primary and secondary diagnoses for which patients were receiving home care services and were computed as specified for the CMS quality monitoring reports (CMS, 2005).

Two additional variables represented baseline integumentary status: (1) status of the most problematic stasis ulcer and (2) status of the most problematic pressure ulcer. Each variable was based on a 0-3 scale, with larger values reflecting more serious lesions. These variables were computed for all patients, not just those with reported skin lesions or open wounds. Patients assessed as having no skin lesions or open wounds were coded as having a "0" for ulcer status.

Finally, three variables representing patients' baseline experience of pain were controlled in all risk-adjusted analyses: (1) a dichotomous variable indicating whether the patient suffered from chronic pain (yes=1, no=0; CMS, 2005); (2) a dichotomous variable indicating whether a patient suffered from intractable pain (i.e., daily pain that was not easily relieved and that affected the patient's activities, relationships, and mental status; yes=1, no=0); and (3) the baseline score indicating the degree to which pain interfered with activity and movement at the beginning of the episode of care (0-3 scale, with larger scores reflecting more frequent interference).

Data Analysis

Descriptive analyses explored unadjusted differences between White patients and their Black and Hispanic counterparts, respectively, with regard to the dependent variables and covariates. For all continuous and ordinal variables, the mean, maximum, minimum, and standard deviation were computed. For categorical variables, frequencies were computed. To identify whether White patients differed from Black or Hispanic patients in unadjusted analyses, ordinary least squares (OLS) regression models were conducted for continuous and ordinal variables and chi-squared tests were conducted for categorical variables. Because of the large size of the study sample, a more stringent p value was used to determine the significance of analytic results. P values less than or equal to .01 were considered to be statistically significant, whereas p values greater than .01 and less than or equal to .05 were considered to be marginally significant.

Racial and ethnic disparities in pain outcomes were examined using logistic regression models controlling for the 22 risk factors described previously. Separate risk-adjusted analyses compared the pain outcomes of White patients to those of Black and Hispanic patients. In these analyses, the race/ethnicity variable was coded such that White was equal to 1 and Black (or Hispanic) was equal to 0. Therefore, an odds ratio greater than 1.0 indicates that White patients had a higher rate on the outcome of interest (i.e., improvement in pain frequency, hospitalization for uncontrolled pain) than did the minority comparison group. Odds ratios less than 1.0 indicate that minorities "achieved" these outcomes at a higher rate than did Whites.

RESULTS

Descriptive Analyses

Table 1 provides information about the demographic characteristics and baseline health status of the sample, by race and ethnicity. The constructs included in the table reflect those variables used as covariates in risk-adjusted analyses. The results of unadjusted analyses examining the relationship between race/ethnicity and pain outcomes also are included. Some of the descriptive analyses presented in Table 1 were reported in an earlier study of racial and ethnic disparities in the functional outcomes of elderly home care recipients (Brega et al., 2005).

White patients differed from Blacks and Hispanics in a number of respects. Demographically, White patients in the sample were slightly, but significantly older than Black and Hispanic patients and were significantly less likely to be female than were Black patients. Per capita income was significantly higher in the counties in which White patients resided than in the counties of residence of Black and Hispanic patients. This finding suggests that county-level income data do reflect the lower SES of minorities, who are more likely than Whites to be poor (Proctor and Dalaker, 2002).

As expected, unadjusted racial/ethnic differences in insurance coverage also were apparent. Although the vast majority of patients in the sample were covered by Medicare, Whites were slightly, but significantly more likely than the other two racial/ethnic groups to have Medicare as a payer source for home health services. Whites were substantially less likely than minority patients to be covered by Medicaid. This latter finding is consistent with previous research in this area (e.g., Peng et al. 2003), and reflects racial and ethnic differences in the financial status of elderly Americans.

A number of studies have shown racial and ethnic differences in the support networks of elderly Americans. Minority patients have been found to receive more informal health-related assistance from friends and family members than do their White counterparts (Tennstedt and Chang 1998). Small, but significant differences in the frequency with which patients received assistance from their primary informal caregivers were apparent in the unadjusted analyses. Whereas Blacks received significantly less frequent assistance from informal caregivers than did Whites, Hispanics received significantly more frequent assistance.

Unadjusted analyses identified some racial and ethnic differences in the baseline medical complexity of patients in the sample, with minority patients (particularly Blacks) appearing to have somewhat more complex cases in comparison with Whites. Black and Hispanic patients had a slightly, but significantly larger number of chronic medical conditions than did Whites and were significantly more likely than White patients to have been discharged from the hospital within 14 days of the beginning of their home health care episodes. In addition, Blacks had slightly, but significantly fewer acute medical conditions than did Whites. Although recovery and rehabilitative prognosis did not differ between White and Hispanic patients, Blacks were significantly less likely than Whites to be rated as having (1) a good probability of improvement in functional status over the course of the episode of care and (2) a good/fair chance of recovering from the current bout of illness. Whereas Black patients were significantly more likely than Whites to be rated as having six or fewer months to live, Hispanics were marginally less likely to be judged as terminal. Finally, Black patients were significantly more likely and Hispanic patients were marginally more likely than their White counterparts to be on service for more than a month.

Table 1. Baseline Patient Characteristics and Unadjusted Pain Outcomes by Race and Ethnicity [a]

	White (N=90,924)	Black (N=9,277)	Hispanic (N=3,247)
Demographic Characteristics			
Age (mean)	78.97	77.08[‡]	76.67[‡]
Sex (% female)	64.3	68.4[‡]	64.4
Per Capita Income (mean)	31,141.54	29,291.93[‡]	29,766.90[‡]
Insurance Coverage			
Medicare as a Payer for Home Care Services (%)	95.5	92.0[‡]	91.2[‡]
Medicaid as a Payer for Home Care Services (%)	3.1	17.0[‡]	19.5[‡]
Support Network			
Frequency of Informal Assistance (mean, 0-6 scale)	4.25	4.15[‡]	4.51[‡]
Medical Complexity			
Number of Acute Medical Conditions (mean)	2.21	2.13[‡]	2.25
Number of Chronic Medical Conditions (mean)	1.65	2.03[‡]	1.77[‡]
Hospital Discharge within 14 Days of Start of Care (%)	63.1	65.6[‡]	69.6[‡]
Good Rehabilitative Prognosis (%)	81.5	78.0[‡]	80.2
Good/Fair Recovery Prognosis (%)	93.4	92.2[‡]	92.8
Terminal Condition (%)	3.3	4.2[‡]	2.6[†]
Length of Stay Greater than 31 Days (%)	36.0	45.1[‡]	37.9[†]
Diagnoses			
Neoplasms (%)	10.8	10.1[†]	9.8
Digestive System Diseases (%)	11.8	10.5[‡]	12.7
Musculoskeletal System Diseases (%)	36.3	32.6[‡]	30.1[‡]
Fractures (%)	12.1	5.0[‡]	10.7[†]
Integumentary Status			
Status of Most Problematic Stasis Ulcer (mean, 0-3 scale)	0.04	0.05[†]	0.05
Status of Most Problematic Pressure Ulcer (mean, 0-3 scale)	0.10	0.11[*]	0.10
Experience of Pain at Start of Care			
Chronic Pain (%)	5.2	4.7	4.7
Intractable Pain (%)	12.1	10.9[‡]	10.0[‡]
Pain Interfering w/ Activity/Movement (mean, 0-3 scale)	1.18	1.00[‡]	1.11[‡]
Unadjusted Pain Management Outcomes			
Improvement in Pain Interfering w/ Activity/Movement (%)	58.6	60.3[†]	60.8
Hospitalization for Treatment of Uncontrolled Pain (%)	0.9	0.7[†]	0.8

[a] For continuous variables, Whites were compared separately with Blacks and Hispanics using ordinary least squares regression. For dichotomous variables, Whites were compared separately with Blacks and Hispanics using chi-squared tests.

[†] $p \leq .05$; [*] $p \leq .01$; [‡] $p \leq .001$

Minority patients, particularly Blacks, appeared to be less likely than White patients to be diagnosed with specific medical conditions commonly associated with pain. In comparison with Whites, Black patients were marginally less likely to be diagnosed with neoplasms and were significantly less likely to be diagnosed with digestive system diseases and musculoskeletal system diseases. Although statistically significant, these differences were small. Black patients also were substantially less likely to be diagnosed as having a fracture, a finding consistent with the literature indicating that elderly Blacks are less likely than elderly Whites to suffer broken bones (Baron et al., 1996; Bohannon, 1999). In comparison with Whites, Hispanics were marginally less likely to be diagnosed with a fracture. Consistent with previous literature examining the incidence of hip fracture across races and ethnicities (Lauderdale et al., 1998), Hispanics had a fracture rate between that of Whites and Blacks. Hispanic patients were significantly less likely than Whites to be diagnosed with musculoskeletal system diseases.

Integumentary problems are an important concern for elderly home health care recipients. Although a relatively small proportion of patients suffer from stasis and pressure ulcers, these conditions can be difficult to treat and often result in significant pain. Whereas Hispanic patients did not differ from Whites in ulcer status, Black patients had stasis and pressure ulcers of a slightly more serious status than did Whites. The status of the most problematic stasis ulcer was marginally worse in Black than White patients, and the status of the most problematic pressure ulcer was significantly worse in Black than White patients.

White patients in the sample were rated as having more severe pain at the start/resumption of care than were patients of the other racial/ethnic groups. Although no racial and ethnic differences were identified in the rate of chronic pain, Whites were slightly, but significantly more likely than their minority counterparts to be rated as having intractable pain and had significantly worse scores at baseline on the OASIS item reflecting the frequency with which pain interfered with activity or movement.

In unadjusted analyses, White patients appeared to fare worse than patients of minority racial/ethnic backgrounds on pain outcomes. Black patients were marginally more likely than White home health care recipients to improve in the frequency with which pain interfered with activity or movement over the course of their episodes of care. Further, Whites were marginally more likely than their Black counterparts to be admitted to the hospital for the treatment of uncontrolled pain. (Although the proportion of affected patients was small - less than 1% - a total of 1,266 patient episodes included in the analysis sample ended in hospitalization for the treatment of uncontrolled pain.) Unadjusted analyses identified no significant difference between Hispanics and Whites on either outcome variable.

Risk-Adjusted Regression Analyses

Logistic regression was used to examine racial/ethnic differences in the two pain outcome measures: (1) improvement in pain frequency and (2) hospitalization for uncontrolled pain. Separate regression models compared the outcomes of White patients to those of Black and Hispanic patients, respectively. All models controlled for the 22 covariates described previously.

Angela G. Brega

Table 2. Risk-Adjusted Effect of Race/Ethnicity on Improvement in Pain Frequency [a]

	White vs. Black		White vs. Hispanic	
	OR	95% CI	OR	95% CI
Demographic Characteristics				
Race/Ethnicity	$0.85^{\ddagger}$	0.80 – 0.91	0.93	0.84 – 1.02
Age	$1.01^{\ddagger}$	1.01 - 1.01	$1.01^{\ddagger}$	1.01 - 1.01
Sex	$0.86^{\ddagger}$	0.83 - 0.89	$0.86^{\ddagger}$	0.83 - 0.89
Per Capita Income	1.00	1.00 - 1.00	1.00	1.00 - 1.00
Insurance Coverage				
Medicare as a Payer for Home Care Services	1.05	0.96 - 1.14	1.06	0.97 - 1.15
Medicaid as a Payer for Home Care Services	0.93	0.86 - 1.02	0.97	0.88 - 1.06
Support Network				
Frequency of Informal Assistance	1.00	1.00 - 1.01	1.00	1.00 - 1.01
Medical Complexity				
Number of Acute Medical Conditions	$1.02^{\dagger}$	1.00 - 1.03	$1.02^{\dagger}$	1.00 - 1.04
Number of Chronic Medical Conditions	$0.96^{\ddagger}$	0.95 - 0.97	$0.96^{\ddagger}$	0.95 - 0.97
Hospital Discharge within 14 Days of Start of Care	$1.14^{\ddagger}$	1.09 - 1.18	$1.14^{\ddagger}$	1.10 - 1.19
Good Rehabilitative Prognosis	$1.26^{\ddagger}$	1.20 - 1.33	$1.27^{\ddagger}$	1.20 - 1.34
Good/Fair Recovery Prognosis	$1.19^{\ddagger}$	1.10 - 1.30	$1.18^{\ddagger}$	1.08 - 1.29
Terminal Condition	$0.82^{\ddagger}$	0.74 - 0.90	$0.78^{\ddagger}$	0.71 - 0.87
Length of Stay Greater than 31 Days	$1.21^{\ddagger}$	1.17 - 1.26	$1.22^{\ddagger}$	1.17 - 1.26
Diagnoses				
Neoplasms	$0.94^{\dagger}$	0.88 - 0.99	$0.93^{\dagger}$	0.88 - 0.99
Digestive System Diseases	1.03	0.98 - 1.09	1.03	0.98 - 1.09
Musculoskeletal System Diseases	$0.64^{\ddagger}$	0.62 - 0.66	$0.64^{\ddagger}$	0.62 - 0.67
Fractures	$0.78^{\ddagger}$	0.75 - 0.82	$0.78^{\ddagger}$	0.75 - 0.82
Integumentary Status				
Status of Most Problematic Stasis Ulcer	$0.92^{\ddagger}$	0.88 - 0.96	0.93^{*}	0.89 - 0.98
Status of Most Problematic Pressure Ulcer	0.99	0.96 - 1.03	1.00	0.96 - 1.04
Pain Experience at Start of Care				
Chronic Pain	$0.85^{\ddagger}$	0.79 - 0.92	$0.85^{\ddagger}$	0.78 - 0.92
Intractable Pain	$0.84^{\ddagger}$	0.79 - 0.89	$0.84^{\ddagger}$	0.80 - 0.89
Pain Interfering w/ Activity/Movement	$1.97^{\ddagger}$	1.90 - 2.04	$1.99^{\ddagger}$	1.92 - 2.06

[a] The odds ratio (OR) with significance level and the 95% confidence interval (95% CI) are presented.
$^{\dagger}p \leq .05$; $^{*}p \leq .01$; $^{\ddagger}p \leq .001$.

Improvement in Pain Frequency

Analyses examining the rate of improvement in pain frequency showed different results depending on the racial/ethnic comparison involved. (Table 2 provides the odds ratios [ORs] and 95% confidence intervals [CIs] for all variables included in the models related to this outcome measure.) Although Whites had a marginally lower rate of improvement than Black patients in unadjusted analyses, this difference became significant when potentially confounding factors were included as covariates. Improvement rates among Whites did not differ from those of Hispanic patients in unadjusted or adjusted analyses.

Hospitalization for Uncontrolled Pain

Risk-adjusted analyses of the rate at which patients' home care episodes ended in hospitalization for the treatment of uncontrolled pain showed no racial or ethnic differences (see Table 3). Although in unadjusted analyses, White patients were marginally more likely than Black patients to be transferred to a hospital for the treatment of uncontrolled pain, the relationship between race and hospitalization rate became nonsignificant when patient demographic characteristics and baseline health status were controlled. There were no significant differences between Whites and Hispanics in the rate of hospitalization in either the unadjusted or adjusted analyses.

Influence of Covariates

Controlling for all other covariates, many of the variables included as predictors in the logistic regression models had a strong impact on pain outcomes (see Tables 2 and 3). Whereas patient age was not a significant predictor of hospitalization outcomes, it was related to improvement in pain frequency. However, although the bivariate correlation between age and improvement rate showed a weak (but significant), negative relationship, with older patients experiencing a lower rate of improvement, the effect of age on pain frequency outcomes reversed direction in the risk-adjusted regression models. Previous research has suggested that older patients report less pain than do younger patients (Desbiens et al., 1996). It may be that, once other factors were controlled, older patients were less likely (or less able) to communicate regarding the severity and ongoing nature of their pain, leading providers to believe that pain relief had been achieved to a larger extent than was actually the case.

Patient sex showed a consistent effect on both pain outcome measures. Women were significantly less likely to show improvement in the frequency of pain and marginally more likely to be hospitalized for the treatment of uncontrolled pain during their home care episodes. This finding is consistent with studies that have shown female patients to have a greater likelihood of being undertreated for pain, in comparison with their male counterparts (Cleeland et al., 1997; McDonald, 1994).

Variables reflecting patient financial status and insurance coverage exerted surprisingly little influence on pain outcomes. Neither Medicare coverage nor Medicaid coverage was a significant predictor of pain outcomes. Because the vast majority of the patients in the sample were covered by Medicare (95.0%), access to health care services was likely to be quite similar across patients, perhaps muting the potential impact of insurance coverage. Per capita income, included in all models as a proxy for patient SES, also was not a strong predictor of pain outcomes. This variable was not significantly related to improvement in pain frequency and was only marginally related to hospitalization for uncontrolled pain when White patients were compared with Black patients.

Involvement of the patient's social support network did not have a major impact on pain outcomes. The frequency of assistance provided by the primary informal caregiver was not related to improvement in pain frequency. However, the frequency of informal assistance was marginally associated with hospitalization outcomes. The more frequently a patient received assistance from his/her primary informal caregiver, the less likely he/she was to be hospitalized for the treatment of uncontrolled pain. Although the effect of the family support network was not strong, it does appear that the availability of an informal caregiver may reduce the chances of very severe pain-related outcomes.

Table 3. Risk-Adjusted Effect of Race/Ethnicity on Hospitalization for Uncontrolled Pain [a]

	White vs. Black		White vs. Hispanic	
	OR	95% CI	OR	95% CI
Demographic Characteristics				
Race/Ethnicity	1.18	0.94 – 1.47	1.06	0.74 – 1.51
Age	1.00	1.00 - 1.01	1.00	1.00 - 1.01
Sex	1.16[†]	1.02 - 1.32	1.18[†]	1.03 - 1.35
Per Capita Income	1.00[†]	1.00 - 1.00	1.00	1.00 - 1.00
Insurance Coverage				
Medicare as a Payer for Home Care Services	1.08	0.80 - 1.45	1.15	0.84 - 1.58
Medicaid as a Payer for Home Care Services	1.20	0.93 - 1.54	1.14	0.86 - 1.50
Support Network				
Frequency of Informal Assistance	0.97[†]	0.94 - 0.99	0.97[†]	0.94 - 1.00
Medical Complexity				
Number of Acute Medical Conditions	1.02	0.96 - 1.08	1.02	0.97 - 1.08
Number of Chronic Medical Conditions	1.01	0.98 - 1.05	1.02	0.98 - 1.05
Hospital Discharge within 14 Days of Start of Care	1.00	0.88 - 1.14	0.98	0.86 - 1.12
Good Rehabilitative Prognosis	0.65[‡]	0.55 - 0.76	0.63[‡]	0.54 - 0.75
Good/Fair Recovery Prognosis	0.83	0.67 - 1.02	0.85	0.69 - 1.05
Terminal Condition	1.04	0.81 - 1.34	1.12	0.87 - 1.45
Length of Stay Greater than 31 Days	0.58[‡]	0.51 - 0.67	0.60[‡]	0.52 - 0.69
Diagnoses				
Neoplasms	1.85[‡]	1.57 - 2.17	1.75[‡]	1.48 - 2.07
Digestive System Diseases	1.38[‡]	1.17 - 1.62	1.39[‡]	1.18 - 1.64
Musculoskeletal System Diseases	1.31[‡]	1.16 - 1.49	1.30[‡]	1.15 - 1.49
Fractures	1.50[‡]	1.27 - 1.78	1.42[‡]	1.19 - 1.69
Integumentary Status				
Status of Most Problematic Stasis Ulcer	1.18[†]	1.03 - 1.35	1.18[†]	1.03 - 1.36
Status of Most Problematic Pressure Ulcer	1.10	1.00 - 1.21	1.09	0.98 - 1.20
Pain Experience at Start of Care				
Chronic Pain	1.07	0.87 - 1.32	1.06	0.86 - 1.30
Intractable Pain	1.91[‡]	1.61 - 2.27	1.89[‡]	1.58 - 2.26
Pain Interfering w/ Activity/Movement	1.54[‡]	1.43 - 1.66	1.54[‡]	1.43 - 1.66

[a] The odds ratio (OR) with significance level and the 95% confidence interval (95% CI) are presented.
[†] $p \leq .05$; [*] $p \leq .01$; [‡] $p \leq .001$

Patient medical complexity was an important predictor of pain outcomes. As expected, patients with a larger number of chronic conditions were significantly less likely than other patients to improve in the frequency of pain interfering with activity or movement. Patients with a larger number of acute medical conditions (i.e., conditions of a short-term nature from which recovery is expected), were marginally more likely to improve in pain frequency over the course of their episodes of care. Patients discharged from a hospital within 14 days prior to the start/resumption of home care services were significantly more likely than other patients to improve in pain frequency. This effect may reflect the greater prevalence of acute medical needs (as opposed to chronic illnesses) among patients recently discharged from the hospital. Bivariate correlations showed that patients discharged from the hospital just prior to starting/resuming home care had a larger number of acute conditions ($r = 0.24$, $p < .001$) and a smaller number of chronic conditions ($r = -0.20$, $p < .001$) than did other patients.

Prognosis was significantly related to pain outcomes. Patients with a good rehabilitative prognosis, reflecting the home care provider's assessment that improvement in functional status was likely, were significantly more likely to improve in the frequency of pain and significantly less likely to be hospitalized for the treatment of uncontrolled pain. Patients rated as having a good/fair prognosis for recovering from the current episode of illness were significantly more likely than other patients to improve in the frequency of pain interfering with activity or movement over the course of their episodes of care. Patients rated as having six months or fewer to live were significantly less likely to improve in pain frequency over the course of their episodes of care.

Patients with home care episodes lasting more than 31 days had significantly higher rates of improvement in pain frequency and significantly lower rates of hospitalization for uncontrolled pain. It may be that patients receiving home health care services for less than a month (63.2% of the sample) were not on service long enough for their analgesic needs to be thoroughly investigated and successfully addressed. Further, patients with more lengthy episodes may have been undergoing treatment for chronic conditions, some of which may be less likely to result in significant, uncontrollable pain than more acute conditions (e.g., congestive heart failure versus hip fracture). Bivariate correlations confirmed that patients on service for more than 31 days had a significantly higher number of chronic conditions ($r = .15$, $p < .001$).

Four diagnoses that often result in significant pain were controlled in the risk-adjusted analyses. Patients diagnosed with musculoskeletal system diseases or fractures were significantly less likely to improve in pain frequency over the course of their episodes of care than were patients without these diagnoses. Being diagnosed with a neoplasm was associated with a marginally lower rate of improvement. Those patients suffering from neoplasms, digestive system diseases, musculoskeletal system diseases, or fractures were significantly more likely than other patients to be hospitalized for the treatment of uncontrolled pain.

Integumentary status, a critical treatment focus in home health services for the elderly, also influenced pain outcomes. Although the status of the most problematic pressure ulcer did not predict pain outcomes, the status of the most problematic stasis ulcer did. Patients with more severe stasis ulcers had significantly lower rates of improvement in pain frequency and marginally higher rates of hospitalization for uncontrolled pain.

As expected, baseline pain scores were an important predictor of pain outcomes. Patients with chronic pain were significantly less likely to improve in pain frequency over the course of their episodes of care. Those identified as having intractable pain at baseline had significantly lower rates of improvement in pain frequency as well as significantly higher rates of hospitalization for uncontrolled pain. Patients with a higher frequency of pain interfering with activity or movement at the start/resumption of care were significantly more likely to be hospitalized for uncontrolled pain, but also had a significantly higher rate of improvement in pain frequency. This latter relationship was consistent with the bivariate correlation between baseline pain frequency and improvement in pain frequency, which showed that a higher frequency of pain at baseline was associated with a higher rate of improvement over the course of the episode of care ($r = .14$, $p < .001$). It may be that providers are less likely to focus significant attention on the analgesic needs of patients with a fairly low frequency of pain at the start/resumption of care and that these patients have less potential for improvement than those patients experiencing severe pain at the beginning of their episodes of care.

CONCLUSION

Although studies examining racial and ethnic disparities in pain management provide inconsistent findings, the majority of work in this area suggests that minorities are more likely than Whites to be undertreated for pain. The current study provides no evidence of a higher rate of oligoanalgesia among minorities and little evidence of any racial/ethnic differences in the pain outcomes of elderly home health care recipients. In risk-adjusted analyses, White, Black, and Hispanic patients were equally likely to be hospitalized for the treatment of uncontrolled pain during the course of their home care episodes. White and Hispanic patients also did not differ with regard to the rate of improvement in the frequency of pain interfering with activity or movement. Contrary to studies suggesting that White patients receive better analgesic care than minorities, the White sample in this study showed a significantly lower rate of improvement in pain frequency than did Black patients. However, this difference was quite small. Whereas 60.3% of Blacks improved in pain frequency during their home care episodes, 58.6% of Whites improved. Although this difference was statistically significant in this large sample, even using a stringent alpha value, it is unlikely to be of clinical importance.

The significant difference between the pain frequency outcomes of Blacks and Whites may have resulted from racial differences in baseline pain severity. Descriptive analyses indicated that, at start/resumption of care, the frequency with which pain interfered with activity or movement was slightly, but significantly higher for White than Black patients. White patients also were significantly more likely to be rated by home care providers as having intractable pain and to be diagnosed with medical conditions known to be associated with pain (i.e., digestive system diseases, musculoskeletal system diseases, fractures). Although multiple variables reflecting the pain experience of patients at start/resumption of care were included in the risk-adjusted regression models, it is possible that racial differences in baseline pain were not completely controlled and thus continued to influence pain outcomes.

While experiencing more frequent and severe pain, White patients also had shorter home care episodes than did their Black counterparts. Whereas 45.1% of Blacks were on service longer than a month, only 36.0% of White patients received care for more than 31 days. The higher degree of baseline pain, in combination with shorter home care episodes, may have constrained the potential for improvement in the pain experience of White patients.

There are a number of reasons that clinically significant differences in pain outcomes may not have been found in this study. Home care represents a unique health care "setting," in comparison with the ED, inpatient, and outpatient settings examined in previous studies of racial/ethnic disparities in analgesic care. In some settings, a patient may be seen at only a single time point (e.g., ED) or may be seen on more than one occasion, but several weeks or months apart (e.g., primary care, specialty cancer practices). In home care, providers interact with their patients many times over a period of weeks or months. This repeated exposure to a patient and his/her style of communication may enhance the provider's ability to interpret the patient's pain expressions, perhaps reducing the barriers in communication between providers and minority patients that have been hypothesized to lead to disparities in pain management (Bonham, 2001; Green et al., 2003; Tait and Chibnall, 2005; Tamayo-Sarver et al., 2003b).

It is possible that the patient assessment process employed in home care also diminishes the influence of communication barriers on pain management decisions. In conducting his/her comprehensive assessment, the home care provider obtains information about the patient's pain experience through interview and observation. In addition to obtaining the patient's direct report of pain, the provider observes the patient engaging in his regular daily activities (e.g., preparing meals, walking to the bathroom). The impact of pain on the patient's ability to move around the home and complete necessary activities may be noted by the provider even when barriers in communication hinder the provider's ability to accurately interpret the patient's direct report of pain. The ability to observe the debilitating effect of pain, and to do so repeatedly over time, may reduce the impact of communication barriers between providers and minority patients.

In addition to becoming quite familiar with the patient, the home care provider often has the opportunity to get to know the members of the patient's family. Family members may be present for home care visits and often become an integral component of the care plan (e.g., an agency may provide fewer home health aide visits for a patient who has family caregivers assisting him/her with personal care and functional activities). Family members may be an important secondary source of information about a patient's experience of pain. Feedback from multiple sources may reduce the chances that race-related communication barriers will result in the undertreatment of pain among minority patients. Although the role of the patient's support network in facilitating the appropriate treatment of pain has not been studied directly (Todd et al., 1993), the results of the current study suggest the possibility that family members and friends may serve a protective function. Controlling for other potentially confounding factors, more frequent involvement by the primary informal caregiver was associated with a marginally lower rate of hospitalization for uncontrolled pain.

In 2002, Fuentes and her colleagues suggested that racial/ethnic differences in the treatment of pain may not have been identified in their study because clinical decision making in the San Francisco General Hospital ED is shared by multiple providers. The same can be said for home health care. A patient may be seen by multiple home care providers (i.e., nurses, therapists, social workers, home health aides) over the course of his/her home care episode. The availability of input from multiple providers about the patient's experience of pain may reduce the likelihood that one provider's ineffective communication with a patient will negatively impact that patient's analgesic care.

Although evidence of clinically significant disparities in the pain outcomes of White and minority home care recipients was not found in this study, evidence that pain is a serious concern for a large percentage of elderly home health care recipients was present. Although 39.9% of patients experienced no pain or only pain that was not severe enough to interfere with activity or movement, 48.6% experienced interference from pain on a daily (40.9%) or constant (7.7%) basis at the start or resumption of care. At baseline, 5.5% of patients were assessed as having chronic pain and 12.8% as having intractable pain.

Although some degree of pain relief was achieved in many patients, a substantial percentage of elderly home care recipients continued to experience serious pain symptoms at the conclusion of their home care episodes. Across the sample, 58.9% of patients experienced some improvement in the frequency with which pain interfered with activity or movement. The remaining 41.1% of patients in pain at the start or resumption of care experienced no relief (and potentially even decline). A full 29.0% continued to experience daily (26.2%) or constant (2.8%) interference from pain. Although nearly half of the patients assessed as having intractable pain at baseline improved over the course of their episodes of care, 5.8% continued to experience pain that was difficult to treat and that affected patients' physical and emotional functioning. As in many other health care settings, the treatment of pain in home health care appears to be suboptimal.

Study Limitations and Strengths

It is important to note that the methods employed in this study differ substantially from those of other studies addressing racial and ethnic disparities in pain management. Critically, the dependent variables examined in the current work focused on pain outcomes (i.e., improvement in pain frequency, hospitalization for uncontrolled pain) rather than on the prescription of analgesic medications, which is the usual focus of studies in this area. Although reviewing patient medications is an important component of the comprehensive patient assessment conducted in home health care, information about medications is not collected as part of the OASIS data set and thus is not available on a national basis. Further, as the OASIS data set does not contain information about the care provider's recommendations and clinical actions to address patient pain, this study cannot establish that the pain of White and minority patients received equivalent attention, just that their ultimate outcomes were essentially the same.

Although the inability to directly examine the pain management decisions of home care providers is a limitation of the study, the focus on patient outcomes is a strength. Prior research in this area focuses heavily on racial/ethnic differences in the prescription of analgesics. Few studies have attempted to examine the quality of the care provided. Cleeland and his colleagues (1994, 1997) stand out in this regard. These investigators assessed the adequacy of pain treatment, examining the degree to which analgesic care complied with World Health Organization guidelines for the management of cancer pain. Likewise, the current study focused on the ultimate outcomes of care, rather than the process of managing pain. Although it is critical to understand how provider's pain management decisions are influenced by patient race/ethnicity, the quality of care provided rests in the degree to which patient pain is relieved as a result of the decisions made.

As the first known examination of racial and ethnic disparities in the pain outcomes of elderly home health care recipients, this study provides important insight into the management of pain in home health care. The study results suggest that pain is a serious clinical concern for many elderly home care patients, but that racial/ethnic disparities in pain outcomes are not present to any clinically significant degree. Although the study did not directly examine the mechanisms underlying disparities, the results suggest that the unique style of interaction between the patient and provider in home health care may reduce the chances that minority patients will be undertreated for pain. Specifically, it is hypothesized that repeated interaction between patient and provider over many weeks or months; feedback from members of the patient's social support network regarding the patient's experience of pain; and input from multiple health care providers may diminish the degree to which communication barriers between providers and minority patients may influence analgesic care. Future research should be conducted to directly examine the impact of these factors on the clinical assessment and treatment of pain.

REFERENCES

Anderson, K. O., Mendoza, T. R., Valero, V., Richman, S. P., Russell, C., Hurley, J., DeLeon, C., Washington, P., Palos, G., Payne, R., and Cleeland, C. S. (2000). Minority cancer patients and their providers: Pain management attitudes and practice. *Cancer, 88*(8), 1929-1938.

Anderson, K. O., Richman, S. P., Hurley, J., Palos, G., Valero, V., Mendoza, T. R., Gning, I., and Cleeland, C. S. (2002). Cancer pain management among underserved minority outpatients: Perceived needs and barriers to optimal control. *Cancer, 94*(8), 2295-2304.

Atherton, M. J., Feeg, V. D., and El-Adham, A. F. (2004). Race, ethnicity, and insurance as determinants of epidural use: Analysis of a national sample survey. *Nursing Economics, 22*(1), 6-13.

Bach, P. B., Guadagnoli, E., Schrag, D., Schussler, N., and Warren, J. L. (2002). Patient demographic and socioeconomic characteristics in the SEER-Medicare database applications and limitations. *Medical Care, 40*(8 Suppl), IV-19-25.

Baron, J. A., Karagas, M., Barrett, J., Kniffin, W., Malenka, D., Mayor, M., and Keller, R. B. (1996). Basic epidemiology of fractures of the upper and lower limb among Americans over 65 years of age. *Epidemiology, 7*(6), 612-618.

Bartfield, J. M., Salluzzo, R. F., Raccio-Robak, N., Funk, D. L., and Verdile, V. P. (1997). Physician and patient factors influencing the treatment of low back pain. *Pain, 73*(2), 209-211.

Bass, D. M., and Noelker, L. S. (1987). The influence of family caregivers on elder's use of in-home services: An expanded conceptual framework. *Journal of Health and Social Behavior, 280*(2), 184-196.

Bates, M. S., Edwards, W. T., and Anderson, K. O. (1993). Ethnocultural influences on variation in chronic pain experience. *Pain; 52(1)*, 101–12.

Baxter, J., Bryant, L. L., Scarbro, S., and Shetterly, S. M. (2001). Patterns of rural hispanic and non-hispanic white health care use. *Research on Aging, 23*(1), 37-60.

Beebe, K., Lawrence, T., and Lintzeris, G. (1985). Medicare admissions and length of stay for short-stay hospitals. *Health Care Financing Review, 7*(1), 117-119.

Bernabei, R., Gambassi, G., Lapane, K., Landi, F., Gatsonis, C., Dunlop, R., Lipsitz, L., Steel, K., and Mor, V. (1998). Management of pain in elderly patients with cancer. *Journal of the American Medical Association, 279*(23), 1877-1882.

Bohannon, A. D. (1999). Osteoporosis and AA women. *Journal of Women's Health and Gender-Based Medicine, 8*(5), 609-615.

Bonham, V. L. (2001). Race, ethnicity, and pain treatment: Striving to understand the causes and solutions to the disparities in pain treatment. *Journal of Law, Medicine, and Ethics*, *29*(1), 52-68.

Brega, A. G., Goodrich, G. K., Powell, M. C., and Grigsby, J. (2005). Racial and ethnic disparities in the outcomes of elderly home care recipients. *Home Health Care Services Quarterly*, *24*(3), 1-21.

Brega, A. G., Schlenker, R. E., Hijjazi, K., Neal, S., Belansky, E. S., Talkington, S., Jordan, A. K., Bontrager, J., and Tennant, C. (2002). *Final Report*. Denver, CO: Center for Health Policy Research.

Cagney, K. A. and Agree, E.M. (1999). Racial differences in skilled nursing care and home health use: The mediating effects of family structure and social class. *Journal of Gerontology Series B-Psychological Sciences and Social Sciences, 54*(4), S223-S236.

Centers for Medicare and Medicaid Services (CMS), U. S. Department of Health and Human Services. (2005). *Outcome-Based Quality Monitoring Reports: Technical Documentation of Measures, August*. Retrieved March 8, 2006 from http://new.cms.hhs.gov/apps/hha/measures.pdf

Chadiha, L. A., Proctor, E. K., Morrow-Howell, N., Darkwa, O. K., and Dore, P. (1995). Post-hospital home care for African-American and White elderly. *The Gerontologist, 35*(2), 233-239.

Chen, I., Kurz, J., Pasanen, M., Faselis, C., Panda, M., Staton, L. J., O'Rorke, J., Menon, M., Genao, I., Wood, J., Mechaber, A. J., Rosenberg, E., Carey, T., Calleson, D., and Cykert, S. (2005). Racial differences in opioid use for chronic nonmalignant pain. *Journal of General Internal Medicine*, *20*(7), 593-598.

Chibnall, J. T., Tait, R. C., and Ross, L. R. (1997). The effects of medical evidence and pain intensity on medical student judgments of chronic pain patients. *Journal of Behavioral Medicine*, *20*(3), 257-271.

Cleeland, C. S., Gonin, R., Baez, L., Loehrer, P., and Pandya, K. J. (1997). Pain and treatment of pain in minority patients with cancer: The Eastern Cooperative Oncology Group Minority Outpatient Pain Study. *Annals of Internal Medicine*, *127*(9), 813-816.

Cleeland, C. S., Gonin, R., Hatfield, A. K., Edmonson, J. H., Blum, R. H., Stewart, J. A., and Pandya, K. J. (1994). Pain and its treatment in outpatients with metastatic cancer. *New England Journal of Medicine*, *330*(9), 592-596.

Collins, K. S., Hall, A., and Neuhaus, C. (1999). *U.S. Minority Health: A Chartbook*. New York: The Commonwealth Fund.

Cooper-Patrick, L., Gallo, J. J., Gonzales, J. J., Vu, H. T., Powe, N. R., Nelson, C., and Ford, D. E. (1999). Race, gender, and partnership in the patient-physician relationship. *Journal of the American Medical Association, 282*(6), 583-589.

Desbiens, N. A., Wu, A. W., Broste, S. K., Wenger, N. S., Connors, A. F., Lynn, J., Yasui, Y., Phillips, R. S., and Fulkerson, W. (1996). Pain and satisfaction with pain control in seriously ill hospitalized adults: Findings from the SUPPORT research investigations. For the support investigators. Study to understand prognoses and preferences for outcomes and risks of treatment. *Critical Care Medicine, 24*(12), 1953-1961.

Dunlop, D. D., Manheim, L. M., Song, J., and Chang, R. (2002). Gender and ethnic/racial disparities in health care utilization among older adults. *Journal of Gerontology Series B-Psychological Sciences and Social Sciences*, *57*(3), S221-S233.

Edwards, R. R., Doleys, D. M., Fillingim, R. B., and Lowery, D. (2001). Ethnic differences in pain tolerance: Clinical implications in a chronic pain population. *Psychosomatic Medicine, 63*(2), 316-323.

Feder, J., Hadley, J., and Zuckerman, S. (1987). How did Medicare's Prospective Payment System affect hospitals? *New England Journal of Medicine, 317*(14), 867-873.

Friedland, L. R., and Kulick, R. M. (1994). Emergency department analgesic use in pediatric trauma victims with fractures. *Annals of Emergency Medicine, 23*(2), 203-207.

Fuentes, E. F., Kohn, M. A., and Neighbor, M. L. (2002). Lack of association between patient ethnicity or race and fracture analgesia. *Academic Emergency Medicine, 9*(9), 910–915.

Green, C. R., Anderson, K. O., Baker, T. A., Campbell, L. C., Decker, S., Fillingim, R. B., Kaloukalani, D. A., Lasch, K. E., Myers, C., Tait, R. C., Todd, K. H., and Vallerand, A. H. (2003). The unequal burden of pain: Confronting racial and ethnic disparities in pain. *Pain Medicine, 4*(3), 277-294.

Green, C. R., Wheeler, J. R., LaPorte, F., Marchant, B., Guerrero, B. (2002). How well is chronic pain managed? Who does it well? *Pain Medicine, 3*(1), 56-65.

Greene, V. L., and Monahan, D.J. (1984). Comparative utilization of community based long term care services by hispanic and anglo elderly in a case management system. *Journal of Gerontology, 39*(6), 730-735.

Gregory, K., Wells, K. B., and Leake, B. (1987). Medical students' expectations for encounters with minority and nonminority patients. *Journal of the National Medical Association, 79*(4), 403-408.

Grossman, S. A., Sheidler, V. R., Swedeen, K., Mucenski, J., and Piantadosi, S. (1991). Correlation of patient and caregiver ratings of cancer pain. *Journal of Pain and Symptom Management, 6*(2), 53-57.

Health Care Financing Administration (HCFA) Office of Statistics and Data Management. (1986) *Medical data current utilization tabulations.* Washington, DC: Department of Health and Human Services, 4.

Hittle, D. F., Shaughnessy, P. W., Crisler, K. S., Powell, M. C., Richard, A. A., Conway, K. S., Stearns, P. M., and Engle, K. (2003). A study of reliability and burden of home health assessment using OASIS. *Home Health Care Services Quarterly, 22*(4), 43-63.

Hostetler, M. A., Auinger, P., and Szilagyi, P. G. (2002). Parenteral analgesic and sedative use among ED patients in the United States: Combined results from the National Hospital Ambulatory Medical Care Survey (NHAMCS) 1992-1997. *American Journal of Emergency Medicine, 20*(3), 139-143.

Jackson, S. A., Shiferaw, B., Anderson, R.T., Heuser, M.D., Hutchinson, K.M., and Mittelmark, M.B. (2002). Racial differences in service utilization: The Forsyth County Aging Study. *Journal of Health Care for the Poor and Underserved, 13*(3), 320-333.

Jenkins, C. L., and Laditka, S.B. (2003). A comparative analysis of disability measures and their relation to home health care use. *Home Health Care Services Quarterly, 22*(1), 21-37.

Jordan, M. S., Lumley, M. A., and Leisen, C. C. (1998). The relationships of cognitive coping and pain control beliefs to pain and adjustment among African-American and Caucasian women with rheumatoid arthritis. *Arthritis Care and Research, 11*(2), 80–8.

Juarez, G., Ferrell, B., and Borneman, T. (1998). Influence of culture on cancer pain management in Hispanic patients. *Cancer Practice, 6*(5), 262-9.

Juarez, G., Ferrell, B., and Borneman, T. (1999). Cultural considerations in education for cancer pain management. *Journal of Cancer Education, 14*(3), 168-73.

Karpman, R. R., Del Mar, N., and Bay, C. (1997). Analgesia for emergency centers' orthopaedic patients: Does an ethnic bias exist? *Clinical Orthopaedics and Related Research, 334*, 270–275.

Kemper, P. (1992). The use of formal and informal home care by the disabled elderly. *Health Services Research, 27*(4), 421-451.

Lauderdale, D. S., Jacobsen, S. J., Furner, S. E., Levy, P. S., Brody, J. A., and Goldberg, J. (1998). Hip fracture incidence among elderly Hispanics. *American Journal of Public Health, 88*(8), 1245-1247.

Lee, W. W., Burelbach, A. E., and Fosnocht, D. (2001). Hispanic and Non-Hispanic White patient pain management expectations. *American Journal of Emergency Medicine, 19*(7), 549-550.

Liu, K., and Manton, K. G. (1988). *Effects of Medicare's Hospital Prospective Payment System (PPS) on Disabled Medicare Beneficiaries: Final Report.* Washington, DC: Urban Institute.

Mauser, E., and Miller, N. A. (1994). A profile of home health users in 1992. *Health Care Financing Review, 16*(1), 17-33.

McCracken, L.M., Matthews, A. K., Tang, T. S., and Cuba, S.L. (2001). A comparison of Blacks and Whites seeking treatment for chronic pain. *Clinical Journal of Pain, 17*(3), 249-255.

McDonald, D. D. (1994). Gender and ethnic stereotyping and narcotic analgesic administration. *Research in Nursing and Health, 17*(1), 45-49.

Meghani, S. H. (2005). Leveling the playing field: Does pain disparity literature suffer from a reporting bias? *Pain Medicine, 6*(3), 269-270.

Miller, B., Campbell, R. T., Davis, L., Furner, S., Giachello, A., Prochaska, T., Kaufman, J. E., Li, L., and Perez, C. (1996). Minority use of community long-term care services: A comparative analysis. *Journal of Gerontology Series B-Psychological Sciences and Social Sciences, 53*(2), S70-S81.

Miller, B., McFall, S., and Campbell, R. T. (1994). Changes in sources of community long-term care among Blacks and White frail older persons. *Journal of Gerontology, 49*(1), S14-S24.

Mindel, C. H., Wright, R., and Starrett, R. A. (1986). Informal and formal health and social support systems of Black and White elderly: A comparative cost approach. *The Gerontologist, 26*(3), 279-285.

Morrison, R. S., Wallenstein, S., Natale, D. K., Senzel, R. S., and Huang, L. (2000). We don't carry that" - Failure of pharmacies in predominantly nonwhite neighborhoods to stock opioid analgesics. *New England Journal of Medicine, 342*(14), 1023-1026.

Morrow-Howell, N., Chadiha, L. A., Proctor, E. K., Hourd-Bryant, M., and Dore. P. (1996). Racial differences in discharge planning. *Health and Social Work, 21*(2), 131-139.

Mui, A. C., and Burnette, D. (1994). Long-term care service use by frail elders: Is ethnicity a factor? *The Gerontologist, 34*(2), 190-198.

Murray, L. A. (2000). Racial and ethnic differences among Medicare beneficiaries. *Health Care Financing Review, 21*(4), 117-127.

Netzer, J. K., Coward, R. T., Peek, C. W., Henretta, J. C., Duncan, R. P., and Dougherty, M.C. (1997) Race and residence differences in the use of formal services by older adults. *Research on Aging, 19*(3), 300-332.

Neu, C.R. and Harrison, S.C. (1988) *Posthospital care before and after the Medicare prospective payment system.* Santa Monica, CA: Rand.

Ng, B., Dimsdale, J. E., Rollnik, J. D., and Shapiro, H. (1996a). The effect of ethnicity on prescriptions for patient-controlled analgesia for post-operative pain. *Pain, 66*(1), 9–12.

Ng, B., Dimsdale, J. E., Shragg, G. P., Deutsch, R. (1996b). Ethnic difference in analgesic consumption for postoperative pain. *Psychosomatic Medicine, 58*(2), 125-129.

Norgard, T. M., and Rodgers W. L. (1997). Patterns of in-home care among elderly Black and White Americans. *Journal of Gerontology Series B-Psychological Sciences and Social Sciences, 52,* S93-101.

Obst, T. E., Nauenberg, E., and Buck, G. M. (2001). Maternal health insurance coverage as a determinant of obstetrical anesthesia care. *Journal of Health Care for the Poor and Underserved,* 12(2), 177-191.

Peng, T. R., Navaie-Waliser, M., and Feldman, P. H. (2003). Social support, home health service use, and outcomes among four racial-ethnic groups. *The Gerontologist,* 43(4), 502-513.

Petrack, E. M., Christopher, N. C., and Kriwinsky, J. (1997). Pain management in the emergency department: Patterns of analgesic utilization. *Pediatrics, 99*(5), 711-714.

Pfefferbaum, B., Adams, J., and Aceves, J. (1990). The influence of culture on pain in Anglo and Hispanic children with cancer. *Journal of the American Academy of Child and Adolescent Psychiatry.* 29(4),642-647.

Proctor, B. D. and Dalaker, J. (2002). *Poverty in the United States: 2001.* In: U.S. Census Bureau (ed.). Current Population Reports, 60-219. Washington, DC, Government Printing Office.

Schore, J. (1994). *Patient, agency, and area characteristics associated with regional variation in the use of Medicare home health services.* Princeton, NJ: Mathematica Policy Research, Inc.

Selbst, S. M., and Clark, M. (1990). Analgesic use in the emergency department. *Annals of Emergency Medicine, 19*(9), 1010-1013.

Shaughnessy, P. W., and Kramer, A. M. (1990). The increased needs of patients in nursing homes and patients receiving home health care. *New England Journal of Medicine, 322*(1) 21-27.

Sleath, B., Roter, D., Chewning, B., and Svarstad, B. (1999). Asking questions about medication: Analysis of physician-patient interactions and physician perceptions. *Medical Care, 37*(11), 1169-1173.

Smedley, B. D., Stith, A. Y., and Nelson, A. R. (Eds.) (2003). *Unequal Treatment: Confronting Racial and Ethnic Disparities in Health Care.* Washington, DC: National Academies Press.

Stern, R. S., and Epstein, A. M. (1985). Institutional responses to prospective payment based on diagnosis-related groups: Implications for cost, quality, and access. *New England Journal of Medicine, 312*(10), 621-627.

Stjernsward, J. (1988). WHO cancer pain relief programme. *Cancer Surveys, 7*(1), 195-208.

Streltzer, J., and Wade, T. C. (1981). The influence of cultural group on the undertreatment of postoperative pain. *Psychosomatic Medicine, 43*(5), 397-403.

Sullivan, L. W., and Eagel, B. A. (2005). Leveling the playing field: Recognizing rectifying disparities management of pain. *Pain Medicine, 6*(1), 5–10.

Tait, R. C., and Chibnall, J. T. (1997). Physician judgments of chronic pain patients. *Social Science and Medicine, 45*(8), 1199-1205.

Tait, R. C., and Chibnall, J. T. (2001). Work injury management of refractory low back pain: Relations with ethnicity, legal representation, and diagnosis. *Pain, 91*(1-2), 47-56.

Tait, R. C., and Chibnall, J. T. (2005). Racial and ethnic disparities in the evaluation and treatment of pain: Psychological perspectives. *Professional Psychology: Research and Practice, 36*(6), 595-601.

Tamayo-Sarver, J. H., Dawson, N. V., Hinze, S. W., Cydulka, R. K., Wigton, R. S., Albert, J. M., Ibrahim, S. A., and Baker, D. W. (2003a). The effect of race/ethnicity and desirable social characteristics on physicians' decisions to prescribe opioid analgesics. *Academic Emergency Medicine, 10*(11), 1239-1248.

Tamayo-Sarver, J. H., Hinze, S. W., Cydulka, R. K., and Baker, D. W. (2003b). Racial and ethnic disparities in emergency department analgesic prescription. *American Journal of Public Health, 93*(12), 2067–2073.

Tennstedt, S., and Chang, B. (1998). The relative contribution of ethnicity versus socioeconomic status in explaining differenes in disability and receipt of informal care. *Journal of Gerontology Series B-Psychological Sciences and Social Sciences, 53B*(2), S61-S70.

Thomason, T. E., McCune, J. S., Bernard, S. A., Winer, E. P., Tremont, S., and Lindley, C. M. (1998). Cancer pain survey: Patient-centred issues in control. *Journal of Pain and Symptom Management, 15*(5), 275-284.

Todd, K. H. (2001). Influence of ethnicity on emergency department pain management. *Emergency Medicine, 13*(3), 274-278.

Todd, K. H., Samaroo, N., and Hoffman, J. R. (1993). Ethnicity as a risk factor for inadequate emergency department analgesia. *Journal of the American Medical Association, 269*(12), 1537–1539.

Todd, K. H., Deaton, C., D'Adamo, A. P., and Goe, L. (2000). Ethnicity and analgesic practice. *Annals of Emergency Medicine, 35*(1), 11–16.

Todd, K. H., Lee, T., and Hoffman, J. R. (1994). The effect of ethnicity on physician estimates of pain severity in patients with isolated extremity trauma. *Journal of the American Medical Association, 271*(12), 925–928.

U.S. Department of Health and Human Services, Public Health Services, Agency for Health Care Policy and Research (1992). *Clinical Practice Guideline. Acute Pain Management: Operative or Medical Procedures and Trauma.* Publication Number 92-0032. Silver Springs, MD: Center for Research Dissemination and Liaison.

U.S. General Accounting Office (GAO), Health, Education, and Human Services Division (HEHS). (1998). *Medicare Home Health Benefit: Impact of Interim Payment System and Agency Closures on Access to Services,* Publication No. GAO/HEHS-98-238, Washington, DC: GAO.

Van Ryn, M., and Burke, J. (2000). The effect of patient race and socio-economic status on physicians' perceptions of patients. *Social Science and Medicine, 50*(6), 813-828.

Von Roenn, J. H., Cleeland, C. S., Gonin, R., Hatfield, A. K., and Pandya, K. J. (1993). Physician attitudes and practice in cancer pain management: A survey from the Eastern Cooperative Oncology Group. *Annals of Internal Medicine, 119*(2), 121-126.

Wallace, S. P., Levy-Storms, L., and Ferguson, L. R. (1995). Access to paid in-home assistance among disabled elderly people: Do latinos differ from non-latino whites?" *American Journal of Public Health, 85*(7), 970-975.

Wallace, S. P., Levy-Storms, L., Kington, R.S., and Andersen, R. M. (1998). The persistence of race and ethnicity in the use of long-term care. *Journal of Gerontology Series B-Psychological Sciences and Social Sciences, 53*(2), S104-S112.

Weisenberg, M., Kreindler, M. L., Schachat, R., and Werboff, J. (1975). Pain: Anxiety and attitudes in black, white, and Puerto Rican patients. *Psychosomatic Medicine, 37*(2), 123–35.

Weisse, C. S., Sorum, P. C., and Dominguez, R. E. (2003). The influence of gender and race on physicians' pain management decisions. *Journal of Pain, 4*(9), 505-510.

Weisse, C. S., Sorum, P. C., Sanders, K. N., and Syat, B. L. (2001). Do gender and race affect decisions about pain management? *Journal of General Internal Medicine, 16*(4), 211-217.

White-Means, S. I., and Rubin, R. M. (2004). Is there equity in the home health care market? Understanding racial patterns in the use of formal home health care. *Journal of Gerontology Series B-Psychological Sciences and Social Sciences, 59B,* (4), S220-S229.

Wolff, B. B. (1985). Ethnocultural factors influencing pain and illness behavior. *Clinical Journal of Pain, 1,* 23-30.

Woodrow, K. M., Friedman, G. D., Siegelaub, A. B., and Collen, M. F. (1972). Pain tolerance: Differences according to age, sex, and race. *Psychosomatic Medicine, 34*(6), 548–56.

Yen, K., Kim, M., Stremski, E. S., and Gorelick, M. H. (2003). Effect of ethnicity and race on the use of pain medications in children with long bone fractures in the emergency department. *Annals of Emergency Medicine, 42*(1), 41-47.

Zalon, M. L. (1993). Nurses' assessment of postoperative patients' pain. *Pain, 54*(3), 329-334.

Zatzick, D. F., and Dimsdale, J. E. (1990). Cultural variations in response to painful stimuli. *Psychosomatic Medicine, 52*(5), 544-557.

Zborowski, M. (1969). *People in Pain.* San Francisco: Jossey-Bass.

In: Racial and Ethnic Disparities in Health and Health Care   ISBN 1-60021-268-9
Editor: Elene V. Metrosa, pp. 41-52   © 2006 Nova Science Publishers, Inc.

Chapter 2

CHRONIC CONDITIONS, HOSPITAL ADMISSIONS, AND THEIR RELATIONSHIP TO ED CROWDING: IMPROVING QUALITY OF CARE AND UTILIZATION WHILE REDUCING DISPARITIES

Jay J. Shen[*]

Department of Health Care Administration and Policy, School of Public Health
University of Nevada at Las Vegas, Las Vegas, NV

Elmer L. Washington

Aunt Martha's Youth Service Center, Chicago Heights, IL

ABSTRACT

Context

Limited research has been done to examine emergency department (ED) admissions as a percentage all hospital admissions and to assess the trends in ED utilization over time.

Objective

To examine relationships between ED utilization, race, insurance status and access to care. To identify priority conditions upon which to explore implications for access and quality improvement efforts.

---

[*] Corresponding Author. (702) 895-5410 (Phone); (702) 895-5573 (Fax)

Design, Setting, and Participants

Cross-sectional data of over 19 million patients hospitalized in the 1995-2001 National Inpatient Sample were weighted to reflect national totals.

Main Outcome Measures

Percent and likelihood of ED admission among all hospital admission in general and as related to race, insurance status, specific clinical conditions, length of stay, and mortality rates.

Results

Percentages of hospital admissions through the ED has progressively increased over time; specifically as related to 16 clinical conditions, mostly chronic. Decreased utilization has been noted for diseases that have been focal points of improvement efforts (e.g., heart failure, acute myocardial infarction, asthma, and cerebral occlusion) while other conditions have shown increased utilization. Disparities of constant magnitude were noted with respect to race and most categories of insurance status. Disparities of increasing magnitude were observed with respect to the uninsured. While trends regarding mortality and length of stay have shown improvements, disparities persisted, especially with respect to the uninsured. Access to care was a significant etiologic factor with areas having higher provider to population ratios showing reduced ED utilization.

Conclusions

Quality improvement efforts need to promote evidence based approaches to chronic conditions where increased ED utilization has been demonstrated including diabetes mellitus and affective psychosis. Access to care by promoting optimal provider to population ratios needs to be prioritized as a cost effective, quality improvement measure. Access to care for uninsured populations should be improved by expansion of availability of insurance benefits.

INTRODUCTION

Challenges facing the health care system and strategies for meeting the challenges have been described in a compelling fashion in the Institute of Medicine's report "Crossing the Quality Chasm." This report emphasizes the need to improve the quality of care for chronic conditions, improve continuity of care, and make care systems responsive to individual patient preferences. [1] By studying patterns of utilization of the emergency department (ED), we propose to assess whether the health care system is moving in this direction. The ED is a setting that is meant for acute, not chronic conditions by its very nature. It is not designed for the primary purpose of promoting continuity of care for most patients. While the ED is an appropriate care source for life threatening acute conditions and some acute exacerbations of chronic conditions, over utilization in inappropriate circumstances potentially diverts resources from patients who need them. [2] Nevertheless, the hospital-based ED also serves as a safety-net for socioeconomically vulnerable persons who lack access to regular care sources resulting in preventable ED visits and hospitalization. [3-4]

Challenges related to ED crowding became increasingly recognized during the 1990s. These challenges have been fueled by a reduction in the number of emergency departments with a concomitant increase in the volume of patients presenting to the ED. [5] As ED crowding has progressed, potential compromises to cost effectiveness and quality of care abound. [6,7] While multiple efforts to address ED crowding have focused on factors intrinsic to the ED, [8-11] few have focused on chronic diseases and factors extrinsic to the ED. [4,12] Based upon our review of the literature, limited research has evaluated the relative contribution of chronic diseases as demonstrated using a national data base. While delays related to inpatient bed availability have been documented as a causative factor, [13] we found few reports that assessed ED admissions as a percentage of all admissions for varying chronic conditions over time and variance over time of the relative contribution of these chronic conditions to ED admissions as a proportion of all hospital admissions. By analyzing these trends, areas in need of improvement can be prioritized.

The Institute of Medicine report, "Crossing the Quality Chasm," recommends that health care leaders prioritize improving the quality of care as related to chronic conditions that cause a disproportionate share of adverse outcomes, medical expenditures, and pain and suffering. [1] Since ED crowding is a major factor that jeopardizes quality of care through reduced access while simultaneously increasing cost, we sought to analyze the nature of the contribution of chronic conditions to ED crowding.

Based on national datasets, we analyzed hospital admissions through the ED. First, we estimated the magnitude of hospital admissions through the ED as a proportion of total hospital admissions. Second, we compared the general trend of ED admissions for specific clinical conditions analyzing the relative frequencies of the most common conditions resulting in hospitalization by way of the ED. Third, we ascertained the trend of disparities as a contributing factor to ED crowding. Finally, we examined relative frequencies of specific diagnoses related to hospital admissions through the ED between 1995 and 2001 and analyzed changes in the relative contribution of varying diagnoses over time prioritizing areas for future improvement efforts.

METHODS

Data

Our main data source was the five year National Inpatient Sample (NIS), 1995, 1997, 1999, 2000 and 2001. The NIS is maintained by the Healthcare Cost and Utilization Project (HCUP) of Agency for Healthcare Research and Quality. Through stratified sampling, the NIS contained about 20% of the total hospital discharges from U.S. community hospitals and can be used to estimate national findings. [14] In addition, the 2000 ARF (Area Resource File) county-based data, which include 2000 Census information, were also used. We excluded delivery discharges since obstetric care has limited relevance to the purpose of our study. After data cleaning, the total numbers of the sample size were, 3,792,803 in 1995,

3,990,087 in 1997, 3,882,261 in 1999, 3,929,320 in 2000 and 3,907,528 in 2001, respectively. Due to the nature of the sampling design of the NIS, we used the SUDAAN software to account for the hospital clustering factor.

Measures

The main dependent variable was hospitalization through ED during the seven-year period (every other year from 1995 through 2001). The percent of ED admission was used in descriptive statistics while the likelihood of ED admission was estimated in multivariate analysis. We also examined hospital mortality during the period to see if the severity of illness (and/or quality of / access to care) had changed as reflected by a change in mortality. In addition, trends of length of stay (LOS) were examined. Finally, focusing on the ED admission measure, we also examined racial disparities and disparities related to patients' health insurance status. Race/ethnicity was categorized as white (the reference group, 77%), African American (13%), Hispanic (7%), Asian/Pacific Islander (1.7%) and Native American (0.3%). Health insurance status, based on payment source, was grouped as Medicare (50%), Medicaid (12%), private insurance including prepaid health plans (the reference group, 33%), and uninsured (i.e., self-paid and no charge, 5%).

Analysis

We combined the trend analyses with the "snap-shot" analysis. The 1995, 1997, 1999 and 2001 NIS data were used to examine the trend of hospitalizations through the ED, while the 2000 NIS data were used to link other data sources for the "snap shot" analysis. The snap-shot analysis enabled us to examine the potential association between physician distribution and ED admission. We merged the 2000 ARF (Area Resource File) county-based data, which includes the 2000 Census information, with the two previous datasets to test the possible effects of health care provider distribution. We calculated a county-based provider-population ratio: the number of primary care providers (including general practice, family practice and pediatric care) per 100,000 population. We hypothesized that the ED admission of a hospital was negatively associated with the population-based numbers of primary care providers in the county where the hospital was located.

In addition, we adjusted covariates available in our datasets in multiple logistical regression analysis in SUDAAN when using ED admission ("yes" or "no") and in hospital death ("yes" or "no") as response variables, respectively. At the patient level, we included age, gender, and median income level (i.e., four levels: <$25,000 (the reference level), $25,000-$34,999, $35,000-$44,999, and >= $45,000) by zip code of the patient's residence. We divided the age into nine groups: 0–4, 5-17, 18-19, 30-39 (the reference group), 40-49, 50-59, 60-69, 70-79, and 80 and older. At the hospital level, we controlled for hospital discharge volume, bed size, teaching hospital status, MSA(metropolitan statistical area) or non-MSA status to indicate rural or non-rural areas, and the region (Northeast, Midwest, South (the reference group) and West) the hospital located.

RESULTS

Through merging the 2000 ARF data we found that the number of primary care providers per 100,000 population was negatively associated with the frequency of ED admissions (regression coefficient, -0.001; p = 0.0004). This negative relationship, however, did not significantly change disparities in ED admission frequencies across racial and health insurance subgroups, based on findings of the multivariate analysis. As compared to whites, African Americans (odds ratio (OR) = 1.50, p < 0.001), Hispanics (OR = 1.41, p < 0.001) and Asians (OR = 1.40, p < 0.001) were more likely to be admitted through ED, while Native Americans had comparable likelihood of being admitted through ED (OR [95% confidence interval (CI)] = 1.33 [0.93, 1.89], p = 0.12). As compared to patients with private insurance coverage, both Medicaid patients (OR = 1.65, p < 0.001) and uninsured patients (OR = 2.48, p < 0.001) were more likely to be admitted through ED.

Table 1 presents the trend of hospital admissions through the ED from 1995 to 2001. While the number of emergency departments declined continuously and the total number of hospital admissions increased continuously, both the total number of hospital admissions through ED and the percentage of admissions through the ED gradually increased, with the latter figures being 46.6% in 1995, 47.9% in 1997, 50.6% in 1999 and 52.5% in 2001. Compared to the year of 1995, the likelihood of being admitted through ED had also become higher, with odds ratios and the 95% confidence intervals being 1.06 [1.05, 1.07], 1.23 [1.21, 1.24] and 1.28 [1.26, 1.29] in 1997, 1999 and 2001, respectively.

Table 1. Trend of Non-Obstetric Hospital Admissions through Emergency Department in NIS

	1995	1997	1999	2001
Number of emergency departments (national total)*	4,923	4,813	4,679	4,621
Total number of admissions	3,792,803	3,990,087	3,882,261	3,907,528
Total number of admissions through ED	1,767,446	1,911,252	1,960,542	2,051,452
Percent of admissions through ED	46.6	47.9	50.5	52.5
OR (95% CI) of getting admitted through ED †	1.00 (reference)	1.06 (1.05, 1.07)‡	1.23 (1.21, 1.24)‡	1.28 (1.26, 1.29)‡

ED = emergency department, OR = odds ratio, CI = confidence interval

* Source: American Hospital Association: http://www.hospitalconnect.com/aha/resource_center/ statistics/statistics.html

† The four year data were pooled. Adjusted for age, gender, race/ethnicity, health insurance status, the median income level by zip code and hospital characteristics.

‡ p< 0.001

Table 2 presents sociodemographic characteristics, as well as length of stay and hospital mortality related to ED admissions between 1995 and 2001. The average age of patients who were admitted through ED markedly increased from 1995 (58.0 years old) to 1997 (59.2 years old) and has slightly increased since then. A similar pattern can be seen with regard to the percentage of female patients admitted through ED. Among all hospital admissions, percentages of ED admissions demonstrated an increasing trend across all racial and insurance subgroups. Percentages of ED admissions increased from 44.5% in 1995 to 50.6% in 2001 for white patients, from 57.3% in 1995 to 60.8% in 2001 for African Americans, and from 48.9% in 1995 to 56.6% in 2001 for Hispanics. The trends for Asians and Native Americans were somewhat different; both increased from 1995 (44.6% and 46.8% for Asians and Native Americans, respectively) to 1999 (54.1% and 54.7% for Asians and Native Americans, respectively) but came down from 1999 to 2001 (51.7% and 50.6% for Asians and Native Americans, respectively). The ED admission rate for all four payment groups gradually increased during that period of time, with the rate for Medicare patients increasing from 48.1% in 1995 to 54.3% in 2001, the rate for Medicaid patients increasing from 53.3% in 1995 to 57.6% in 2001, the rate for privately insured patients increasing from 39.4% in 1995 to 45.3% in 2001, and the rate for uninsured patients increasing from 59.6% to 70.2%. Among those who were admitted through the ED, the length of stay decreased from 6.5 days to 5.2 days and in-hospital mortality declined from 4.6% to 3.9% during the period between 1995 and 2001.

Table 2. Trend of Percents of Admissions Through ED among All Admissions by Patient Sociodemographic Characteristics, and LOS and Mortality among Admissions through ED[*]

	1995	1997	1999	2001
Mean age, year [†‡]	58.0	59.2	59.2	59.3
Female [‡]	52.6	53.4	53.4	53.9
Race/ethnicity				
White	44.5	45.5	48.2	50.6
African American	57.3	58.6	60.9	60.8
Hispanic	48.9	54.6	56.4	56.6
Asian/Pacific Islander	44.6	48.2	54.1	51.7
Native American	46.8	47.2	54.7	50.6
Payment source				
Medicare	48.1	49.2	52.8	54.3
Medicaid	53.3	54.6	57.3	57.6
Private	39.4	41.2	43.0	45.3
Uninsured	59.6	64.2	66.4	70.2
Length of stay, day [†‡]	6.5	5.5	5.2	5.2
Discharge status as death [‡]	4.6	4.3	4.2	3.9

ED = emergency department.
[*] Data are expressed as percentage.
[†] Mean.
[‡] Only among patients admitted through ED.

Table 3 further shows disparities in ED admissions across racial/ethnic and health insurance subgroups. Both African Americans and Hispanics were more likely to be admitted through ED than their white counterparts, and the odds ratios declined slightly between 1995 and 2001. The odds ratios of African Americans over whites were 1.65, 1.72, 1.66 and 1.58 in 1995, 1997, 1999 and 2001, respectively. The odds ratios of Hispanics over whites were 1.37,

1.33 and 1.26 in 1997, 1999 and 2001, whereas the odds ratio of 1.18 in 1995 was not statistically significant with a 95% of confidence interval (CI) ranging between 0.96 and 1.45. No consistent disparities in ED admissions were observed between Asians and whites and between Native Americans and whites from 1995 to 2001. Results related to the payment source revealed more clear disparities in likelihood of getting ED admission. As compared to patients covered by private insurance, Medicaid patients showed consistently higher but relatively stable likelihood of being admitted through the ED (odds ratios around 1.60) over the period, whereas the higher likelihood of being admitted through the ED for uninsured patients has become progressively higher (odds ratios, 2.05, 2.33, 2.37 and 2.63 over the four years, respectively).

Racial disparities in mortality were less obvious than those in ED admission rates. In three of the four years (1995, 1997 and 2001), African Americans showed higher mortality odds ratios of around 1.10 than whites. Compared to whites, Asians seemed to experience a higher mortality risk in recent years (ORs, 1.20 in 1999 and 1.18 in 2001) than in previous two years (CIs, [0.95, 1.27] and $p = 0.19$ in 1995, [0.97, 1.27] and $p = 0.12$ in 1997). The payment source related disparities in mortality were much stronger. Although no trend of a widening gap was observed, both Medicaid patients (ORs, 1.55, 1.59, 1.39 and 1.41 in 1995, 1997, 1999 and 2001, respectively) and uninsured patients (ORs, 1.22, 1.36, 1.22 and 1.23 in 1995, 1997, 1999 and 2001, respectively) constantly showed higher mortality risk than their privately insured counterparts between 1995 and 2001.

Table 4 lists the 16 clinical conditions that most frequently contributed to hospitalization through the ED, a list that remained consistent during each of the years studied. In total, the 16 conditions accounted for over 40% of the total number of admissions through the ED with this percentage continuing to increase during the period studied (41.2%, 42.7%, 44.1% and 44.0% in 1995, 1997, 1999 and 2001, respectively). Symptoms involving the respiratory system and other chest systems (3.6%, 3.8%, 4.4% and 5.2% in 1995, 1997, 1999 and 2001, respectively), heart failure (5.2%, 5.2%, 4.9% and 4.9% for the four years, respectively) and unspecified pneumonia (4.0%, 4.1%, 5.4% and 4.7%, respectively) occupied the top three spots during the entire period. As a percentage of total admissions through the ED; heart failure, acute myocardial infarction (3.0%, 2.9%, 2.9% and 2.8% for the four years, respectively), asthma (2.4%, 2.2%, 2.1% and 1.9% for the four years, respectively), and occlusion of cerebral arteries (2.1%, 2.0%, 1.8% and 1.7%, respectively) declined, while rates of admission for symptoms involving respiratory system and other chest symptoms and diabetes mellitus (1.7%, 1.7%, 1.8% and 2.0% in the four years, respectively) increased. Among the 16 most frequent diagnoses, more than half were either a chronic diagnosis or a condition requiring a chronic diagnosis as a necessary etiologic agent.

Table 3. Trends of Disparities in the ED Admission and Related Mortality

Variable	1995 Odds Ratio	1995 95% C.I.	1997 Odds Ratio	1997 95% C.I.	1999 Odds Ratio	1999 95% C.I.	2001 Odds Ratio	2001 95% C.I.
Admission through ED†								
Race/ethnicity								
White (reference)	1.00	-	1.00	-	1.00	-	1.00	-
African American	1.65***	(1.49, 1.82)	1.72***	(1.57, 1.88)	1.66***	(1.53, 1.80)	1.58***	(1.42, 1.76)
Hispanic	1.18	(0.96, 1.45)	1.37***	(1.21, 1.55)	1.33***	(1.18, 1.50)	1.26***	(1.12, 1.41)
Asian/Pacific Islander	1.07	(0.91, 1.26)	1.15**	(1.00, 1.31)	1.25***	(1.06, 1.47)	1.06	(0.88, 1.28)
Native American	1.12	(0.96, 1.31)	1.07	(0.84, 1.36)	1.34***	(1.14, 1.58)	0.99	(0.76, 1.28)
Payment source								
Private (reference)	1.00	-	1.00	-	1.00	-	1.00	-
Medicaid	1.61***	(1.50, 1.73)	1.56***	(1.44, 1.70)	1.61***	(1.51, 1.72)	1.55***	(1.44, 1.67)
Uninsured	2.05***	(1.69, 2.50)	2.33***	(2.13, 2.55)	2.37***	(2.13, 2.65)	2.63***	(2.39, 2.90)
Mortality†‡								
Race/ethnicity								
White (reference)	1.00	-	1.00	-	1.00	-	1.00	-
African American	1.12***	(1.07, 1.18)	1.12***	(1.06, 1.18)	1.05	(0.98, 1.12)	1.10***	(1.03, 1.17)
Hispanic	1.02	(0.93, 1.11)	0.91**	(0.83, 1.00)	0.95	(0.87, 1.03)	0.97	(0.90, 1.05)
Asian/Pacific Islander	1.10	(0.95, 1.27)	1.11	(0.97, 1.27)	1.20***	(1.08, 1.33)	1.18**	(1.01, 1.39)
Native American	0.58**	(0.37, 0.91)	1.16	(0.76, 1.76)	1.17	(0.88, 1.56)	1.11	(0.79, 1.55)
Payment source								
Private (reference)	1.00	-	1.00	-	1.00	-	1.00	-
Medicaid	1.55***	(1.44, 1.67)	1.59***	(1.48, 1.69)	1.39***	(1.29, 1.51)	1.41***	(1.30, 1.52)
Uninsured	1.22***	(1.12, 1.34)	1.36***	(1.24, 1.50)	1.22***	(1.10, 1.36)	1.23***	(1.12, 1.36)

ED = emergency department, CI = confidence interval

* p < 0.10, ** p < 0.05, *** p < 0.01

† adjusted for age, gender, the median income level and hospital characteristics.

‡ Only among patients admitted through ED

Table 4. Top 16 Clinical Conditions as the Percentage of the Total ED Admissions

Clinical Condition	ICD-9 Code of Principle Diagnosis	1995		1997		1999		2001	
		Percent	Rank	Percent	Rank	Percent	Rank	Percent	Rank
Symptoms involving respiratory system and other chest symptoms	786	3.6	3	3.8	3	4.4	3	5.2	1
Heart failure	428	5.2	1	5.2	1	4.9	2	4.9	2
Unspecified pneumonia	486	4.0	2	4.1	2	5.4	1	4.7	3
General symptoms	780	2.8	5	2.8	6	3.0	5	3.1	4
Other forms of chronic ischemic heart disease	414	2.7	6	3.3	4	3.0	6	3.1	5
Cardiac sysrhythmias	427	2.6	7	2.7	7	2.6	8	2.8	6
Acute myocardial infarction	410	3.0	4	2.9	5	2.9	7	2.8	7
Chronic bronchitis	491	1.9	13	2.4	8	3.0	4	2.5	8
Disorders of fluid, electrolyte, and acid-based balance	276	2.2	9	2.2	10	2.3	9	2.5	9
Affective psychoses	296	1.8	14	1.9	14	1.7	15	2.1	10
Diabetes mellitus	250	1.7	15	1.7	15	1.8	12	2.0	11
Asthma	493	2.4	8	2.2	9	2.1	10	1.9	12
Occlusion of cerebral arteries	434	2.1	10	2.0	12	1.8	13	1.7	13
Other disorders of urethra and urinary tract	599	1.4	16	1.6	16	1.6	16	1.7	14
Fracture of lower limb	820	2.0	11	1.9	13	1.9	11	1.6	15
Septicemia	038	2.0	12	2.1	11	1.8	14	1.6	16
Total		41.2		42.7		44.1		44.0	

ED = emergency department

DISCUSSION

Since hospital admissions through the ED account for about 15% of total ED volume, these admissions contribute to ED crowding. In addition, time required to transfer a patient from the ED to a hospital bed further exacerbates the problem. [15] Furthermore, admissions through the ED due to ambulatory sensitive conditions are likely to result from inadequate access to primary care. Multiple etiologic factors could be responsible for inadequate access to care including inadequate health insurance, lack of continuity of care based upon a stable relationship with a primary care physician, and barriers to access including long wait times, large geographic distances to sources of care, and challenges navigating an increasingly complex health care system. [1,16,17] Finally, an aging population with a higher prevalence of chronic disease may be creating a challenge for a health care system that frequently provides sub-optimal care for such conditions. [1] It is interesting to note from our dataset that those conditions which showed a relative decline in percentage of ED admissions were conditions that have drawn a great deal of attention from researchers and other interested stake holders resulting in the increased use of clinical guidelines and critical pathways for these conditions including heart failure, asthma, acute myocardial infarction, and stroke (represented by cerebral occlusion). While one might argue that these guidelines are often implemented in the hospital setting and therefore not relevant for preventing presentation to the ED, the counter argument is that high quality of care implemented in the hospital with appropriate follow up decreases the likelihood of presentation to the ED. Since more than half of the diagnoses among ED admissions were either chronic conditions or problems that were likely to have a chronic condition as a necessary predisposing etiologic factor, such as diabetes mellitus and affective psychoses, more needs to be done to ensure that high standards of care with emphasis on prevention and early treatment are made available for these conditions as well. Specific conditions that have shown increased rates of ED utilization include diabetes mellitus, affective psychoses, other disorders of urethra and urinary tract, and general symptoms. It should also be noted that these conditions are more likely to be impacted by critical pathways and guidelines that are implemented on the outpatient side rather than conditions like heart failure which are clearly impacted by inpatient guidelines and protocols.

The role of disparities related to ethnicity and insurance status also plays a significant factor causing the trend of increased admissions through the ED. Most studies have found that socioeconomically vulnerable populations, such as minorities, Medicaid patients and the uninsured, use the ED as part of a safety net compensating for inadequate access to ambulatory primary care. [3,4] While our data showed racial/ethnic disparities and disparities related to health insurance status with regard to ED admission, generally, we did not observe an increase in the magnitude of the disparity, the only exception being uninsured patients who have become increasingly likely to be admitted through ED as compared to those covered by private insurance. The increasing magnitude of this disparity most likely is an indication of the cost sensitivity of this group in the face of rapid health care price inflation. With respect to other groups, the reason that the magnitude of the disparity did not increase is that rates of ED admissions as a proportion of all hospital admissions have been increasing at a similar rate in all groups studied, with the exception of the uninsured whose rates have been increasing even more rapidly.

This study has limitations. First, the HCUP project for the data collection of the NIS is not mandatory, not all states so far have participated. In addition, among participating state, a few did not provide information about race. As a result, using the weighted NIS data to reflect the national total could contribute to some inaccuracy. Given the consistent pattern of the data over the years studied we do not believe that any potential inaccuracy was sufficient enough to limit the validity of the findings. Second, based on the datasets used, we were unable to divide private insurance into subgroups such as commercial indemnity plan, HMO or PPO plans that may have different effects on primary ambulatory care that, in turn, can affect ED admissions. Third, as suggested by the Institute of Medicine, much research is needed to analyze disparities in care beyond comparisons of African American and white patients. [18] Although we included five major racial/ethnic groups in this study, the small percentages representing Asian/Islander patients and Native American Patients in our data set might partially explain the lack of consistent trends shown in these populations. Finally, since the NIS did not allow linkage with ARF data, the measure of the total number of primary care providers per 100,000 population was based on the county where the hospital was located rather than where the patient resided.

In conclusion, since this trend of increasing ED admissions was observed regardless of race/ethnicity and health insurance status, it is clear that system wide changes in health care delivery are needed. Some of theses changes should build on previous successes by extending the use of clinical guidelines and critical pathways to conditions where the use of these tools has been more limited and to outpatient settings. Other changes may involve improving access by promoting an optimal ratio of primary care physicians/providers to population served and extending insurance benefits so that uninsured patients can have increased access to care. Additional research that further defines nonspecific symptoms such as "respiratory and chest symptoms" and "general symptoms" as a contributor to ED admissions is warranted to determine how to more effectively address these conditions.

ACKNOWLEDGEMENT

This project was supported by grant number 1 R03 HS13056 from the Agency for Healthcare Research and Quality.

REFERENCES

[1]   Institute of Medicine. *Crossing the Quality Chasm: A New Health System for the 21st Century*. Washington, D.C.: The National Academies Press; 2000.

[2]   Schull MJ, Lazier K, Vermeulen M, Mawhinney S, Morrison LJ. Emergency department contributors to ambulance diversion: a quantitative analysis. *Ann Emerg Med.* 2003; 41(4): 467-476.

[3]   Gaskin DJ, Hoffman C. Racial and ethnic differences in preventable hospitalizations across 10 states. *Med Care Res Rev.* 2000;57 Suppl 1:85-107.

[4]   4. Oster A, Bindman AB. Emergency department visits for ambulatory care sensitive conditions: insights into preventable hospitalizations. *Med Care.* 2003;41(2):198- 207.

[5]   Schafermeyer RW, Asplin BR. "Hospital and emergency department crowding in the
       United States." *Emerg Med.* 2003;15(1):22-7.
[6]   Schull MJ, Morrison LJ, Vermeulen M, Redelmeier DA. Emergency department
       gridlock and out-of-hospital delays for cardiac patients. *Acad Emerg Med.* 2003
       Jul;10(7):709-16. Related Articles, Links
[7]   Schull MJ, Morrison LJ, Vermeulen M, Redelmeier DA. Emergency department
       overcrowding and ambulance transport delays for patients with chest pain. *CMAJ.*
       2003; 168(3): 277-283.
[8]   Schneider SM, Gallery ME, Schafermeyer R, Zwemer FL. "Emergency department
       crowding: a point in time." *Ann Emerg Med.* 2003;42(2):167-172.
[9]   Ganapathy S, Zwemer FL Jr. "Coping with a crowded ED: an expanded unique role for
       midlevel providers." *Am J Emerg Med.* 2003;21(2):125-128.
[10]   Cardin S, Afilalo M, Lang E, Collet JP, Colacone A, Tselios C, Dankoff J, Guttman A.
       Intervention to decrease emergency department crowding: does it have an effect on
       return visits and hospital readmissions? *Ann Emerg Med.* 2003;41(2):173-185.
[11]   Miro O, Sanchez M, Espinosa G, Coll-Vincent B, Bragulat E, Milla J. Analysis of
       patient flow in the emergency department and the effect of an extensive reorganization.
       Emerg Med J. 2003;20(2):143-148.
[12]   Amre DK, Infante-Rivard C, Gautrin D, Malo JL. Socioeconomic status and utilization
       of health care services among asthmatic children. *J Asthma.* 2002;29(7):625-631.
[13]   Derlet RW, Richards JR. Emergency department overcrowding in Florida, New York,
       and Texas. *South Med J.* 2002;95(8):846-849.
[14]   Agency for Healthcare Research and Quality. Nationwide Inpatient Sample (NIS)
       Powerful   Database   for   Analyzing   Hospital   Care.   Available   at:
       http://www.ahrq.gov/data/hcup/hcupnis.htm. Accessed November 10, *2003.*
[15]   Richards JR, Navarro ML, Derlet RW. Surevey of directors of emergency departments
       in California on ED overcrowding. *West J. Med.* 2000;172(6):385-388.
[16]   Weinick RM, Drilea SK. Usual sources of health care and barriers to care, 1996. *Stat
       Bull Metrop Insur Co.* 1998;79(1):11-17.
[17]   Weinick RM, Zuvekas SH, Cohen JW. Racial and ethnic differences in access to and
       use of health care services, 1977 to 1996. *Med Care Res Rev.* 2000;57 Suppl 1:36-54.
[18]   Institute of Medicine. *Unequal Treatment: Confronting Racial and Ethnic Disparities
       in Healthcare.* Washington, D.C.: The National Academies Press; 2003.

In: Racial and Ethnic Disparities in Health and Health Care
Editor: Elene V. Metrosa, pp. 53-72
ISBN 1-60021-268-9
© 2006 Nova Science Publishers, Inc.

Chapter 3

RACIAL/ETHNIC DISPARITIES IN HYPERTENSION AND DIABETES ASCRIBED TO DIFFERENCES IN OBESITY RATE

Ike S. Okosun[*]

Associate Professor of Public Health, Institute of Public Health, Georgia State University, Atlanta, Georgia

John M. Boltri[†]

Professor of Family Medicine, Department of Family Medicine, Mercer University School of Medicine, Macon, Georgia

ABSTRACT

Context

American ethnic minorities, particularly those of African and Hispanic descent have a greater risk of developing hypertension and type 2 diabetes compared to American Whites. Despite the consistency of the epidemiologic evidence of the racial/ethnic variation for these diseases, relatively little is known with confidence about the causes of the non-White dilemma.

Objective

To determine how much of the relative difference in the rates of hypertension and type 2 diabetes between high-risk Blacks and Hispanics and low-risk Whites is attributable to their differences in obesity.

---

[*] Phone: (404) 651-4249: Fax: (404) 651-1559: Email: iokosun@gsu.edu
[†] Phone: (478) 633-5758: Fax: (478) 784-5496: Email: Boltri.john@mccg.org

Methods

Data (n=5531) from the 1999-2002 U.S. National Health and Nutrition Examination Surveys were utilized for this analysis. Gender-specific proportions of White to non-White differences in odds of hypertension and diabetes that were due to their relative differences in the prevalence of obesity were estimated using relative attributable risk derived from multiple logistic regression modeling. Statistical adjustment was made for age, education, alcohol intake, education, and physical activity.

Results

50.2% and 30.6% of differences in odds of hypertension between White men and Black men and between White men and Hispanic men, respectively, are attributable to their differences in rates of obesity. The analogous values for diabetes were 70.7% and 57.4% for Black men and Hispanic men. Also, 30.6 % and 13.4% of differences in odds of hypertension between White women and Black women and between White women and Hispanic women, respectively, are associated with their differences in rates of obesity. The analogous values for diabetes are 62.2% and 83.7% for Black women and Hispanic women when compared with White women.

Conclusion

The magnitude of racial/ethnic differences in hypertension and diabetes due to their differences in obesity provides an encouraging reason to continue to implement public health obesity prevention programs in the United States' minority groups. Aggressive programs to reduce obesity and increase physical activity in Blacks and Hispanics may prove useful in reducing racial/ethnic disparities in hypertension and diabetes.

Key words: Obesity, Hypertension, Diabetes, Ethnicity and disease, Population attributable risk, Relative attributable risk

INTRODUCTION

American ethnic minorities, particularly those of African and Hispanic descent have greater risks of developing hypertension and non-insulin dependent diabetes mellitus (type 2 diabetes) compared to American Whites [1-6]. Despite the consistency of the epidemiologic evidence of the racial/ethnic variation for these diseases, relatively little is known with confidence about the causes of the non-White dilemma. The two most common factors explaining racial/ethnic disparities for these diseases are access to health care and treatment [7-8]. However, healthcare access and treatment disparities do not totally explain racial/ethnic differences for these diseases. Understanding reasons for the non-White disadvantage for these diseases is critical for developing effective public health programs in eliminating racial/ethnic disparities as proposed by the United States Healthy People 2010 objective [9].

Racial/Ethnic Differences in Hypertension

The prevalence of hypertension in African Americans is among the highest in the world [10]. The prevalence of hypertension is estimated to be about 37% for African Americans, compared with 20%-25% for non-Hispanic whites [1-2, 10]. African Americans have earlier age of onset and increased rates of consequences of hypertension, including stroke, cardiovascular disease, and renal failure compared to Whites [11]. The estimated prevalence of hypertension is about 28.7% for Hispanic Americans [13]. A review of the recent studies of genetic epidemiology has not exposed unique genotypes that explain hypertension or the disparate impact endured by African and Hispanic Americans [13]. However, the emerging consensus is that environmental factors predominate in their effect and are mutable [3]. Epidemiologic literature has shown that racial/ethnic minorities with hypertension receive less aggressive treatment for their high blood pressure compared to Whites. Indeed, a recent review of medical records of about 1200 patients who had a minimum of two hypertension-related outpatient visits to one of twelve general internal medicine clinics during one year period showed that 80.3% Whites were likely to have therapy intensified compared with 71.5% Latinos [14]. The ethnic differences in therapy intensification from the study were largely due to differences in frequency of clinic visits and in the prevalence of diabetes [14]. The U.S. Veterans Administration study to investigate the contribution of differential access to health care to lower blood pressure control rates in African American compared with White hypertensive patients showed that the ethnic disparity in blood pressure control between Blacks and Whites was approximately 40% less at VA than at non-VA health care sites (6.2% vs 10.2%; P<.01) [4].

Racial/Ethnic Differences in Type 2 Diabetes

Type 2 diabetes in the United States is increasing in adolescents, young adults and in the elderly and there are significant disparities in diabetes with Whites having the lowest rates [15-19]. The prevalence of diabetes is estimated to be 8.4-8.7% for non-Hispanic Whites, 13.3-15.0% for non-Hispanic Blacks, and 9.5-13.8% for Mexican Americans [16, 17]. Diabetes is estimated to be 1.7 to 1.8 times as prevalent in Hispanics and blacks, compared to whites [16]. There is also evidence that Whites with diabetes have better control of their illness compared with Blacks and Hispanics as evidenced by hemoglobin A1c levels [20].

Racial/Ethnic Differences in Obesity

Obesity is increasing dramatically in the United States and most likely contributes substantially to the burden of many chronic health conditions. The National Health and Nutrition Examination Survey (NHANES) data indicate continuing disparities between U.S. adults of racial/ethnic groups in the prevalence of obesity. A similar increasing prevalence of overweight has been observed in U.S. children and adolescents [21]. The prevalence of overweight in US children, defined as a body mass index exceeding the 95th percentile for age and sex increased between 1986 and 1998 [21]. Between the study periods of 1986 and 1998, overweight prevalence increased to 21.5% among African Americans, 21.8% among

Hispanics, and 12.3% among non-Hispanic whites [21]. The trends in increased obesity in the US as demonstrated in this study may be due to the shift of energy intake, food portion size and snacking patterns at the population level [22].

Explanatory Power of Obesity for Racial/Ethnic Variations in Hypertension and Diabetes

Obesity has consistently been shown as an important risk factor for racial/ethnic differences in hypertension, since mean body mass index (BMI) levels are higher among these American minorities compared to American Whites [23-29]. In a multi-state screening project examining the relationship between obesity and cardiovascular risk factors in the United States, compared to non-overweight respondents, SBP increased by 13.2 mmHg for severely obese (p < 0.001); by 8.9 mmHg for obese (p < 0.001), and by 5.2 mmHg (p < 0.001) for overweight respondents, respectively [12]. Increases in diabetes have also been observed in conjunction with the rise in obesity [30-32]. The decrease in many cardiovascular risk factors, including high blood cholesterol and high blood pressure at all BMI levels that have been observed in the US is not applicable to what has been observed for diabetes [33]. Unlike these cardiovascular risk factors, the prevalence of diabetes has increased in Whites, Blacks and Hispanics, for the periods between 1976 and 2000 [34]. The increase was concentrated among individuals with BMI of 35 or greater in whom the proportion of cases that were diagnosed increased from approximately 41% to 83% [34].

METHODOLOGIC ISSUES ASSOCIATED WITH STUDYING OBESITY AND RACIAL/ETHNIC VARIATIONS IN DISEASES

The basic methodological issues that are associated with studying racial/ethnic differences in the association of obesity with diseases include lack of consensus in three ways; (1) how to measure and quantify obesity, (2) how to quantify the association of obesity with diseases, and (3) how to measure the impact of obesity on diseases.

Obesity Measurement

One of the unsettled methodological areas in comparing obesity across racial/ethnic groups is the lack of agreement of the BMI cutpoint for obesity. BMI is a height adjusted measure of generalized obesity. It is an anthropometric surrogate measure of body fat that is easy to measure and interpret. Although its cutpoint is critical for triggering public health or clinical action on obesity, the current cutpoint for obesity (BMI of 30 kg/m2 or greater) is somewhat subjective. A BMI of 30 or higher has a different meaning for body fat across racial/ethnic groups [35]. Hence comparing the association of obesity defined by BMI of 30 kg/m^2 or greater with various disorders such as hypertension and diabetes is a subject of disagreement [36]. Indeed, many studies have shown differential predictive values of BMI of 30 kg/m^2 or greater for many cardiovascular and coronary disease risk factors [35, 37].

However, BMI is highly correlated with body fat determined using other methods such as underwater weighing, deuterium dilution, dual-energy X-ray absorptiometry, magnetic resonance and computed tomography [38].

Quantifying Obesity Risk

Studies quantifying the association of obesity risk with diseases are not consistent. Odds ratios and relative risks are the most common statistics seen in epidemiologic literature. In retrospective designs, odds ratios often approximate relative risks if the disease under study is rare. For hypertension that is relatively common in the US, the use of odds ratio in estimating relative risk is questionable. In cross-sectional studies, prevalence odds ratios are often used to quantify the association of obesity with hypertension.

Estimation of Odds Ratio

The odds ratio compares whether the probability of a certain event is the same for two groups (cases and controls). An odds ratio of 1 implies that the event is equally likely in both groups. An odds ratio that is greater than one implies that the event is more likely in the first group. An odds ratio less than one implies that the event is less likely in the first group. For a dichotomous response variable with outcomes event and nonevent, a dichotomous risk factor variable X takes the value 1 if the risk factor is present and 0 if the risk factor is absent. According to the logistic regression model, the log odds function, $g(X)$, is given by:

$$g(X) = \log \Pr(\text{event} \mid X) \div \Pr(\text{noevent} \mid X) = \beta_0 + \beta_1 X \qquad [1]$$

The odds ratio φ is defined as the ratio of the odds for those with the risk factor ($X=1$) to the odds for those without the risk factor $(X=0)$. The log of the odds ratio is given by:

$$\log(\varphi) = \log(\varphi(X=1, X=0)) = g(X=1) - g(X=0) = \beta_1 \qquad [2]$$

The parameter, β_1, associated with X represents the change in the log odds from $X = 0$ to $X = 1$. Thus, the odds ratio is obtained simply by exponentiation of the value of the parameter that is associated with the risk factor. The odds ratio indicates how the odds of the event changes when X changes from 0 to 1. For instance, an odds ratio of 3 means that the odds of an event when $X=1$ is three times the odds of an event when $X=0$.

Estimation of Relative Risk

In a cohort study individuals with differing exposures to a risk factor are identified and then observed for the occurrence of outcomes over some time period. The incidence rates of the disease of interest are measured and related to estimated exposure levels. Incidence can be measured as a proportion or rate. When measured as a proportion, incidence is identical with risk. It is often regarded as absolute risk. Incidences from two groups can be contrasted in absolute terms (subtracting one incidence from the other) or in relative terms (by division). The absolute comparison of incidence proportions is termed the risk difference while the relative comparison of incidences is called the risk ratio. In simple terms, proportions from two independent groups can be compared using notation for a cross tabulation:

	Disease+	Disease-	Total
Exposure+	A_1	B_1	N_1
Exposure -	A_0	B_0	N_0
Total	M_1	M_0	N

where, A indicates "case" and B indicates "noncase." Subscript 1 denotes "exposed" and subscript 0 denotes "nonexposed." For example, A1 indicates the number of exposed cases, A0 indicates the number of nonexposed cases, and so on. There are N1 exposed subjects and N0 nonexposed subjects. There are N subjects.

To determine the risk ratio, let P_1 represent the incidence proportion (risk) estimate in the exposed group, and let P_0 represent the risk estimate in the nonexposed group. Thus,

$$P_1 = A_1/N_1 \text{ and } P_0 = A_0/N_0 \qquad\qquad [3]$$

The risk ratio (RR), also called relative risk is calculated as:

$$RR = P_1/P_0 \qquad\qquad [4]$$

RR represents the incidence rate in the exposed group divided by the incidence rate in the unexposed group. The above RR formula can be applied to prevalences, and hence the prevalence ratio can be calculated. The prevalence ratio is equal to the risk ratio when the average duration of disease is the same in the groups, the disease is rare, and the disease does not influence the presence of the exposure.

The risk ratio is a multiplier of risk. For example, a risk ratio of 3.99 is about 4, indicating that the risk in the exposed group is 4 times that of the non-exposed group. The risk ratio can also be viewed as measuring the effect of the exposure in relative terms. The risk ratio above (or below) 1 quantifies the relative increase (or decrease) in risk associated with the exposure. Cohort studies can either be performed prospectively or retrospectively from historical records.

Quantifying Obesity Impact

Population Attributable Risk

The most commonly used statistical and epidemiologic measure of impact of a risk factor on an outcome is population attributable risk [39]. Population attributable (PAR) risk is defined as a population's disease rate that would not occur if the risk factor(s) of interest had been absent [39-41]. Population attributable risk is the portion of the incidence of a disease in the population (exposed and nonexposed) that is due to exposure. The PAR is calculated by subtracting the incidence in the unexposed (Iu) from the incidence in total population (exposed and unexposed) (Ip):

$$PAR = Ip - Iu \qquad\qquad [5]$$

Population attributable risk percent (PAR%) is the percent of the incidence of a disease in the population (exposed and nonexposed) that is due to exposure. It is the percent of the incidence of a disease in the population that would be eliminated if exposure were eliminated. The PAR% is calculated by dividing the PAR by the incidence in the total population and then multiplying the product times 100 to obtain a percentage:

$$PAR\% = \frac{Ip - Iu}{Ip} * 100, \text{ or } \frac{PAR}{Ip} \qquad\qquad [6]$$

In a retrospective study, population attributable risk is often estimated as [40, 41]:

$$\frac{P_E (OR-1)}{1+P_E (OR-1)} * 100 \qquad\qquad [7]$$

where P_E is the prevalence of risk factor, and OR is the odds ratio comparing individuals with disease with those who do not have disease. The analogous formula for a prospective study is:

$$\frac{I_E (RR-1)}{1+I_E (RR-1)} * 100 \qquad\qquad [8]$$

where I_E is the incidence of the risk factor, and RR is the relative risk comparing individuals with the disease with those who do not have the disease. Indisputably, estimating the population attributable risk is necessary because it provides the basis for public health disease prevention programs.

Relative Attributable Risk

An important but often overlooked question in determining the contribution of risk factors to racial/ethnic differences in diseases is, "What fraction of the difference in the rates of disease between high-risk and low-risk groups is due to their differences in the prevalence of the risk factor?" The answer to this question requires the use of a rarely used statistical measure called the relative attributable risk (RAR). First described by Cornfield [42], and subsequently by Breslow and Day [43], RAR is defined as the proportion of the excess disease rate in the high-risk group that would disappear if the high-risk group had the same prevalence of risk factor(s) as the low risk population. RAR is based on the assumption that the relationship between the risk factor(s) and the disease in the high-risk population is causal [42-45]. RAR as a percentage can be estimated using the following formula [44-45]:

$$RAR = \frac{[AR_2 - AR_1] \div [1 - AR_1]}{[R - 1] \div [R]} * 100 \qquad\qquad [9]$$

where AR_2 and AR_1 denote attributable risks of disease in the high-risk and the low-risk group, respectively. R is the overall prevalence rate of disease and is calculated as:

$$R = [\lambda_2 \sum_{i=0}^{k} P_{2k} \Gamma_k] \div [\lambda_1 \sum_{i=0}^{k} P_{1k} \Gamma_k] = R_0 w \qquad [10]$$

where λ_1 and λ_2 are prevalence rates of the disease for the non-exposed in low and high risk populations, respectively. $\Gamma_0 = 1$, Γ_1, ... Γ_k denotes the associated odds ratio which is assessed to apply equally to the high risk and the low risk populations. P_{1k} is the proportion of the low risk population exposed to the risk factor, and P_{2k} for the high risk population. The ratio may be decomposed into the product of t terms, the ratio of rates, $R_0 = [\lambda_2] \div [\lambda_1]$, which would persist if the high and low risk populations have the same pattern of exposure, and a multiplicative factor $w = [\sum P_{2k} \Gamma_k] \div [\sum P_{1k} \Gamma_k]$, which denotes how much R_0 is changed by exposure differences. Termed as a confounding risk ratio, w measures the degree to which the effect of one factor on the prevalence of disease is confounded by the effects of the other factors [46-48].

OBJECTIVE OF STUDY

Many studies investigating the contribution of obesity to racial/ethic differences in deaths or diseases such as hypertension and type 2 diabetes are often restricted to conceptual frameworks where population attributable risks are often estimated in quantifying the role of obesity [49-50]. To our knowledge the use of relative attributable risk to quantify the contribution of obesity to racial/ethnic variation in hypertension and diabetes is rare. Hence, this study sought to determine how much of the relative difference in the rates of hypertension and type 2 diabetes between Blacks and Hispanics and Whites is attributable to differences in their obesity rates.

METHODS

Data from the 1999-2001 National Health and Nutrition Examination Survey (NHANES) collected by the National Center for Health Statistics of the Center for Disease Control and Prevention (CDC) were used for this analysis. The measurement and sampling procedures have been previously described [51-52]. Briefly, the NHANES 1999-2001 is a national, cross-sectional, multistage probability sample of the US civilian, non-institutionalized population, selected using a complex, stratified, multistage probability cluster sampling design. This sample is considered to be highly representative of the U.S. civilian population. Consent was obtained from all subjects for the interview (which included collection of demographic data) and for the physical examination and laboratory testing.

Variables that are used for this analysis include race/ethnicity, age, height, weight, waist circumference, diastolic and systolic blood pressures, total cholesterol, physical activity and alcohol use status. Only adults who were identified as non-Hispanic White, non-Hispanic

Black and Hispanic Americans between 18 to 85 years old were included in this investigation. Height, weight, diastolic (DBP) and systolic (SBP) blood pressures were measured and laboratory samples were obtained in the mobile examination center [53]. All techniques and equipment were standardized. Height was measured in meters to the nearest 0.1 cm using a stadiometer against a vertical wall with a rigid headboard and an inelastic tape measure [53]. Weight was measured in the upright position using a Toledo self-zeroing scale (Seritex, Carlstadt, New Jersey) and recorded to the 0.01 kg. Waist measurements were made at the natural waist midpoint between the lowest aspect of the rib cage and highest point of the iliac crest, and to the nearest 0.1 cm. The technique used to obtain blood pressure was similar to the latest recommendations of the American Heart Association [54]. Three and sometimes four blood pressure measurements were taken on all eligible individuals using a mercury sphygmomanometer. Participants who are 50 years and older who were unable to travel to the mobile examination units were offered an abbreviated examination in their homes. Total cholesterol was measured enzymatically in serum or plasma in a sequence of coupled reactions that hydrolyze cholesteryl esters and oxidize the 3-OH group of cholesterol [53]. The concentration of total cholesterol is proportional to the color intensity of the reaction.

Definition of Terms

Diabetes was defined based on the answer to the question: *Has a doctor ever told you that you have diabetes? Hypertension* was defined as SBP $\geq$ 140 or DBP $\geq$ 90 mmHg, or current use of anti hypertension medication. *Education* reported in years of schooling was classified as less than high school, high school and greater than high school for this analysis. Questions on alcohol use in NHANES covered lifetime and recent (past 12 months) use of alcohol. In this analysis alcohol use was defined as current if the subject indicated having used alcohol for at least one time in the past 12 months. Subjects who reported moderate *physical activity* over the past 30 days were classified as those who are currently engaged in physical activity. In terms of variables we did not consider for our analysis, those who were excluded due to missing variables of interest were not different from the population examined in our study.

Statistical Analysis

Statistical programs available in SAS for Windows [55] and SUDAAN [56] were utilized for this analysis. To account for disproportionate probabilities of selection, over sampling, and non-response, appropriate sample weights provided by NHANES were used for the analysis. Estimates of standard errors were computed using the SUDAAN statistical program by means of the delete 1 jackknife method, partitioning the sample into 52 replicates by deleting one unit at a time [57].

Racial/ethnic differences in continuous and categorical variables were evaluated using one-way analysis of variance (ANOVA) and chi-squared statistics, respectively. Prevalences of hypertension and diabetes were age-adjusted by direct methods using the 2000 U.S. population census data. Gender-specific associations of obesity with hypertension and diabetes was determined using odds ratios from the logistic regression analysis in which dummy variables were used to compare Whites with non-Whites. In the regression models statistical adjustments were made for age, education, alcohol use, total cholesterol, and physical activity. In order to determine whether obesity had the same effect for hypertension and diabetes in the three racial/ethnic groups, we fitted the gender-specific interaction term between obesity and race/ethnicity (Model II) in the logistic regression model.

Public health consequences of hypertension and diabetes were quantified using population attributable risk (PAR) expressed as a percentage (Model I) using odds ratio comparing individuals with the disease (hypertension and diabetes) with those who do not have the disease.

To estimate the fraction of White to non-White differences in the rates of the disease (hypertension and diabetes) that was due to their relative differences in the prevalence of obesity, we estimated the RAR. In all analyses, P <0.05 and 95% confidence intervals were used to indicate statistical significance.

RESULTS

The basic characteristics of men (n=2626) and women (n=2905) who were eligible for this study are shown in Tables 1 and 2, respectively. Overall, there were significant racial/ethnic differences for all variables studied (P <.05). White men and women were older than their Black and Hispanic counterparts (P <.01). White men had larger waist girth and higher prevalences of abdominal obesity, physical activity and alcohol use than Black and Hispanic men (P <.001). Black men had higher mean values of BMI and DBP compared with their White and Hispanic counterparts. Black men also had higher prevalences of hypertension, diabetes and obesity compared to White and Hispanic men (P <.001). Black women had larger waist girth and had higher mean values of DBP and SBP than White and Hispanic women (P <.001). Black women also had higher prevalences of abdominal obesity, hypertension and diabetes compared with White and Hispanic women (<.001). The mean values of serum cholesterol and the prevalences of physical activity and alcohol intake were higher in White women compared to Black and Hispanic women (P <.001).

The association of obesity with hypertension and diabetes in men as determined from multiple logistic regression models is shown in Table 3 (Model I). As shown, obesity was associated with increased odds of hypertension (OR: 2.22; 95% CI: 1.77-2.77) and diabetes (OR: 2.04; 95% CI: 1.46-2.87), adjusting for age, education, alcohol intake, education, physical activity and race/ethnicity. Compared with Whites, Black race/ethnicity was associated with 112% increased odds of hypertension and 129% increased odds of diabetes. Compared with Whites, Hispanic race/ethnicity was associated with 37% decreased odds of hypertension and 135% increased odds of diabetes. Table 3 (Model II) also shows multiple logistic regression models of the associations of obesity with hypertension and diabetes that included fitting the interaction between race/ethnicity and obesity. As shown, there were significant interactions between race/ethnicity and obesity in models testing the association of obesity with hypertension and diabetes.

Table 1. Characteristics of studied variables in men

Variables	Whites	Blacks	Hispanics	P-value
N	1414	575	637	
Age (years)	52.1 ± 20.7	43.2 ± 18.9	40.6 ± 18.7	<.001
Weight (kg)	86.4 ± 18.1	84.6 ± 20.7	79.2 ± 17.6	<.001
Height (cm)	176.4 ± 7.4	176.9 ± 6.9	169.7 ± 7.2	<.001
Body mass index (kg/m^2)	24.8 ± 5.3	27.8 ± 6.2	27.4 ± 5.3	.019
Waist circumference (cm)	100.4 ± 14.3	93.6 ± 17.2	95.9 ± 13.7	.003
Blood Pressures (mmHg)				
Diastolic	71.4 ± 14.4	73.6 ± 16.3	68.9 ± 13.5	<.001
Systolic	125.0 ± 17.4	128.2 ± 19.0	128.2 ± 19.0	<.001
Total Cholesterol (mg/dl)	196.6 ± 45.5	192.7 ± 43.6	196.8 ± 41.8	.040
Prevalences (%)				
Abdominal obesity	67.8	42.1	49.8	<.001
Hypertension	38.6	43.7	41.8	<.001
Type 2 diabetes	8.0	9.6	9.4	<.001
Obesity	22.8	29.4	26.1	<.001
Physical activity	55.1	37.5	32.0	<.001
Alcohol intake	82.2	75.1	75.2	<.001

Table 2. Characteristics of studied variables in women

Variables	Whites	Blacks	Hispanics	P-value
N	1613	628	664	
Age (years)	51.1 ± 21.7	43.6 ± 19.6	40.4 ± 18.8	<.001
Weight (kg)	72.9 ± 18.2	79.9 ± 21.7	70.2 ± 16.2	<.001
Height (cm)	162.5 ±6.8	162.9 ±6.3	157.2 ±6.4	<.001
Body mass index (kg/m2)	27.6 ±6.6	30.0 ±7.8	28.5 ±6.2	<.001
Waist circumfcrcncc (cm)	93.2 ± 15.6	95.9 ± 17.2	93.9 ± 14.5	.003
Blood Pressures (mmHg)				
Diastolic	68.4 ± 13.3	70.7 ± 14.9	67.1 ± 12.2	<.001
Systolic	124.1 ± 23.4	125.9 ± 23.5	118.8 ± 21.3	<.001
Total Cholesterol (mg/dl)	208.8 ± 42.1	197.5 ± 42.8	197.8 ± 43.3	<.001
Prevalences (%)				
Abdominal obesity	24.4	29.4	22.7	<.001
Hypertension	35.9	43.6	40.0	<.001
Type 2 diabetes	5.6	10.0	8.3	<.001
Obesity	31.2	45.5	34.1	<.001
Physical activity	56.5	34.2	35.7	<.001
Alcohol intake	91.2	80.8	83.1	<.001

Table 3. Multivariate odds ratio for association of obesity with hypertension and type 2 diabetes in men

| | Model I | | | Model II | | | Model I | | | Model II | | |
| | Hypertension | | | | | | Type 2 diabetes | | | | | |
Variable	OR	95%	CI	OR	95%	CI	OR	95%	CI	OR	95%	CI
Obesity	2.22	1.77	2.77	1.93	1.44	2.58	2.04	1.46	2.87	3.83	2.37	6.19
Age	1.05	1.04	1.06	1.05	1.04	1.06	1.05	1.04	1.06	1.06	1.04	1.07
Education												
High school	0.73	0.55	0.98	0.72	0.54	0.97	1.07	0.68	1.68	1.15	0.73	1.81
College	0.65	0.50	0.85	0.65	0.50	0.84	0.81	0.53	1.20	0.83	0.55	1.26
Alcohol intake	1.89	1.21	2.94	1.87	1.20	2.90	3.73	1.13	12.24	3.88	1.18	12.76
Total cholesterol	1.00	0.99	1.01	1.01	0.99	1.02	0.99	0.98	1.00	0.99	0.98	1.00
Physical activity	1.04	0.85	1.29	1.04	0.84	1.28	1.14	0.81	1.61	1.16	0.83	1.64
Race**												
Black	2.12	1.62	2.76	1.75	1.27	2.40	2.29	1.49	3.51	3.56	2.06	6.17
Hispanic	0.63	0.46	0.83	0.62	0.44	0.88	2.35	1.51	3.64	4.17	2.43	7.16
Race*obesity												
* Black	--	--	--	1.95	1.10	3.46	--	--	--	0.36	0.15	0.83
* Hispanic	--	--	--	0.99	0.56	1.77	--	--	--	0.21	0.14	0.53

OR, Odds ratio; CI, Confidence intervals from the logistic regression analysis; **, Reference group is White

The association of obesity with hypertension and diabetes in women as determined from multiple logistic regression models is shown in Table 4 (Model I). As revealed, obesity was associated with increased odds of hypertension (OR: 2.46; 95% CI: 1.96-3.09) and diabetes (OR: 3.28; 95% CI: 1.32-4.63), adjusting for age, education, alcohol intake, education, physical activity and race/ethnicity. Similar to the findings in men, being a Black woman was associated with 133% increased odds of hypertension and 111% increased odds of diabetes. Relative to White, Hispanic race/ethnicity was associated with 21% decreased odds of hypertension and 192% increased odds of diabetes. As shown (Model II), by significant interaction terms in regression models, the responses of obesity for hypertension and diabetes in women are different across race/ethnicity.

Because of the significant interaction between race and obesity we fitted race/ethnic specific multiple logistic regression models for men and women in Table 5 and Table 6, respectively. In men obesity was associated with increased odds of hypertension in Whites (OR: 1.89; 95% CI: 1.42-2.83), Blacks (OR: 3.76; 95% CI: 2.25-6.28) and Hispanics (OR: 1.98; 95% CI: 1.18-2.31), adjusting for age, education, alcohol intake, education, and physical activity. In men obesity was also was associated with an increased odds of diabetes in Whites (OR: 2.46; 95% CI: 2.19-3.47), Blacks (OR: 3.21; 95% CI: 1.03-3.99) and Hispanics (OR: 2.78; 95% CI: 1.33-3.00), after adjusting for the independent variables. In women obesity was associated with increased odds of hypertension in Whites (OR: 3.00; 95% CI: 2.18-4.14), Blacks (OR: 2.12; 95% CI: 1.25-3.35) and Hispanics (OR: 1.72; 95% CI: 1.05-2.78), adjusting for the other independent variables. In women obesity was also was associated with an increased odds of diabetes in Whites (OR: 3.98; 95% CI: 2.33-6.08), Blacks (OR: 2.48; 95% CI: 1.36-4.86) and Hispanics (OR: 3.33; 95% CI: 1.81-6.26), after adjusting for the other independent variables. Moderate physical activity was associated with decreased odds of hypertension and obesity in both White men and White women.

Table 4. Multivariate odds ratio for association of obesity with hypertension and type 2 diabetes in women

	Model I			Model II			Model I			Model II		
	Hypertension						Type 2 Diabetes					
Variable	OR	95% CI		OR	95% CI		OR	95% CI		OR	95% CI	
Obesity	2.46	1.96	3.09	3.03	2.21	4.16	3.28	1.32	4.63	3.89	2.31	6.57
Age	1.08	1.07	1.09	1.08	1.07	1.09	1.05	1.04	1.06	1.05	1.04	1.06
Education												
High school	0.92	0.67	1.27	0.91	0.67	1.27	0.92	0.58	1.45	0.92	0.58	1.45
College	0.75	0.57	1.00	0.75	0.57	1.00	0.73	0.48	1.10	0.72	0.47	1.10
Alcohol intake	1.25	0.82	1.88	1.26	0.84	1.89	0.82	0.45	1.50	0.83	0.45	1.52
Total cholesterol	1.00	0.99	1.01	1.00	0.99	1.01	0.99	0.98	1.00	0.99	0.98	1.02
Physical activity	0.99	0.78	1.24	1.00	0.80	1.26	1.02	0.71	1.46	1.02	0.71	1.47
Race**												
Black	2.33	1.75	3.11	2.67	1.83	3.90	2.11	1.35	3.29	2.63	1.34	5.18
Hispanic	0.79	0.59	1.08	0.99	0.68	1.44	2.92	2.87	4.56	3.31	1.81	6.06
Race*obesity												
* Black	--	--	--	0.72	0.42	1.24	--	--	--	0.69	0.29	1.62
* Hispanic	--	--	--	0.57	0.32	1.00	--	--	--	0.79	0.30	1.71

OR, Odds ratio; CI, Confidence intervals from the logistic regression analysis; **, Reference group is White

Table 5. Racial/ethnic specific association of obesity with odds of hypertension and type 2 diabetes in men

	White		Black		Hispanic		White		Black		Hispanic	
	Hypertension						Type 2 Diabetes					
Variable	OR	95% CI	OR	95% CI	OR	95% CI	OR	95% CI	OR	95% CI	OR	95% CI
Obesity	1.89	1.42 - 2.83	3.76	2.25 - 6.28	1.98	1.18 - 2.31	2.46	2.19 - 3.47	3.21	1.03 - 2.99	2.78	1.33 - 3.00
Age	1.05	1.04 - 1.06	1.06	1.04 - 1.07	1.06	1.05 - 1.09	1.04	1.02 - 1.06	1.08	1.01 - 1.11	1.09	1.05 - 1.10
Education												
High school	0.81	0.54 - 1.23	0.67	0.37 - 1.29	0.63	0.31 - 1.27	0.91	0.47 - 2.30	1.82	0.75 – 4.44	1.04	0.35 - 3.08
College	0.76	0.52 - 1.09	0.47	0.27 - 0.81	0.59	0.32 - 1.07	0.63	0.35 - 1.81	1.09	0.44 - 2.41	0.39	0.17 - 1.91
Alcohol intake	1.60	0.81 – 3.15	2.08	0.96 - 4.02	1.97	0.76 - 5.10	1.12	0.22 - 1.43	1.24	0.25 - 6.11	0.99	0.98 - 1.06
Total cholesterol	1.00	0.99 - 1.01	1.00	0.99 - 1.01	1.00	0.99 - 1.01	0.95	0.98 - 1.01	0.99	0.98 - 1.01	0.99	0.98 - 1.01
Physical activity	0.94	0.72 – 0.98	1.13	0.71 - 1.82	1.35	0.81 - 2.24	0.96	0.62 - 0.98	1.02	0.98 - 3.38	1.20	0.60 - 2.44

OR, Odds ratio; CI, Confidence intervals from the logistic regression analysis

Population attributable risks for hypertension and diabetes that are associated with obesity in Whites, Blacks and Hispanics are shown in Table 7. As shown, proportions of odds of hypertension explained by obesity in men were 16.9%, 44.8% and 20.4%, for Whites, Blacks and Hispanics, and 25%, 26.2% and 31.7% for diabetes, respectively. In women, proportions of odds of hypertension explained by obesity were 38.4%, 33.8% and 19.7%, for Whites, Blacks and Hispanics, and 48.2%, 40.2% and 44.3% for diabetes, respectively.

Table 6. Racial/ethnic specific association of obesity with odds of hypertension and type 2 diabetes in women

	White		Black		Hispanic		White		Black		Hispanic	
	Hypertension						Type 2 Diabetes					
Variable	OR	95% CI	OR	95% CI	OR	95% CI	OR	95% CI	OR	95% CI	OR	95% CI
Obesity	3.00	2.18 - 4.14	2.12	1.25 - 3.35	1.72	1.05 - 2.78	3.98	2.33 - 6.08	2.48	1.36 - 4.86	3.33	1.81 - 6.26
Age	1.08	1.07 - 1.09	1.08	1.06 - 1.10	1.08	1.07 - 1.10	1.06	1.04 - 1.08	1.03	1.01 - 1.05	1.06	1.04 - 1.08
Education												
High school	0.98	0.61 - 1.59	0.66	0.35 - 1.22	0.96	0.49 - 1.90	0.99	0.47 - 2.40	0.91	0.38 - 1.81	0.86	0.36 - 2.06
College	0.72	0.47 - 1.18	0.66	0.38 - 1.12	1.03	0.59 - 1.80	0.83	0.43 - 1.72	1.06	0.50 - 2.23	0.39	0.17 - 0.90
Alcohol intake	1.21	0.62 - 2.35	1.58	0.82 - 3.05	0.95	0.40 - 2.26	0.40	0.15 - 1.68	1.25	0.44 - 3.56	1.11	0.34 - 3.56
Total cholesterol	1.00	0.99 - 1.01	1.00	0.99 - 1.01	1.00	0.99 - 1.01	0.99	0.98 - 1.01	0.99	0.98 - 1.00	0.99	0.98 - 1.01
Physical activity	0.98	0.72 - 0.99	1.14	0.70 - 1.85	0.90	0.54 - 1.51	0.96	0.56 - 0.98	0.73	0.34 - 1.55	1.39	0.73 - 2.66

OR, Odds ratio; CI, Confidence intervals from the logistic regression analysis

Table 7. Population and relative attributable risks for hypertension and type 2 diabetes associated with obesity

	Men			Women		
	White	Black	Hispanic	White	Black	Hispanic
Population attributable risk (%)						
Hypertension	16.9	44.8	20.4	38.4	33.8	19.7
Type 2 diabetes	25.0	26.2	31.7	48.2	40.2	44.3
Relative attributable risk (%)						
Hypertension	Reference	50.2	4.9	Reference	70.7	57.4
Type 2 diabetes	Reference	30.6	13.4	Reference	62.2	83.7

Table 7 also shows relative attributable risks for hypertension and diabetes in Blacks and Hispanics that are associated with their differences in the rates of obesity as compared with Whites. As shown. 50.2% and 4.9% of the differences in odds of hypertension between White men and Black men and between White men and Hispanic men, respectively, are attributed to their differences in rates of obesity. The analogous values for diabetes were 30.6% and 13.4% for comparing Black men and Hispanic men with White men, respectively. Also, 70.7% and 57.4% of differences in odds of hypertension between White women and Black women and between White women and Hispanic women, respectively, are due to higher rates of obesity in non-Whites. The analogous values for diabetes were 602.2% and 83.7% for Black women and Hispanic women when compared with White women.

DISCUSSION

Higher prevalences of hypertension and diabetes among Blacks and Hispanics have been documented since the early part of the last century. In the United States, the prevalence of hypertension between 1988 and 2000 increased by 3.1% and 4.6% for Whites and Blacks, respectively [58]. Recent reports also show that the number of persons with diabetes has increased in the United States in the same time period [59-60].

Although Blacks and Hispanics are socioeconomically disadvantaged compared to Whites based on measures of income and education [61-63], these measures alone, do not completely explain their excesses in hypertension and diabetes. Obesity which is more common in Blacks and Hispanics than Whites, [19, 52, 64] may have explanatory power for the higher prevalences and risks of hypertension and diabetes in these minority groups. Indeed, rates of hypertension and diabetes have risen sharply with increasing obesity in recent years among Blacks and Hispanics in the United States [52, 65-68]. The prevalence of obesity in adults has risen from 13% to 31% in the past 25 years [52]. In the period between 1999 and 2002, the prevalence of obesity among adults with diagnosed diabetes was 57.9% for non-Hispanic whites, 63.0% for non-Hispanic blacks, and 59.5% for Mexican Americans [19]. Hence, there is a need to completely clarify the role of obesity in racial/ethnic variations for diseases, including hypertension and diabetes.

In this study we used a different approach to examine the contribution of the excess rates of obesity in Blacks and Hispanics that are associated with their higher prevalences for hypertension and diabetes. We utilized the 1999-2001 United States National Health and Nutrition Examination Surveys. These surveys are highly respected because the sampling schemes are representative and national in scope. The training program and quality control measures that were instituted in the surveys provide an added level of credibility to the data.

The results of this analysis showed significant racial/ethnic differences in the odds of hypertension and diabetes attributable to rates of obesity. In men, obesity was associated with increased odds of 89%, 276% and 98% for hypertension and 146%, 221% and 178% increased odds of diabetes in Whites, Blacks and Hispanics, respectively. The population attributable risk of hypertension due to obesity in these groups were 16.9%, 44.8% and 20.4%, and 25%, 26.2% and 31.7% for diabetes in Whites, Blacks and Hispanics, respectively. In women, obesity was associated with increased odds of 200%, 112% and 72% for hypertension and 298%, 148% and 233% increased odds of diabetes in Whites, Blacks and Hispanics, respectively. The population attributable risk of hypertension due to obesity in women were 38.4%, 33.8% and 19.7%, and 48.2%, 40.2% and 44.3% for diabetes in Whites, Blacks and Hispanics, respectively.

The results of this study also showed that in both men and women the relative differences in the odds of hypertension and diabetes between Whites and non-Whites are attributable to their differences in the prevalence of obesity. Approximately 50% and 31% of the differences in odds of hypertension and diabetes, respectively, between White men and Black men are due to their differences in the rates of obesity. The corresponding values comparing White women and Black women were approximately 71% and 62% for hypertension and diabetes, respectively. Also, approximately 5% and 13% of the differences in odds of hypertension and diabetes, respectively, between White men and Hispanic men are due to their differences in the rates of obesity. The corresponding values comparing White women and Hispanic women with White women were approximately 57% and 84%, respectively.

PUBLIC HEALTH IMPLICATIONS OF FINDINGS

The results of this study have significant implications in terms of obesity prevention at population-based levels. In this study, the prevalence of obesity in White men, Black men and Hispanic men were 22.8%, 29.4% and 26.1%, respectively. The corresponding values in White women, Black women and Hispanic women were 31.2%, 45.5% and 34.1%, respectively. Accordingly, if the prevalences of obesity in Blacks and Hispanics were reduced to the levels seen in Whites, hypertension and diabetes rates would also be reduced to rates seen in Whites. This has significant implications for racial/ethnic disparities in the prevalence of hypertension and diabetes between Blacks, Hispanics and Whites. These results suggest that much of disparity could be reduced by reducing obesity in Blacks and Hispanics. However, a major limitation of this study must be taken into account in the interpretation of results from this study. As a cross-sectional study, directionality of the associations of obesity with hypertension and diabetes cannot be clearly established. The replication of this study using a prospective epidemiologic approach is needed to add credibility to the result of this study.

CONCLUSION

The contribution of obesity to racial/ethnic variations for the prevalence odds of hypertension and diabetes in this study is noteworthy, and may provide an explanation for racial/ethnic differences for hypertension and diabetes. The results of this study indicate that there would be a significant reduction in hypertension and diabetes if obesity prevalence in minority groups is reduced to the levels seen in Whites. This indicates that obesity reduction strategies in ethnic minorities should be a major health policy imperative in addressing racial/ethnic disparities for hypertension and diabetes in the United States. There is a need to investigate the role of obesity in racial/ethnic variations for other obesity-associated sequalae.

REFERENCES

[1]   Centers for Disease Control and Prevention (CDC). Racial/ethnic disparities in prevalence, treatment, and control of hypertension--United States, 1999-2002. *MMWR* 2005;54:7-9.

[2]   Burt VL, Cutler JA, Higgins M, Horan MJ, Labarthe D, Whelton P, Brown C, Roccella EJ. Trends in the prevalence, awareness, treatment, and control of hypertension in the adult US population. Data from the health examination surveys, 1960 to 1991. *Hypertension.* 1995;26:60-69.

[3]   Cooper RS, Liao Y, Rotimi C. Is hypertension more severe among U.S. blacks, or is severe hypertension more common? *Ann Epidemiol.* 1996;6:173-180.

[4]   Rehman SU, Hutchison FN, Hendrix K, Okonofua EC, Egan BM. Ethnic differences in blood pressure control among men at Veterans Affairs clinics and other health care sites. *Arch Intern Med.* 2005;165:1041-1047.

[5]   Harris MI, Flegal KM, Cowie CC, Eberhardt MS, Goldstein DE, Little RR, Wiedmeyer HM, Byrd-Holt DD. Prevalence of diabetes, impaired fasting glucose, and impaired glucose tolerance in U.S. adults. The Third National Health and Nutrition Examination Survey, 1988-1994. *Diabetes Care.* 1998;21:518-524.

[6]   Ahluwalia IB, Mack KA, Murphy W, Mokdad AH, Bales VS. State-specific prevalence of selected chronic disease-related characteristics--Behavioral Risk Factor Surveillance System, 2001. *MMWR Surveill Summ.* 2003;52:1-80.

[7]   Adams AS, Zhang F, Mah C, Grant RW, Kleinman K, Meigs JB, Ross-Degnan D. Race Differences in Long-Term Diabetes Management in an HMO. *Diabetes Care.* 2005;28:2844-2849.

[8]   Lin SX, Larson E. Does provision of health counseling differ by patient race? *Fam Med.* 2005;37:650-654.

[9]   US Department of Health and Human Services. Healthy people 2010: understanding and improving health. 2nd ed. Washington, DC: US Department of Health and Human Services; 2000.

[10] Kearney PM, Whelton M, Reynolds K, Whelton PK, He J. Worldwide prevalence of hypertension: a systematic review. *J Hypertens.* 2004;22:11-19.

[11] Gadegbeku CA, Lea JP, Jamerson KA. Update on disparities in the pathophysiology and management of hypertension: focus on African Americans. *Med Clin North Am.* 2005;89:921-33.

[12] Joshi AV, Day D, Lubowski TJ, Ambegaonkar A Relationship between obesity and cardiovascular risk factors: findings from a multi-state screening project in the United States. *Curr Med Res Opin.* 2005;21:1755-1761.

[13] Fields LE, Burt VL, Cutler JA, Hughes J, Roccella EJ, Sorlie P. The burden of adult hypertension in the United States 1999 to 2000: a rising tide. *Hypertension.* 2004;44:398-404.

[14] Hicks LS, Shaykevich S, Bates DW, Ayanian JZ. Determinants of racial/ethnic differences in blood pressure management among hypertensive patients. *BMC Cardiovasc Disord.* 2005;5:16.

[15] Brown AF, Gregg EW, Stevens MR, Karter AJ, Weinberger M, Safford MM, Gary TL, Caputo DA, Waitzfelder B, Kim C, Beckles GL. Race, ethnicity, socioeconomic position, and quality of care for adults with diabetes enrolled in managed care: the Translating Research Into Action for Diabetes (TRIAD) study. *Diabetes Care.* 2005;28:2864-2870.

[16] National Institute of Diabetes and Digestive and Kidney Diseases. National Diabetes Statistics: Total prevalence of diabetes by race/ethnicity among people aged 20 years or older United States, 2005. [monograph on the Internet]. Bethesda, MD: National Diabetes Information Clearinghouse.http://diabetes.niddk.nih.gov/dm/pubs/statistics/index.htm#10.

[17] Lethbridge-Cejku M, Vickerie J. Summary health statistics for U.S. adults: National Health Interview Survey. 2003. National Center for Health Statistics. Tables 7 and 8. *Vital Health Stat* 10 (225). 2005. p 28-31.

[18] Center for Disease Control and Prevention. Prevalence of Diabetes and Impaired Fasting Glucose in Adults-United States, 1999-2000. *MMWR* 2003;52:833-7.

[19] Eberhardt MS. Prevalence of overweight and obesity among adults with diagnosed diabetes--United States, 1988-1994 and 1999-2002. *MMWR* 2004;53:1066-1068.

[20] Boltri J, Okosun I, Davis-Smith Y, Vogel R. Hemoglobin A1c levels in diagnosed and undiagnosed Black, Hispanic, and White persons with diabetes: results from NHANES 1999-2000. *Ethnicity and Disease 2005;* 15: 562-567.

[21] Strauss RS, Pollack HA. Epidemic Increase in Childhood Overweight, 1986-1998. *JAMA.* 2001;286:2845-2848.

[22] McCrory MA, Suen VM, Roberts SB. Biobehavioral influences on energy intake and adult weight gain. *J Nutr* 2002;132:3830S-3834S.

[23] Okosun IS. Racial differences in rates of type 2 diabetes in American women: how much is due to differences in overall adiposity? *Ethn Health.* 2001;6:27-34.

[24] Okosun IS, Chandra KM, Choi S, Christman J, Dever GE, Prewitt TE. Hypertension and type 2 diabetes comorbidity in adults in the United States: risk of overall and regional adiposity. *Obes Res.* 2001;9:1-9.

[25] Bermudez OI, Tucker KL. Total and central obesity among elderly Hispanics and the association with Type 2 diabetes. *Obes Res.* 2001;9:443-451.

[26] Resnick HE, Valsania P, Halter JB, Lin X. Differential effects of BMI on diabetes risk among black and white Americans. *Diabetes Care.* 1998;21:1828-1835.

[27] Flegal KM, Carroll MD, Ogden CL, Johnson CL. Prevalence and Trends in Obesity Among US Adults, *1999-2000 JAMA,*2002; 288: 1723 -1727.

[28] Hedley AA, Ogden CL, Johnson CL, Carroll MD, Curtin LR, Flegal KM. Prevalence of Overweight and Obesity Among US Children, Adolescents, and Adults, *1999-2002 JAMA,* 2004; 291: 2847 – 2850.

[29] David S. Freedman; Laura Kettel Khan; Mary K. Serdula; Deborah A. Galuska; William H. Dietz. Trends and Correlates of Class 3 Obesity in the United States From 1990 Through 2000. *JAMA,*2002; 288: 1758 - 1761.

[30] Laurencin MG, Goldschmidt R, Fisher L. Type 2 diabetes in adolescents. How to recognize and treat this growing problem. *Postgrad Med.* 2005;118:31-36.

[31] Centers for Disease Control and Prevention (CDC), Prevalence of diabetes and impaired fasting glucose in adults-United States, 1999–2000, *MMWR* 2003;52:833–837.

[32] Brosnan CA, Upchurch S, Schreiner B. Type 2 diabetes in children and adolescents: an emerging disease. *J Pediatr Health Care.* 2001;15:187-193.

[33] Gregg EW, Cheng YJ, Cadwell BL, Imperatore G, Williams DE Flegal KM *et al.,* Secular trends in cardiovascular disease risk factors according to body mass index in US adults, *JAMA* 293 (2005) (15), pp. 1868–1874.

[34] Gregg EW, Cadwell BL, Cheng YJ, Cowie CC, Williams DE, Geiss L, Engelgau MM, Vinicor FTrends in the Prevalence and Ratio of Diagnosed to Undiagnosed Diabetes According to Obesity Levels in the U.S. *Diabetes Care 2004;*27:2806-2812.

[35] Henderson RM. The bigger the healthier: are the limits of BMI risk changing over time? *Econ Hum Biol.* 2005;:339-366.

[36] Deurenberg P, Yap M, van Staveren WA. Body mass index and percent body fat: a meta analysis among different ethnic groups. *Int J Obes Relat Metab Disord.* 1998;22:1164-1171.

[37] Shiwaku K, Anuurad E, Enkhmaa B, Nogi A, Kitajima K, Yamasaki M, Yoneyama T, Oyunsuren T, Yamane Y. Predictive values of anthropometric measurements for multiple metabolic disorders in Asian populations. *Diabetes Res Clin Pract.* 2005:52-62.

[38] Bhansali A, Nagaprasad G, Agarwal A, Dutta P, Bhadada S. Does Body Mass Index Predict Overweight in Native Asian Indians? A Study from a North Indian Population. *Ann Nutr Metab.* 2005;50:66-73.

[39] Dictionary of Epidemiology. Last JM (ed). *International Epidemiological Association* 2001, Oxford University Press, New York, NY.

[40] Leon Gordis. *Epidemiology.* Elsevier Saunders Publishing 2004.

[41] Encyclopedia of Epidemiologic Methods. Gail MH, and Benichou J (eds.). 2000. John Wiley & Son, Ltd. New York, NY.

[42] Cornfield J. A method of estimating comparative rates from clinical data. Applications to cancer of the lung, breast and cervix. *J National Cancer Institute* 1951;11:1269-1275.

[43] Breslow NE, Day NE. Statistical Methods in Cancer Research. Vol 1-Analysis of case-control studies. IARC Scientific Publications, Lyon, France 1980.

[44] Lele C, Whittemore AS. Different disease rates in two populations: how much is due to differences in risk factors? *Stat Med* 1997;16:2543–2554.

[45] Gefeller O. Relative attributable risks. *Epidemiology* 1996;7:217- 218.

[46] Mietiinen OS. Component of crude odds ratio. *American Journal of Epidemiology.* 1972;96:168-172.

[47] Eyigou A, McHugh R. On the factorization of the crude relative risk. *American Journal of Epidemiology.* 1977;106:188-193.

[48] Schlesselman JJ. Assessing the effect of confounding variables *American Journal of Epidemiology.* 1982;108:3-8.

[49] Mark DH. Deaths attributable to obesity. *JAMA.* 2005;293:1918-1919.

[50] Flegal KM, Graubard BI, Williamson DF, Gail MH. Excess deaths associated with underweight, overweight, and obesity. *JAMA.* 2005;293:1861-1867.

[51] Williams DE, Cadwell BL, Cheng YJ, Cowie CC, Gregg EW, Geiss LS, Engelgau MM, Narayan KM, Imperatore G. Prevalence of impaired fasting glucose and its relationship with cardiovascular disease risk factors in US adolescents, 1999-2000. *Pediatrics.* 2005;11:1122-1126.

[52] Gregg EW, Cheng YJ, Cadwell BL, Imperatore C, Williams DE, Flegal KM, Narayan KM, Williamson DF. Secular Trends in Cardiovascular Disease Risk Factors According to Body Mass Index in U.S. Adults. *Obstet Gynecol Surv.* 2005;60:660-661

[53] *www.cdc.gov/nchs/nhanes.*

[54] Pickering TG, Hall JE, Appel LJ, Falkner BE, Graves JW, Hill MN, Jones DH, Kurtz T, Sheps SG, Roccella EJ; Council on High Blood Pressure Research Professional and Public Education Subcommittee, American Heart Association. Recommendations for blood pressure measurement in humans: an AHA scientific statement from the Council on High Blood Pressure Research Professional and Public Education Subcommittee. *J Clin Hypertens (Greenwich).* 2005;7:102-109.

[55] SAS Release 8.02. SAS Institute, Cary, NC.

[56] Shah BV, Barnwell BG, Bieler GS, SUDAAN User's manual. Research Triangle Institute. Research Triangle Park, NC.

[57] Wolter KM. Introduction to variance estimation. Springer-Verlag, New York, NY (1990).

[58] Hajjar I, Kotchen TA. Trends in prevalence, awareness, treatment, and control of hypertension in the United States, 1988-2000. *JAMA.* 2003;290:199-206.

[59] Mokdad AH, Bowman BA, Ford ES, Vinicor F, Marks JS, Koplan JP. The Continuing Epidemics of Obesity and Diabetes in the United States. *JAMA,* 2001; 286: 1195 - 1200.

[60] Cowie CC. Prevalence of Diabetes and Impaired Fasting Glucose in Adults—United States, 1999-2000. *JAMA,* 2003; 290: 1702 – 1703.

[61] Chang VW, Lauderdale DS. Income disparities in body mass index and obesity in the United States, 1971-2002. *Arch Intern Med.* 2005;165:2122-2128.

[62] Lewis TT, Everson-Rose SA, Sternfeld B, Karavolos K, Wesley D, Powell LH. Race, education, and weight change in a biracial sample of women at midlife. *Arch Intern Med.* 2005 ;165:545-551.

[63] Gordon-Larsen P, Adair LS, Popkin BM. The relationship of ethnicity, socioeconomic factors, and overweight in US adolescents. *Obes Res.* 2003;11:121-129.

[64] Boardman JD, Saint Onge JM, Rogers RG, Denney JT. Race differentials in obesity: the impact of place. *J Health Soc Behav.* 2005;46:229-243.

[65] Kimm SY, Barton BA, Obarzanek E, McMahon RP, Sabry ZI, Waclawiw MA, Schreiber GB, Morrison JA, Similo S, Daniels SR. Racial divergence in adiposity during adolescence: The NHLBI Growth and Health Study. *Pediatrics.* 2001;107:E34.

[66] Liao Y, Tucker P, Okoro CA, Giles WH, Mokdad AH, Harris VB. REACH 2010 Surveillance for Health Status in Minority Communities – United States, 2001--2002. *MMWR Surveill Summ.* 2004;53:1-36.

[67] Klein DJ, Aronson Friedman L, Harlan WR, Barton BA, Schreiber GB, Cohen RM, Harlan LC, Morrison JA. Obesity and the development of insulin resistance and impaired fasting glucose in black and white adolescent girls: a longitudinal study. *Diabetes Care.* 2004;27:378-383.

[68] Qureshi AI, Suri MF, Kirmani JF, Divani AA. Prevalence and trends of prehypertension and hypertension in United States: National Health and Nutrition Examination Surveys 1976 to 2000. *Med Sci Monit.* 2005;11:403-409.

In: Racial and Ethnic Disparities in Health and Health Care   ISBN 1-60021-268-9
Editor: Elene V. Metrosa, pp. 73-100   © 2006 Nova Science Publishers, Inc.

Chapter 4

BIOLOGICAL BASIS OF THE RACIAL DISPARITIES IN HEALTH AND DISEASES: AN EVOLUTIONARY PERSPECTIVE

Windsor Mak, * *Raymond T. F. Cheung and Shu Leong Ho*

Department of Medicine, Queen Mary Hospital, University of Hong Kong, P.R.C.

ABSTRACT

The genetic constituents of all human races are exceedingly similar, and racial diversity only accounts for less than 5 % of the overall genetic variations within our entire species. Nevertheless, this subtle difference is associated with an apparent asymmetry in health-related problems across the races. This chapter focuses on the biological basis for the racial disparities in health and diseases, which will be interpreted from an evolutionary perspective. Firstly, the uneven distribution of genetic diseases among different ethnic groups can be attributed to some chance events in human history. This is illustrated by the aggregation of certain uncommon mutations in Ashkenazi Jews. Conversely, racially or geographically circumscribed diseases may merely reflect the pathogenic influences from environmental or cultural factors, rather than genuine race-specific biological differences. The examples used are haemorrhagic stroke in East Asians, megaloblastic anaemia in South Asians, kuru, and Japanese encephalitis. To enhance survival in the natural environment, our ancestors evolved adaptive mechanisms against the various environmental threats through natural selection. Therefore, the genetic compositions of different population groups may be modified by the specific selection pressures within their habitats. Relevant examples include the "anti-AIDS gene" *CCR5-Δ32* and the population pattern of pharmacogenetic polymorphisms. However, besides promoting successes in survival and reproduction, adaptive traits may be associated with tradeoffs that can result in human diseases. Moreover, relaxation of selection pressures upon urbanization can produce discordance between our biological makeup and the modern lifestyle. Such maladaptations are manifested as the so-called "diseases of civilization" or

---

* Correspondence to: Dr. W. Mak, M.B.Ch.B., M.B.A., M.R.C.P., Associate Consultant in Neurology. University Department of Medicine, 4/F, Professorial Block, Queen Mary Hospital, Hong Kong, P.R.C.Tel: (852) 2855 3315; Fax: (852) 2974 1171; Email: makwaiwo@hotmail.com

"afflictions of affluence". This is illustrated by the propensity for hypertension in African Americans and ethnic differences in susceptibility to diabetes mellitus.

INTRODUCTION

Phylogenetic studies using haploid markers have repeatedly confirmed the fact that all human populations share a common ancestry. Estimations by analysing mitochondrial DNA polymorphisms traced our origin back to a single ancestor, popularly known as the "mitochondrial Eve", that lived in East Africa between 120 to 250 thousand years before present [Cann *et al*. 1987, Vigilant *et al*. 1991, Ingman *et al*. 2000]. Studies applying non-recombining Y-chromosomal markers (i.e., the "Adam" side) also coalesced all human lineages back to a common African origin, but at a more recent date of about 60,000 years ago [Underhill *et al*. 2001].

During the Upper Palaeolithic and Mesolithic Periods, our ancestors dispersed within as well as out of Africa and extended their geographical range to all major regions of the world except the Antarctic. The entire pre-Neolithic human population was less than one million [Biraben 1979]. These Stone Age hunter-gatherers scattered around in small settlements typically of twenty-five to a hundred members [Mithen 1994]. Gene flow between different tribes was probably minimal. The amount of forage resources available within exploration distance of each campsite, which ranged from 80 to 300 kilometres, was only sufficient to sustain a population density of 0.005 to 0.05 persons per kilometre square [Gamble 1999]. This constraint was lifted about ten thousand years ago when agriculture was adopted. Successes in food production favoured expansion of farming tribes over the hunter-gatherers. As a result, the previous population structure, a *status quo* that had been maintained for several thousand generations, was reorganized, with formation of huge regional clusters that overflowed into territories of other indigenous groups.[1] This produced, within less than two hundred generations, an exaggerated asymmetry among the Neolithic populations; a few underwent disproportionate expansions while the others perished down to extinction or became absorbed. New social networks and group identities were also created, which cultivated the eventual emergence of nations, races, and ethnicities. Ancestral histories or phylogeographical affiliations of contemporary populations can now be inferred objectively

---

[1] Demic diffusion is a population replacement process caused by mass movement of people into territories with previous occupants. The natives are either expelled or dominated by the newcomers. The many episodes of demic diffusion recorded in human history can now be tested with molecular techniques. For example, Wen *et al*. [2004] demonstrated a tight clustering of Y-chromosome haplogroups among the Hans from all regions of China, while the mitochondrial markers showed an apparent geographical differentiation, indicating a male-driven demic diffusion in ancient time. This is concordant with the Han legends and historical records. Analysis of ancestral markers in Indian populations also confirmed the several waves of demic diffusion, as speculated by historians [Basu *et al*. 2003]; the earliest inhabitants were the Austro-Asiatic tribals, followed by the Dravidians, who then retreated southwards upon arrival of the Indo-European-speaking nomads from the mid-Asian steppes. Prior to the employment of molecular techniques, population groups were commonly classified under a system using linguistic families as surrogates for ancestral inference. For instance, most modern European languages belong to the Indo-European family. The conventional inference was that the indigenous settlers of the continent had been replaced by Indo-European-speaking colonizers (who migrated from Asia during the Neolithic period), and the Basque-speaking groups (who lived at the border of Spain and France) were the last European natives. However, this demic diffusion model was disproved by molecular evidence; about 80 % of West Europeans possess phylogenetic signatures that can be traced back to the Upper Palaeolithic period [Richards *et al*. 1996, 1998, and 2000, Semino *et al*. 2000], indicating that most people from this region are actually aboriginal.

by analysing their genetic polymorphisms or haplotype markers[2] [Bamshad *et al.* 2003, Rosenberg *et al.* 2003].

The concepts of race as well as ethnicity have always been controversial and confusing in human history. Population groups are typically differentiated by their external physical appearances, such as skin colour, hair texture, shape of nose and eyes, and the geographical location that they live in or originated from. Moreover, people under the same nation are divided into various ethnic groups by incorporating sociological or political elements, like language, culture, presumed ancestry, and religion, on top of their external traits. For example, the number of official ethnic groups in the People's Republic of China amounts to fifty-six (plus seventeen, if those from Taiwan are also counted). It is well known that an individual's racial or ethnic label does not accurately reflect his or her underlying genetic or biological constituent. In the United States, for instance, different population groups were conventionally classified under ethnic labels such as whites, African Americans, Hispanics, Asians, Native Americans, and Pacific Islanders, etc. Similar schemes are still routinely used in biomedical research for categorized the demographic data of patients. However, such classification schemes are often vague and non-scientific. For example, a study looking at the ancestral DNA markers in Hispanics showed that the proportions of European, Native American, and African contributions were dissimilar across the Hispanic communities from different states [Bertoni *et al.* 2003]. Therefore, it is scientifically unsound to group them indiscriminately under a single ethnic stock. The same problem applies to "Asians" as well, which loosely encompasses all population groups migrated from the entire continent of Asia. Among the world's major geographical regions, Asia has one of the most complex and diversified population structures. Analysis of multilocus polymorphisms demarcated within Asia four main population clusters (i.e., Middle East, Central Asia, South Asia, and East Asia) that had distinctive allelic frequencies [Rosenberg *et al.* 2002], implying that "Asians" is just a convenient label arbitrarily tagged onto an admixture of genetically heterogeneous individuals.

On the other hand, the actual magnitude of genetic variations attributable to racial differentiation is subtle and only belongs to a small fraction of the entire diversity within our species. While more than 90 % of the human genetic differences represent race non-specific, within-population variations, only 3 to 5 %[3] are accounted for by inter-racial plus inter-regional dissimilarities [Dean *et al.* 1994, Rosenberg *et al.* 2002]. This would translate into an absolute genetic difference of 0.03 % or less among the human races (assuming the overall genetic divergence within the human lineage is 0.6 % [Carroll 2003]). Nevertheless, this close genetic affinity is paradoxically linked with apparent racial disparities in health-related problems, which include incidence and severity of diseases as well as outcome of medical care.

Genetic diseases distribute unevenly from one population to another, and individual groups often exhibit their distinctive patterns and frequencies of genetic mutations. Burchard *et al.* [2003] estimated that disease-associated genes with allelic frequencies of less than 2 %

---

[2] This is not equivalent to the delineation of racial boundaries. Even molecular techniques cannot serve the purpose of assigning an individual precisely into a particular pre-defined population group.

[3] This small difference is exceptional for large mammals, the animal class to which humans belong. In African elephants or North American grey wolves, the inter-group genetic difference represents 40 % or 75 %, respectively, of the total within-species variation [Olson 2002]. This probably reflects our relatively recent and rapid dispersion around the globe and our long generation cycle (i.e., fifteen to twenty-five years per generation).

(in the respective populations) are nearly always race or ethnic specific, and mutations with frequencies of between 2 and 20 % typically affect single or certain population groups more than the others. Besides the less common single-locus genetic diseases, susceptibility to complex degenerative and polygenic disorders, such as hypertension, diabetes mellitus, atherosclerosis, stroke, and malignancies, and their manifestations may also follow a racial pattern.

However, the biological variations used for defining human races, whether historical or novel, cannot adequately explain these disparities. External physical features are the results of natural selection during human dispersion; our ancestors evolved morphological variations in order to enhance adaptation to environmental pressures, such as climate, altitude, amount of sunlight, and type of food, in their respective geographical locations. The expression of physical traits is encoded by a relatively small number of genes, which are unlikely to be relevant when diseases are concerned. The phylogenetic signatures used for making ancestral inferences, which are assumed to be neutral mutations, also do not correspond to our inherent biological dissimilarities in connection with health and diseases.

To account for the racial disparities in health-related problems, other biological as well as social factors are to be held responsible. This chapter focuses on the evolutionary perspectives of the former, which will be discussed under three sections: 1) isolation and genetic diseases, 2) non-genetic factors and diseases, and 3) health and diseases associated with natural selection or relaxation of selection pressures.

ISOLATION AND GENETIC DISEASES

Firstly, the asymmetrical distribution of genetic diseases can be attributed to a series of historical chance events, which were mediated by geographical isolation coupled with a founder effect and the subsequent endogamous reproduction.

Biological and Non-biological Isolating Mechanisms

It is widely accepted that geographical isolation and allopatric speciation are essential for the emergence of novel species [Mayr 1976]. In the beginning, several members of an established species split off from the parent pool to form an aberrant segregate that enlarges into a separate population if the founders can survive and proliferate. Geographical or environmental barriers, if adequate, will interrupt gene flow between the two clusters of the initially identical species. At the same time, evolution in the isolated colony deviates from the parent pool because of 1) random mutations that are selectively neutral, and 2) natural selection if the new habitat is ecologically different from the original one. The gradual accumulation of genetic divergence will eventually result in the formation of an incipient species with morphological and physiological alterations, which prohibit reproduction between the new and parent species.

The most recently coexisting hominid subspecies were *Homo sapiens sapiens* (HSS), or anatomically modern human, and *Homo sapiens neanderthalensis*. It is commonly believed that both of these hominid subspecies were descendants of *Homo heidelbergensis* [Tattersall and Schwartz 2001]. While HSS evolved directly from the parent pool of East African *Homo heidelbergensis*, Neanderthals probably stemmed from an isolated population outside Africa. Before the two hominid subspecies encountered when HSS spread to the Middle East at approximately 50,000 years ago [Underhill *et al.* 2000 and 2001], they had been separated from each other for at least half a million years [Kring *et al.* 1997]. Fossil records as well as analysis of parental haploid markers in contemporary humans failed to show any evidence that HSS and Neanderthals had ever interbreed successfully during their coexistence of over 20,000 years in Europe and West Asia. Therefore, half a million years of separation and genetic divergence may already be adequate to create a reproduction barrier in hominids.[4]

Among all the contemporary human populations, the maximum genetic distance exists between the sub-Saharan Africans and aboriginal Australians [Bowcock *et al.* 1994, Cavalli-Sforza *et al.* 1994], with an estimated separation of up to three thousand generations or fifty to seventy-five thousand years [Mountain and Cavalli-Sforza 1997]. Similar to other species, geographical barriers and physical distance were the most important forces that had influenced human genetic differentiation [Burchard *et al.* 2003]. Theoretically, endogamous mating within geographically isolated human groups, if sufficiently extended, would lead to accumulation of genetic mutations, allopatric speciation, and eventually diversification into incipient species. However, members of all human populations are able to "interbreed". Therefore, the duration of isolation (i.e., at most three thousand generations) and the degree of genetic divergence produced within this period are inadequate to create an effective biological reproduction barrier between the various human populations. However, the isolation is sufficient to generate and retain an uneven occurrence of disease-associated genetic mutations (see next subsection).

Besides geographical isolation, other non-biological isolating mechanisms[5] had also conferred an effective "reproduction barrier" among the ethnic groups. For many centuries, non-biological factors such as language, religion, social attitudes, rules, policies, and other sources of group identity, had prevented intermarriages between, as well as within, human populations. These social and cultural restrictions, which were prominent in the past, still remain relatively important in some of the present day societies.

Founder Effect, Random Drift, and Endogamous Reproduction: Genetic Diseases in Ashkenazi Jews and Samaritans

Endogamous reproduction within an isolated population, which may be geographical or cultural, can shield off the effects of gene flow from neighbouring groups on its genetic composition. As a result, the genetic characteristics of its founders can be largely preserved.

---

[4] Some authors hold alternative hypotheses. Diamond [1992] suggested that although it might be biologically feasible for Neanderthals and HSS to hybridise, a cultural or moral barrier would stop them from interbreeding, like a human would never mate with a chimpanzee naturally. Conversely, Klawans [2000] proposed a biological explanation that the HSS birth canal was incompatible with passage of a hybrid from a Neanderthal male, and a different schedule of brain maturation would render the offspring between an HSS male and Neanderthal female severe mental incapacity.

[5] The term "*isolating mechanisms*" was originally defined by Mayr [1963] as *biological properties of individuals which prevent the interbreeding of populations that are actually or potentially sympatric*. However, social and cultural factors, which are non-biological, were and still are important barriers of gene flow among different ethnic groups.

Most populations began with a few individuals. If a number of the founders were carriers of a particular allele, which may be rare in the global gene pool, that allele will be represented in an unusually large proportion of their descendants. This founder effect is applicable to populations that proliferated from: 1) isolated settlements at new geographical sites, or 2) major demographical bottlenecks leaving a small number of survivors. Moreover, during the early phase of population expansion, the allelic frequency can be further amplified by random genetic drift.

In a preponderantly inbreeding population, the force of a founder phenomenon plus the subsequent random drift and allopatric isolation may be strong enough to overcome or limit the effects of natural selection [Cavalli-Sforza et al. 1994, Stearns 1999]. Therefore, disease-associated genes may escape elimination and continue to perpetuate, which is particularly true for recessively-inherited conditions. Even though the homozygote state may not be compatible with survival or reproduction, heterozygote carriers can still persist and multiply, thereby maintaining the disease mutation at a certain population frequency. This explains why some lethal, or selectively-adverse, hereditary conditions happen to aggregate in specific ethnic groups but seldom affect others, as illustrated by the propensity for familial breast cancer and a number of very rare autosomal recessive metabolic syndromes in Ashkenazi Jews (Table 1).

Table 1. Some hereditary diseases that are commoner in Ashkenazi Jews than other population groups [Motulsky 1995, Rubinstein 2004]

Disease	Overall heterozygote frequency in Ashkenazi Jews
Tay Sachs disease	3 – 4 %
Gaucher disease	4 – 6 %
Canavan disease	1.7 – 2 %
Neimann-Pick disease	1 – 2 %
Mucolipoidosis IV	~ 1 %
Bloom syndrome	~ 1 %
Idiopathic torsion dystonia	0.1 – 0.3%
Familial dysautonomia	3 %
Factor XI deficiency	8.1%
Pentosuria	2.5 – 3 %
Breast cancer (BRCA1 and 2)	2.5 %

Ashkenazi Jews are the descendents of Jewish immigrants who settled along the Rhine River in the Ninth Century. Historically, they formed an isolated ethnic cluster that had restricted gene flow with the outside groups. The current Ashkenazim population is over ten million, which accounts for approximately 80 % of the entire Jewry. They were believed to originate from just a few thousand individuals whom belonged to the wealthier fraction of the early Ashkenazim community [Motulsky 1995]. There was probably an incidental preponderance of rare genetic mutations in these founders. With a prominent founder effect and subsequent endogamous reproduction, those uncommon monogenic hereditary diseases could be maintained and transmitted down the generations.

The Samaritans had a similar phylogeographical background as the Jews, although the cultural backgrounds of these two ethnic groups were very different. Analysis of phylogenetic markers suggested that most of the Samaritan and Jewish patrilineages were identical and can be traced back to a common ancestry at the time of the Assyrian conquest of the kingdom of Israel [Shen *et al*. 2004]. Similar to the Jews, Samaritans were also severely oppressed throughout their history. By the early Twentieth Century, the entire Samaritan population contracted down to a bottleneck of five families, or less than a hundred and fifty individuals [Olson 2002, Shen *et al*. 2004]. Afterwards, they expanded to the current population of approximately six hundred. The Samaritans practise strict within religion marriage. For more than two thousand years, gene flow between the Samaritans and other populations was essentially negligible, making them the most inbred ethnic group among all the races. But unlike the Ashkenazi Jews, who were also an endogamous population and related to them through a common group of ancient ancestors, the Samaritans rarely have monogenic hereditary diseases other than Usher syndrome, an autosomal dominant disorders which causes congenital deafness and progressive visual loss. This probably indicates that the 146 individuals who founded the contemporary Samaritan population were by chance a healthy group who did not carry too many disease-associated mutations. Therefore, what determines the frequency of hereditary diseases in a population is the genetic composition of its founders rather than the subsequent degree of endogamous mating.

NON-GENETIC FACTORS AND DISEASES

Beginning and creation come form the East. Fish and salt are the products of water and ocean and of the shores near the water. The people of the regions of the East eat fish and crave salt; their living is tranquil and their food delicious. Fish causes people to burn within, and the eating of salt defeats the blood. Therefore the people of these regions are all of dark complexion and careless and lax in their principles. Their diseases are ulcers, which are most properly treated with acupuncture by means of a needle of flint. ... Precious metals and jade come from the regions of the West. The dwellings in the West are built of pebbles and sandstone. Nature exerts itself to bring a good harvest. The people in these regions live on hills and, because of the great amount of wind, water, and soil, become robust and energetic. They wear no clothes other than those of coarse woollen stuff or coarse matting. They eat good and variegated food and therefore are flourishing and fertile. Hence pathogens cannot injure their external bodies, and if they get disease they strike at the inner body. These diseases are most successfully cured with poison medicines. ... The North is the region of storing and laying by. The country is hilly, there are biting cold winds, frost and ice. The people of these regions find pleasure in living in the wilderness, and they live on milk products. The extreme cold causes many diseases. These diseases are most fittingly treated with cauterisation by burning the dried tinder of artemisia. ... Nourishment and growth come form the South. The sun makes the life of those who live in the regions of the South plentiful and nourishing. Although there is water beneath the earth, the soil is deficient, it collects dew and mist. The people crave sour food and curd. They are secretive and soft in their ways and attached to the red colour. Their diseases are bent and contracted muscles and numbness. These diseases are most fittingly treated with acupuncture with fine needles. ... The region of the centre, the Earth, is level and moist. Everything is created by the Universe meets in the centre and is absorbed by the Earth. The people of the regions of the centre eat mixed food and do not toil. Their diseases are many: they suffer from complete paralysis and chills and fever. These diseases are most fittingly treated with breathing exercises, massage of skin and flesh, and exercises of hands and feet.

Chapter 12, *Huang Di Nei Jing* [translated by Veith, 2002]

Huang Di Nei Jing (*The Yellow Emperor's Cannon of Medicine*) has been a fundamental text in Traditional Chinese Medicine for over 2,000 years. The above chapter addresses the importance of environmental factors and diet in shaping the distinctive regional pattern of diseases. This insight is mandatory when interpreting health-related problems in different population groups. The presence of geographically or racially circumscribed variations may merely reflect environmental or cultural (i.e., lifestyle) influences rather than the biological attributes independently associated with racial origins. The following examples are used to illustrate this phenomenon: 1) The effect of diet on stroke subtypes and mortality in East Asians, 2) Megaloblastic anaemia in South Asians and how living conditions interact with their social customs to produce nutritional deficiencies, 3) Transmission of kuru by a distinctive rite, and 4) Japanese encephalitis in countries practising irrigated rice cultivation.

Diet and Stroke in East Asians

Stroke is the collective term for a constellation of cerebrovascular diseases. There are multiple aetiologies as well as stroke subtypes, and the distribution of which are not the same in different populations. Stroke can be crudely divided into haemorrhagic and ischaemic; the former includes intracerebral haemorrhage (ICH), subarachnoid haemorrhage, and other subtypes of intracranial haemorrhages, while the latter is even more heterogeneous.

Stroke can be considered an aetiologically multifactorial degenerative condition that represents the final outcome of complex gene-gene and gene-environmental interactions. Any race-specific genetic differences are unlikely to be important in the predisposition to stroke. Similar to most of the chronic diseases, susceptibility alleles to stroke are likely to be ancient and imprinted in the genome of all human populations [Cooper *et al.* 2003]. Therefore, it is highly improbable for stroke-prone genotypes to be confined to individual races. Conversely, non-genetic factors, such as diet, lifestyle, socio-economic status, and education, are more relevant in determining the prevalence and manifestations of stroke or other atherosclerotic diseases among different populations or ethnic groups. Therefore, it is inappropriate to use race or ethnicity as an independent variable in epidemiological or related studies without adjusting for socio-economic and the other confounding factors.

Intracerebral haemorrhage carries a higher mortality and is more disabling than ischaemic stroke or other subtypes of haemorrhagic stroke [Broderick *et al.* 1999]; mortality from ICH can be over 50 % and the majority of survivors will never regain functional independence. According to the literature, ICH accounts for about 10 % of all strokes [Shah and Biller 1998]. In Chinese and other East Asians, ICH appears to be more prevalent. Several prospective studies were performed in Hong Kong to define the stroke subtypes in Chinese. The first was carried out from 1984 to 1985 in Queen Mary Hospital [Huang *et al.* 1990]. In this survey, 165 cases (38 %) of ICH and 270 cases of ischaemic strokes were recorded. The subsequent Shatin Stroke Registry (1989) reported 211 cases (28 %) of ICH and 531 cases of ischaemic stroke [Kay *et al.* 1992]. A more recent survey at Queen Mary Hospital (1996 to 1999) found that 23 % of strokes were ICH [Cheung *et al.* 2001]. A high proportion of ICH

(45 %) was also observed in the Eastern Stroke and Coronary Heart Disease Collaborative (ESCHDC) Group Study [1998].

Hypercholesterolaemia is an important risk factor that predisposes to atherosclerosis and its complications, including coronary artery disease, peripheral vascular disease, and ischaemic stroke. In the Seven Countries Study [Menotti et al. 1993], large between-population differences in coronary mortality were observed. The main determinant of coronary mortality was the mean cholesterol level within a given population, rather than the racial factor across the cohorts.

Paradoxically, low cholesterol had been associated with higher incidence of ICH [Yano et al. 1989, Neaton et al. 1992, Iribarren et al. 1996, Segal et al. 1999, ESCHDC Group 1998]. East Asians are well-known to have lower cholesterol levels than westerner; mean cholesterol level was 4.5 mmol/L in both the ESCHDC and Shibata studies [Nakayama et al. 1997] as compared with 5.7 mmol/L in AFCAPS/TexCAPS conducted in Texas [Downs et al. 1998]. The average cholesterol level in Hong Kong Chinese was 5.4 mmol/L [Fong et al. 1994]. This comparison may illustrate an inverse relationship between cholesterol level and haemorrhagic stroke; the proportion of ICH was highest in the ESCHDC study cohort, intermediate in Hong Kong, and lowest in the United States. In the ESCHDC Study, the group with the most elevated cholesterol had the highest risk of ischaemic stroke, but they also had the lowest risk of ICH. This trend was also observed in the Honolulu Heart Study [Yano et al. 1989] and Multiple Risk Factor Intervention Trial [1982]. The biological basis for this relationship is yet to be clarified.

Moreover, low cholesterol level is associated with increased stroke mortality [Iso et al. 1989, Dyker et al. 1997, Roquer et al. 2005]. The prevalence and mortality of stroke was considered to be higher in East Asians. Stroke was the leading cause of death in Japan from 1950 to 1980, and mortality rate was twice of that in western countries [Menotti et al. 1990]. Intracerebral haemorrhage was the predominant stroke subtype. Most researchers attributed these differences to uncontrolled blood pressure and other lifestyle-related risk factors rather than race-specific genetic dissimilarities [Yatsu 1991]. Furthermore, the Ni-Hon-San Study conducted between 1972 and 1976 showed that Japanese men living in Hiroshima and Nagasaki had a twofold increase in incidence of ICH as compared with Japanese American men from Hawaii [Takeya et al. 1984]. In addition to hypertension, a low consumption of fat and protein was suggested to be a risk factor for ICH in Japanese [Tanakan et al. 1982, Kagan et al. 1985], which might also be extrapolated to other East Asians with similar dietary habits. Traditional Japanese diet consisted of a very low level of animal protein. Typically, less than 15 % of their total daily energy intake was derived from animal products, as compared with up to 40 % in western diets [Sauvaget et al. 2004]. With socio-economic developments since the 1970s, eating habits as well as dietary quality of the Japanese had changes remarkably. The Hiroshima/Nagasaki Life Span Study showed a progressively increasing consumption of animal products in the Japanese diet [Sauvaget et al. 2003, 2004]. A parallel upward shift of cholesterol level also occurred during this period [Shimamoto et al. 1989]. At the same time, the incidence and mortality from stroke, ICH in particular, had been continuously declining [Shimamoto et al. 1989, Nakayama et al. 1997], and the present epidemiological pattern of stroke in Japan is close to that in the western countries. (A similar trend of stroke mortality was also observed in Hong Kong [Yu et al. 2000].) Recently, several studies had demonstrated an interesting "dose-dependant" protective effect of dietary animal products against death from stroke [Sauvaget et al. 2003, 2004], and an increased risk of ICH with low intake of saturated fat and animal proteins [Iso *et al.* 2001]. From these observations, it can be speculated that the previous high ICH rate and stroke mortality in East Asian countries were related to an ultra-low consumption of animal products, while the epidemiological changes in the last few decades could be due to improved dietary quality and "normalization" of cholesterol in the populations.

Table 2. Proportion of lacunar infarction in Hong Kong as compared with registries from western countries

	All cases of ischaemic stroke	Lacunar stroke
Queen Mary Hospital (84 – 85)	n = 270	n = 117 (43 %)
Queen Mary Hospital (96 – 99)	n = 608	n = 270 (44 %)
Western registries:		
Lausanne		15 %
Dijon		15 %
Oxfordshire		25 %
NINDS*		13 %

* In the National Institute of Neurological Disorders and Stroke rt-PA Stroke Study [1995], only 5 out of the 606 patients recruited were Asians.

Besides ICH, lacunar infarction, a subtype of ischaemic stroke, is also commoner in Chinese (Table 2). According to Fisher's schema [Caplan *et al.* 1986], both lacunar stroke and ICH are caused by hypertension-related atherosclerotic disease of the small perforating vessels that penetrate and supply the deep cerebral regions, resulting in lipohyalinosis and narrowing of the arterial lumen (which predisposes to lacunar infarction) and, at the same time, microaneurysm formation (hence ICH). Therefore, hypertension is responsible for the pathogenesis of both lacunar infarction and ICH, or the predominant stroke subtypes in East Asians. Adopting a healthy lifestyle, including lowering of salt intake, and better surveillance and control of hypertension might also have contributed to the recent decline in stroke mortality in East Asian countries (please refer to the next section for more discussions on hypertension).

Megaloblastic Anaemia in South Asians

Vitamin B12 and folate deficiencies are the two main causes of megaloblastic anaemia. It is mandatory to distinguish the former from the latter, as replacing folic acid in a vitamin B12 deficient patient can precipitate acute and irreversible neurological complications, which include delirium, spinal cord degeneration, and polyneuropathy.

Megaloblastic anaemia is prevalent in India. The most frequent cause is folate deficiency, which may either be a result of nutritional deprivation from poverty or malabsorption due to tropical sprue. Vitamin B12 deficiency is considered a rare condition because autoimmune pernicious anaemia is uncommon in South Asians, and well-water, which may contain up to 0.1 µg of vitamin B12 per litre from its natural flora [Britt *et al.* 1971], provides an alternative and often adequate source of the vitamin. Therefore, in conventionally medical teaching, the popular notion was that megaloblastic anaemia in a dark-skinned patient is invariably due to folate deficiency. However, if their living condition is altered, this rule of thumb may be totally reversed.

Britt *et al*. [1971] investigated a series of twenty-five Indian immigrants living in London who were diagnosed to have megaloblastic anaemia. Thirteen patients (52 %) had vitamin B12 deficiency, in contrast with only six cases of pure folate deficiency. (If these patients were treated empirically with folic acid replacement basing on the conventional belief, over half of them would end up with detrimental consequences.) Most patients with vitamin B12 deficiency had nutritional deprivation, probably as a result of the interaction between their traditional social customs and a non-traditional living environment. They were either Sikh or Hindu lacto-vegetarians. After moving to London, the milk added for cooking, instead of well-water, became their main source of vitamin B12. However, Indian food is typically prepared by prolonged heating, and this would degrade most of the vitamin. In a recent survey conducted at an Ontario family clinic, vitamin B12 deficiency could still be detected in 46 % of South Asian clients, as compared with less than 5 % in the general population [Gupta *et al*. 2004], and those who consumed a traditional lacto-vegetarian diet were also more likely to have a decreased vitamin level (odds ratio = 2.14).

Kuru in Fore Melanesians

The kuru epidemic decimated a Fore-speaking group of Melanesians in the Mid-Twentieth Century. The disease was confined to a highly localized region at the eastern highland of Papua New Guinea. Kuru, which means shiver in the Fore language, ran an invariably fatal course. The victim usually died within a year after onset of symptoms, which consisted of progressive cerebellar ataxia, myoclonus, dysarthria, dystonia, and dementia. The kuru epidemic peaked in the 1950s. In some villages, up to 10 % of the natives could develop the disease per annum. Gajdusek and Zigas [1957] recorded a death toll of 1,400 over several years, which represented more than 10 % of the entire population. There was a remarkable gender asymmetry in the incidence of kuru; women were affected ten times more than men, and children over the age of five years developed the disease at an intermediate rate.

Kuru is now known to be a kind of transmissible spongioform encephalopathy. It is caused by the accumulation of a protease-resistance aberrant prion protein PrP^{res} in the central nervous system, which leads to its degeneration. Once transmissible particles with this pathogenic isoform enter the system, they can serve as templates to spark off a self-perpetuating cycle, converting the normal structural prion protein PrP^c into further copies of PrP^{res}. A kuru-like syndrome could be induced by inoculated chimpanzees with "infected" human brain tissues. Incubation period in chimpanzees was 18 to 21 months. Other transmissible spongioform encephalopathies that affect humans include sporadic and familial Creutzfeldt-Jakob disease (CJD), iatrogenic CJD (transmitted through contaminated neurosurgical instruments, implants, and pituitary extracts), variant CJD, and a few less common syndromes.

Kuru was transmitted across the Fore Melanesians through ritual endocannibalism, which was practised as a bereavement ceremony for their deceased relatives. This rite started since the late Nineteenth Century. The corpses were ingested after minimal cooking. The muscles were taken up by the men, while women and children shared the brain and viscera. Many of the deceased were victims of kuru, and cannibalism amplified the "recycling" of pathogenic prion proteins within the Fore population. Women and children were more frequently affected because the dose of transmissible pathogens was higher in the parts that they consumed. In addition, they would rub tissues from the corpses over their bodies, which might further facilitate the inoculation of prion pathogens via entry through skin sores, conjunctiva, and nasal passages.

It seems that cannibalism is the only transmitting route of kuru, as no apparent vertical or lateral transmission had ever been documented. Although the neighbouring clans also practised cannibalism, they refrained from eating those who died of kuru, so that they were less afflicted by the epidemic. After banning of cannibalism in New Guinea, the kuru epidemic was rapidly extinguished.

Japanese Encephalitis, an Epidemic Caused by Altered Ecology

Japanese encephalitis (JE), which is prevalent in East and Southeast Asia, the Indian Subcontinent, and some Pacific Rim countries, represents a disease that emerged under the specific ecological setting of a geographical location, rather than from the biological or genetic factors of its inhabitants.

St. Louis encephalitis (SLE), West Nile (WN) encephalitis, Murray Valley encephalitis (MVE), and JE are caused by closely related strains of arthropod-born flaviviruses. Their transmissions involve the complex interplay of viruses, vectors, vertebrate hosts, and the interacting climatic and ecological factors [Solomon 2004, Weaver and Barrett 2004]. In the natural environment, an enzootic cycle is maintained by the transmission of viruses through arthropod vectors among certain hosts that are able to survive a prolonged and high-titre viraemia. The viruses may also infect dead-end hosts inadvertently when they encroach upon the cycle. The latter usually succumb before developing a high-titre viraemia, and the viruses will, therefore, not be able to re-enter the cycle.

With the introduction of agriculture, the original habitats of these natural vectors and hosts were disrupted. The newly created human-friendly niche was then filled up with a whole range of novel organisms, including crops, domesticated animals, as well as human beings. Faced with a drastically altered environment, most of the naturally occurring species would be replaced, but a few that fitted particularly well into the new ecological setting might multiply opportunistically. The original enzootic cycle, which was of a relatively small scale in the natural habitat, might abut on the new agricultural setting and become transformed into a rural epizootic transmission cycle. The vectors would exploit hosts that were either novel to the natural enzootic cycle or familiar ones that had emerged as preponderant members under the new ecological setting. If a large number of intermediate hosts were available, the rural epizootic cycle would be greatly amplified, resulting in a large reservoir of viruses and severe spillover effect to dead-end hosts, which may include humans.

Japanese encephalitis is the most prevalent viral encephalitis worldwide; it accounts for 30,000 to 50,000 cases of infections per year (the actual number of cases is much higher, as the ratio of manifested to subclinical infections is 1:25 to 1:400), which is more than all the other types of arthropod-born flavivirus encephalitides combined. The first major outbreak of JE occurred in 1924. Within a hundred years, JE spread across a vast geographical range, and the number of people at risk now exceeds two billion. In the temperate zone, JE occurs during the summer months, while it is a year-round endemic disease in the tropical areas with an annual incidence of 10 to 100 per 100,000. Japanese encephalitis causes a life-threatening meningoencephalomyelitis or polio-like flaccid paralysis in humans. The case fatality rate is approximately 20 % to 30 %, leading to at least 10,000 to 15,000 deaths per year, and over 50 % of survivors are left with long-term neuropsychiatric sequelae.

Solomon *et al.* [2003] analysed the DNA and amino acid sequences of the encephalitic flaviviruses. By comparing their geographical range and phylogenetic relationships, the authors reconstructed an ancestral African virus from which the various flavivirus families branched off, including firstly the SLE viruses, followed by WN viruses, and eventually a common progenitor group that diverged into the MVE and JE virus families about 350 years ago. For the JE viruses, all the major genotypes as well as the maximum degree of genetic diversity were present in the Indonesia-Malaysia region. These findings suggest that a basal strain of JE virus, which probably originated from this location, evolved and diverged into all the other JE virus lineages. These viruses were initially maintained by small-scale enzootic cycles within the Southeast Asian tropical rain forests. The infection was passed around wild birds, bats, and snakes by more than a dozen of mosquito species. During the Nineteenth Century, the intensification of agriculture and other food production industries in East and Southeast Asia had precipitated the conversion of JE into an epizootic disease. Japan was the first to be afflicted since her agricultural development was ahead of the other countries. The extensive practice of irrigated rice cultivation in the region have provided plenty of breeding grounds for the *Culex* mosquitoes, which are the most frequently incriminated vectors for transmission of JE viruses. The abundant mosquitoes and crops also attract a huge population of migrating birds, such as the black-crowned night heron and the Asiaiatic cattle egret.[6] They are responsible for maintaining the viruses and spreading them across the region. Pigs, horses, and domesticated fowls, which were novel to the natural enzootic cycle, also amplify the rural epizootic cycle very efficiently. Large numbers of these domesticated animals, together with their huge reservoirs of JE viruses, are kept adjacent to human dwellings, so that *Culex* mosquitoes can conveniently transmit the infection to humans. Humans are dead-end hosts for JE viruses. A person infected in the countryside cannot start off an urban epidemic cycle after travelling to the cities even if the right vector is available. However, other epizootic or enzootic infections had been converted into important urban epidemics, provided that a sufficient viraemia can be sustained in human. Examples include AIDS and SARS.

HEALTH AND DISEASES ASSOCIATED WITH NATURAL SELECTION OR RELAXATION OF SELECTION PRESSURES

Besides the barrier effect of geographical isolation, influence from natural selection against environmental threats at different geographical localities was also extremely important in determining the genetic differentiation among human populations. Like all natural organisms, human evolved distinctive adaptive traits to enhance their survival under the specific and often unique climatic, ecological, and other environmental selection pressures

---

[6] The population and geographical range of cattle egret expanded drastically across Asia during the Nineteenth Century, which coincided with the extension of irrigated rice fields as well as spread of JE in the region [Solomon *et al.* 2003].

within their habitats. An obvious example is the association between the amount of sunlight and skin pigmentation. Bowcock *et al.* [1991] estimated that as much as one third of the overall human genetic polymorphisms evolved as a result of natural selection. Polymorphisms that differ in frequency from group to group may have specific effects on health and diseases.

Besides creating solutions for adverse environmental circumstances, natural selection may also create problems that manifest themselves as human diseases. The ultimate aim of natural selection is to maximise an individual's abilities to gain genetic representation in future generations, which may not necessarily be translated into fitness in terms of health or longevity [Williams and Nesse 1991]. Many of the human physiological and anatomical arrangements are vulnerable to diseases because they are shaped as such by natural selection to serve specific adaptive functions. For example, an abnormal gene that confers certain adaptive benefits (i.e., enhance survival or reproductive success or both) may be maintained in the population at a relatively high frequency even though it severely compromises the fitness of some carriers.

Conversely, maladaptation can be produced by relaxation of selection pressures. Two examples, hypertension in African Americans and ethnic differences in susceptibility to diabetes mellitus, are used to illustrate this phenomenon.

CCR5-Δ32 Mutation

Infective pathogens are some of the most important selection pressures in shaping the human genome, because their ancestors co-evolved with ours. The often-quoted examples in medical curriculum, which may also be the only ones quoted, are haemoglobinopathies in the protection against malarial infections. These include sickle-cell disease (five haplotypes, regions of origin corresponding to Senegal, Cameroon, Benin, Central African Republic, and India), and the thalassaemias (α-thalassaemia in Africans and people of Mediterranean origin, β-thalassaemia in Southeast Asians and those of Mediterranean origin). Glucose-6-phosphate dehydrogenase deficiencies[7] (three major variant groups, affecting Africans, Sardinians and Sephardic Jews, and Chinese) might also be selected for their partial protection against malaria.

In the transmission of human immunodeficiency virus type-1 (HIV-1), the β-chemokine receptor CCR5 serves as an entry port for viruses to infect the monocytes and other lymphoid cells, including $CD4^+$ T cells. A 32-basepair deletion (*Δ32*) in the receptor's encoding gene will knockout its expression on cell surface, thereby blocking the entry of HIV-1. Individuals with two copies of *Δ32* are highly resistant to HIV-1, while heterozygote carriers will have a lower level of viraemia after infection and retarded rate of progression to AIDS and death [Ioannidis *et al.* 2001, Mulherin *et al.* 2003]. Unlike the haemoglobinopathies or glucose-6-phosphate dehydrogenase deficiencies, no apparent tradeoffs had yet been associated with *CCR5-Δ32*.

---

[7] Over four hundred mutations for glucose-6-phosphate dehydrogenase deficiency had been identified, which evolved independently but were selected for under the same environmental pressure (i.e., a process of convergence evolution). The molecular diversity of the thalassaemias may also be explained by a similar phenomenon.

Table 3. Frequency of *CCR5-Δ32* allele reported in different population groups
[Libert *et al.* 1998, Stephens *et al.* 1998, Lucotte 2002, Salem 2003]

Population groups	Allelic frequency of *CCR5-Δ32*
Mordvinian	0.163
Finnish	0.091–0.158
Icelander	0.147
Swedish	0.137–0.142
Russian	0.122–0.139
French	0.052–0.135
Estonian	0.133
Polish	0.133
Slovakian	0.133
Danish	0.083–0.123
Belgian	0.092–0.119
British	0.111–0.117
Lithuanian	0.115
Irish	0.045–0.113
German	0.106–0.108
Norwegian	0.105
Czech	0.102
Spanish	0.038–0.098
Austrian	0.089
Italian	0.021–0.087
Hungarian	0.086
Swiss	0.085
Albanian	0.082
Slovenian	0.077
Portuguese	0.052–0.064
Turkish	0.063
Bulgarian	0.045
Greek	0.042–0.044
Sardinians	0.040
Iranian	0.024
Moroccan	0.015
Syrian	0.014
Tunisian	0.010
Egyptian	0.006
Others*	0.00

* Georgian, Lebanese, Saudi, Cheyenne, Pima Indian, Pueblo Indian, Korean, Chinese

CCR5-Δ32 mutation is exceedingly uncommon in non-Europeans. A north-to-south gradient of allelic frequency is also observed among the European populations (Table 3), with the highest frequency in Northern and North-eastern Europe [Libert *et al.* 1998, Stephens *et al.* 1998, Lucotte 2002]. By inference from microsatellite estimates, the founder event from which *CCR5-Δ32* originated could be dated back to around 1,400 to 3,500 years ago [Libert *et al* 1998], and the mutation probably first appeared in North-eastern Europe. Its population frequency was then extended by random drift. During the Ninth to Thirteenth Century, the mutation was disseminated down and across Europe by the Vikings, producing its subsequent clinal pattern.

Some researchers suggested that, given the relatively recent origin of *CCR5-Δ32*, its high prevalence in some populations could not be simply attributed to random drift and gene flow, which are neutral evolutionary mechanisms, and strong selection pressures were essential to produce its rapid extension [Liberts *et al.* 1998, Stephens *et al.* 1998, Galvani and Slatkin 2003]. They speculated that even prior to the emergence of HIV, this "anti-AIDS gene" was already intensely selected for its protection against other devastating infections in history. A significant Darwinian fitness can only be assumed upon two fulfilments: 1) A plausible biological explanation for the protection is available. 2) Intensity of selection pressure is sufficient to drive *CCR5-Δ32* to a population frequency of ≈ 10 % within the given time frame.

Plague was one of the deadliest communicable diseases known to human. Two major outbreaks of pneumonic plague were recorded in European history [Cartwright and Biddiss 2004]; the Black Death pandemic (1346 – 1361) and Great Plague (1665 – 1666) claimed the lives of 25 % to 40 % and 15 % to 20 % of Europeans, respectively. In between and after these pandemics, plague was transmitted through epizootic cycles involving rodents, flea vectors and humans, causing episodic outbreaks in the bubonic form. Before being largely exterminated from Europe by the end of the Seventeenth Century, plague had been maintained within the region for over four hundred years. In addition, chemokine receptors might have a role in Yersinia-induced macrophage apoptosis. Hence, Stephens *et al.* [1998] speculated that the selection pressure imposed by plague had facilitated the extension of *CCR5-Δ32* among European populations.

Alternatively, smallpox could also exert a prominent population selection effect, which might even be more profound than plague because of its continuous rather than fluctuating influence [Galvani and Slatkin 2003]. Smallpox was first introduced to Europe before the Seventh Century [Cartwright and Biddiss 2004]. From then onwards, it persisted as a human-to-human transmitted childhood endemic disease that was associated with a high case fatality. Vaccination against smallpox was experimented on during the Eighteenth Century, but was not widely adopted until more than a hundred years later. Before its eradicated in the Mid-Twentieth Century, smallpox had been maintained in Europe for more than a thousand years, and its cumulative mortality might be much greater than that from plague. Poxviruses also exploit the human immune system through chemokine receptors [Lucotte 2002]. With a mathematical model, Galvani and Slatkin reconstructed the changes in prevalence of *CCR5-Δ32* under the selection pressure from smallpox, and demonstrated that a 10 % population frequency could already be attained within seven hundred years, which is compatible with the current epidemiological observations.

After eradication of plague and smallpox, *CCR5-Δ32* became selectively neutral until the AIDS era. With re-emergence of selection pressure, a further extension of its gene frequency and distribution may be anticipated, which might ultimately reduce the global susceptibility to AIDS. Therefore, *CCR5-Δ32* can be considered a pre-adapted trait; the mutation remained latent prior to being "activated" by the novel environmental threat of AIDS, which would be followed by an increasing population representation in future generations through natural selection.

In some African countries, over 20 % of the adult populations are infected with HIV. Although *CCR5-Δ32* has not yet extended to the Africans, they had independently evolved a distinctive mutation, *CCR2-64I,* that can also reduce the virulence of HIV infection [Gonzalez *et al*, 1999]. Similar to *CCR5-Δ32*, *CCR2-64I* can be viewed as a preadaptation. Instead of plague or smallpox, *CCR2-64I* might be selected historically for its protection against zoonotic retroviruses transmitted from simians. Schliekelman *et al.* [2001] estimated that for those who possess the protective genotype, the capacity of lifetime reproduction is increased by 15 % to 30 %. In endemic regions, this would be translated into a population selection effect comparable to heterozygote haemoglobin S against malaria.

Maladaptations from Relaxation of Selection Pressures

In almost all developed nations, complications from atherosclerosis account for the highest proportion of deaths. Hypertension and diabetes mellitus are two top-ranking, in terms of frequency of occurrence as well as importance, cardiovascular risk factors. The exact pathogenic mechanisms of hypertension and diabetes are not fully understood, but their high prevalence might suggest some underlying adaptive advantages in the ancestral environment that favoured their selection and retention. It is generally accepted that both genetic and environmental factors, as well as their interactions, have major contributory roles to the pathogenesis of hypertension or diabetes. The disease-susceptibility genotypes probably mediate a differential intensity of haemodynamic or glycaemic responsiveness to various environmental stimuli, rather than exert a direct physiological effect. Their inheritances are complex and polygenic, and not uniform across affected individuals of the same population or different populations (i.e., a process of convergence evolution, with multiple mutations all leading to a final common phenotype). Therefore, these susceptibility genotypes and their manifestations can be inherited in a "dose-dependant" manner; a lineage that accumulates a larger dose of mutations might be more predisposed to developing these conditions or exaggerated response to environmental factors.

"Genetic quirks" are defined by Nesse and Williams [1991, 1995] as genes that were of little biological detriments, or possibly some benefits, in the ancestral environment, but would cause diseases when the individual is exposed to certain environmental novelties. Our current living conditions are profoundly different from those under which human evolved. Therefore, many "modern" diseases can be accounted for by the interactions between our innate physiology and novel aspects in the environment.

African Americans have the highest prevalence of hypertension among all the ethnic groups in the United States [Saunders 1991, Douglas et al. 2003, Williams et al. 2004]. They also tend to have a poorer outcome with early target organ damages, including renal failure, cardiomyopathy, and stroke. As a result, their mortality from hypertension-related complications is three to five times that of the whites [Saunders 1991]. Hypertension in African Americans is characterised by a tendency for sodium retention and being more volume dependant [Saunders 1991, Gerber and Crews 1999], so that they may respond differently to "standard" pharmacological interventions. African Americans typically respond well to dietary salt restriction and diuretics, but are relatively resistant to β-adrenergic blockers, angiotensin-converting-enzyme inhibitors, and angiotensin receptor blockers [Douglas et al. 2003, Williams et al. 2004], which may reflect their low renin status and a predisposition to salt sensitivity.

There are postulations that the sodium retaining ability of West Africans evolved as an adaptive trait for enhancing survival in the arid inland regions of Africa [Boaz 2002]. Conservation of electrolytes and extracellular fluid volume are facilitated by a high glomerular filtration rate and an almost complete renal tubular reabsorption of the filtered sodium chloride load [Berlim and Abeche 2001]. This mechanism might have been further amplified in African Americans by the historical bottleneck of slave trade, which began in the early Sixteenth Century and lasted for more than three hundred years. During this largest migration event in human history, over twelve million West Africans were transported across the Atlantic Middle Passage in slave ships to the New World [Olson 2002]. Millions of them died on their way. Dysentery, dehydration, and heat stroke were among the most frequent causes of mortality. The slave ship environment created an intense selection pressure and bottleneck effect; those who could conserve salt and fluid better were more likely to survive [Wilson and Grim 1991], resulting in a disproportionate representation of salt sensitivity in their present day descendants.

Hypertension is exceedingly rare in cultures that are still practising a traditional lithic lifestyle, including natives living in rural West Africa. Therefore, the culprit of hypertension in African Americans is not their salt-retaining ability, but is the interaction of this inherent adaptive function with inappropriate environmental inflictions. The usual sodium intake of a Palaeolithic hunter-gatherer was estimated to be 690 mg per day [Eaton et al. 1988]. In contrast, access to salted food is unlimited under the contemporary westernised lifestyle. Sodium content of a typical American diet can be up to 7,000 mg per day, which is over ten times the amount consumed by our ancestors in the natural environment. Therefore, in the modern society and upon relaxation of selection pressure, the superior sodium-retaining ability in Africans Americans has paradoxically become a disease-driving maladaptation. Similarly, the prevalence of hypertension and related complications are escalating in many urbanizing African nations, as they are now consuming a lot more salted food.

A species' genetic composition is tailored to suit the specific environmental selection pressures under which it evolved. The existing human genome is the end result of several million years' of natural selection, and was constantly shaped by dietary as well as other lifestyle factors of our ancestors. Hominids evolved over at least four million years during the Pliocene and Pleistocene Epochs. Throughout this critical period of human evolution, our ancestors foraged on natural resources in order to survive, and hunting-gathering is considered the lifestyle for which the main bulk of our genome was selected.

The Neolithic period saw a radical transformation of our ancestors' lifestyle through domestication of plants and animals. Since then, the human habitat began to depart from the "Palaeolithically-programmed" human biology [Chakravarthy and Booth 2004]. A ten thousand year-old event, by the standards of evolution, occurred only recently. Therefore, these post-Neolithic lifestyle alterations, despite being profound, only had negligible impacts on the human genome.[8] The Industrial Revolution, followed by technological revolution in the last few decades, further accelerated this discordance. Contemporary humans are like Stone Agers being displaced to the Space Age via a fast lane [Eaton et al. 1988]. Our established genetic constituents are poorly prepared for the modern affluent lifestyle, which is changing too rapidly for our genetic adaptations to keep pace with. As a result of this mismatch, the so-called "diseases of civilization" or "afflictions of affluence", such as diabetes mellitus, obesity, complications from atherosclerosis, and malignancies from novel

---

[8] The acquisition of lactase persistence (to accommodate novel nutritional resources [Cavalli-Sforza et al. 1994]) and mutation for cystic fibrosis (heterozygous carriers may be more resistant to dehydration from infective diarrhoeas [Nesse and Williams 1995], which became prevalent after the Neolithic population expansion, although cholera or dysentery had not reached an epidemic scale in Europe until the Nineteenth Century [Cartwright and Biddiss 2004]) may be some exceptions.

environmental carcinogens, emerged as preponderant causes of mortality and morbidity in the modern world.

The concept of thrifty genotype was first proposed by Neel [1962] to illustrate the evolutionary *raison d'être* of diabetes mellitus. Thriftiness can be considered an adaptive strategy when food is scarce. In the ancestral environment, food shortage posed a major threat to human survival. Therefore, genes that facilitated the efficient intake and utilization of food and energy were favourably selected. Extraction, synthesis and retention of essential nutrients were optimised through various thrifty mechanisms. Together with a craving behaviour for these nutrients or their substrates and a tendency towards minimization of energy expenditure, survival in the natural environment could be enhanced. However, as members of the contemporary affluent societies, our built-in thriftiness might have become a redundancy or even a maladaptation. Nowadays, our lavish meals consist of highly refined, palatable foodstuffs that are fat-laden and concentrated in calories. The majority of people living in industrialized societies rarely have the need to exercise. Leisure activities are also becoming more sedentary. This discordance between our naturally selected thriftiness but unnatural modern lifestyle is considered the culprit for the global epidemic of obesity, insulin resistance, and type 2 diabetes mellitus.

Diabetes mellitus remains an uncommon condition in contemporary lithic societies [Eaton *et al.* 1988], but a rapid upsurge of disease prevalence often coincided with their acculturation to a more westernised lifestyle. It is well recognized that different ethnic groups living in industrialized societies do not exhibit the same susceptibility to diabetes mellitus [Zimmet and Thomas 2003]. Moreover, disease prevalence in natives often surpasses that of the non-indigenous settlers [Strassmann and Dunbar 1999]. The Pima Indians and aboriginal Australians are among the groups that have the highest disease prevalence [Knowler *et al.* 1990, Daniel *et al.* 1999]. Their propensities for developing diabetes mellitus is still significantly elevated as compared with Europeans after adjusted for obesity [Daniel *et al.* 1999, Zimmet and Thomas 2003]. The exact reason for this racial disparity is not fully understood. Some authors suggested that the rapid acculturation of indigenous societies provided little opportunity for them to adapt to a "diabetogenic" lifestyle [Baschetti 1998, Daniel *et al.* 1999] (i.e., a quirk phenomenon activated by abrupt withdrawal of selection pressure). Conversely, non-indigenous settlers were able to develop adaptive mechanisms against the adverse selection effects as they were historically exposed to a diabetogenic diet. However, even for the most modernized nations, the majority of their members were still living under a rudimentary socio-economic setting before the Industrial Revolution, which was less than ten generations ago. Therefore, diabetes mellitus was not a relevant cause of early mortality until recently, and any adaptive traits that protect against diabetes would not confer a significant degree of Darwinian fitness to enable them to prevail in the past.

To account for the pathogenesis of type 2 diabetes mellitus, Hales and Barker [1992] proposed a thrifty phenotype hypothesis, which may also be relevant in explaining the racial differences in disease expression. They speculated that nutritional deprivation around the time of birth would activate the thrifty phenotype, which predisposes an individual to a higher risk of type 2 diabetes mellitus later in life. In countries settled by westerners, a high percentage of indigenous populations are from a socially disadvantageous background, as they are often marginalized as ethnic minorities. Under-nutrition in infancy is a common problem and, according to the thrifty phenotype hypothesis, would switch on their thriftiness. In other words, the variable prevalence of diabetes mellitus across different ethnic groups may be attributed to a biological effect secondary to social inequalities, rather than a genuine racial genetic difference.

Pharmacogenetic Polymorphisms

Clinicians practising in multiethnic communities will realise that patients from different population groups may not have the same response or side-effect profile to standard drug regimens. Moreover, physicians working in non-western countries may also find the drug dosages required by many of their patients are different from those quoted in textbooks, formularies, and even the insert recommendations. A number of trials had specifically explored the relationship between race and effects of pharmacological agents [Zhou et al. 1989, Yancy et al. 2001], although most of these studies only applied empirical racial categories (i.e., without genetic verification).

Besides dietary factors and personal habits, such as smoking and alcohol, which may affect the pharmacokinetic properties of drugs or compromise their therapeutic benefits indirectly, differential drug responses across population groups are frequently attributed to genetic variations of drug metabolising enzymes. Mutations involving the drug metabolising system are common. They are associated with altered pharmacokinetics to various agents, leading to loss of efficacy or unexpected adverse effects in the carriers. Distributions of such polymorphisms are different across the various populations, with some mutations or poor metaboliser phenotypes being more common in certain groups (Table 4). However, it must be stressed that none of the mutations, or the resulting traits, is exclusive for a particular race, and the presence of deviated drug metabolising status is not uniform across all individuals of the same group. In other words, the correlation between race and drug metabolising status is not absolute; some populations contain a bigger proportion of poor metabolisers with certain pharmacological agents than the other groups, so that their members will have a higher probability of developing altered drug responses when given these agents.

The cytochrome P450 (CYP) isoenzymes constitute the largest system for metabolising drugs in human. Within the CYP families, approximately 40 % of the enzymes utilized for this purpose exist in polymorphic forms [Xie et al. 2001]. The P450 genes that encode for these enzymes can be traced back to an ancient prokaryocytic origin. Subsequently, a whole range of CYP isoenzymes emerged from gene duplications. They then diversified and were selected and retained for their abilities to detoxify various biological toxins in the natural environment. Most of them were plant-based toxins, which evolved as a defence against over-consumption by animals, and there might be considerable geographical heterogeneities in both their characters and intensities. As a result, the selection of CYP detoxification system (or polymorphisms) in various animal species, including our ancestors, would be driven by the regional pattern of plant-based toxins. This explains the asymmetrical distribution of pharmacogenetic polymorphisms among the human populations, as many of the commonly used medications still bear some structural similarities with plant-based proteins. Besides, some CYP variants might be responsible for antagonising certain unknown environmental toxins that were historical or no longer existed in the human habitat (i.e., isoenzymes which turned selectively neutral). Their subsequent spread could be mediated through gene flow, resulting in the clinal gradients of polymorphisms observed across neighbouring populations. In addition, CYP enzymes can be protective against some environmental carcinogens and possibly xenobiotics, which may be important in the pathogenesis of neurodegenerative disorders. Nevertheless, their exact roles in disease-protection need to be verified by further experimental or observational data, including those collected from different populations.

Table 4. The proportions of poor metablisers of some drug-metabolising enzymes in different population groups (clinically relevant substrates or medications are in brackets) [Meyer 1999, Wood 2001, Xie *et al.* 2001]

Drug-metabolising enzyme	Percentage of poor metabolizer		
	Blacks	Caucasians	East Asians
CYP2D6	0 – 19 %	5 – 10 %	1 – 2 %
(Antiarrhythmics, antidepressants, neuroleptics, opioids, amphetamines, β-blockers)			
CYP2C9	1 – 3 %	8 – 14 %	1 – 2 %
(Anticoagulants, oral hypoglycaemic agents, non-steroidal anti-inflammatory drugs, phenytoin, losartan, fluvastatin)			
CYPC19	4 %	2.5 – 6 %	14 – 23 %
(Benzodiazepines, barbiturates, phenytoin, tricyclic antidepressants, proton-pump inhibitors, proguanil)			
NAT2	40 – 70%		10 – 30 %
(Sulphonamides, isoniazid, dapsone, caffeine)			

Other than drug metabolising enzymes, polymorphisms in drug transporters and receptors can also give rise to differential therapeutic responses [Meyer 1999, Xie *et al.* 2001].

Most drugs were developed in the western countries. Before international multicentre studies have become popular, therapeutic regimens were usually based on data obtained from just one or two ethnic populations. In a typical drug trial conducted in the United States, the majority of subjects recruited are Caucasians, with a smaller number of African Americans, and a negligible proportion of members from other ethnicities. The results, which mainly represent findings in Caucasians, and recommendations derived are then extrapolated to all population groups without taking into account the racial distribution of pharmacogenetic polymorphisms. Therefore, their applicability may be limited in non-western populations.

Conversely, race or ethnicity is not a reliable proxy for guiding the choice of drugs or treatments, as inter-individual variations within a group can be substantial and must be taken into consideration. Clinical practice should be informed by the available evidence obtained from well-designed trials and understanding of disease mechanisms, rather than a patient's race. Moreover, racial profiling, which is usually based on biased perceptions, cannot replace the comprehensive evaluation of each patient regardless of racial or ethnic backgrounds and tailoring of drug regimens according to individual response. Over-reliance on empirical racial categories runs the risk of fuelling inequities in medical care; members from minority groups may be deprived from receiving the appropriate treatment because of some poorly justified stigmatisations. Moreover, inadequate response after treatment might be erroneously attributed to a patient's "race" instead of failure of clinical judgement.

CONCLUSION

Evolutionary Medicine, or Darwinian Medicine, is a rapidly emerging discipline. Besides medical scientists, clinicians from all specialties will find Darwinian theories relevant and attractive in many areas of their fields. Incorporating the scientific concepts of evolution when interpreting health and diseases will provide new insights into the pathogenesis and epidemiology of many common disorders. Darwinian theories also have a lot of potential applications in preventive medicine, health promotion for the general public, and helping patients to come to terms with their illnesses.

The notion that race is a scientific concept speaks of nothing but an ingrained fallacy. There is no clear-cut or quantifiable definition of what "race" is; classification by external physical characteristics, self-reported ancestry, and even phylogeographical markers cannot provide a satisfactory solution. However, the habitual division of people into mutually exclusive racial or ethnic subpopulations often convey an impression that they carry with them inherent genetic differences that are relevant to health and diseases, which is often misleading. Nevertheless, in public health, biomedical research, as well as clinical practice, racial taxonomies are frequently used for making inferences on an individual's underlying genetic or biological makeup. Unexplained disparities in disease expressions or treatment responses across racial and ethnic groups are almost always loosely attributed to "genetic influences", especially when there is no supporting genetic data.[9]

The assumption that race or ethnicity is an independent clinical variable should be interpreted with caution. When managing an individual patient, other than a handful of hereditary conditions, knowledge on the patient's ancestral background is usually not of major clinical importance. On the contrary, clinicians are often biased by their perceptions or stigmatisations regarding the racial predisposition to certain diseases, which are often unjustifiable at the level of an individual patient. As a result, diagnosis and choice of management may be misguided, thereby undermining the medical care received by some ethnic populations.

Conversely, at the macro-level, certain health-related problems are recognized to be associated with membership of predefined groups, and the correlation can be cultural, social, environmental, geographical, but not necessarily genetic. Group membership actually reflects non-genetic predispositions to diseases much more often than genetic predispositions. Therefore, although race or ethnicity cannot be employed as a surrogate for an individual's genetic biology, it may provide practical clues regarding other "indirect" factors that are relevant in driving the racial disparities in health and diseases, such as socio-economic deprivation, deficient education, and unhealthy lifestyle. These indicators are important when designing screening or health-education programmes and public policies.

---

[9]   Such practice is termed "black box epidemiology" by Fustinoni and Biller [2000].

REFERENCES

Bamshad M.J., Wooding S., Watkins W.S., Ostler C.T., Batzer M.A., Jorde L.B. Human population genetic structure and inference of group membership. *Am J Hum Genet* 2003;72:578-589.

Baschetti R. Diabetes epidemic in newly westernised populations: is it due to thrifty genes or to genetically unknown foods? *J R Soc Med* 1998;91:622-625.

Basu A., Mukherjee N., Roy S., *et al.* Ethnic India: a genomic view, with special reference to peopling and structure. *Genome Res* 2003;13:2277-2290.

Berlim M.T., Abeche A.M. Evolutionary approach to medicine. *South Med J* 2001;94:26-32.

Bertoni B., Budowle B., Sans M., Barton S.A., Chakraborty R. Admixture in Hispanics: distribution of ancestral population contributions in the Continental United States. *Hum Biol* 2003;75:1-11.

Biraben J.N. Essai sur l'évolution du nombre des homes. *Population* 1979;1:13-25.

Boaz N. *Evolving Health. The Origins of Illness and How the Modern World is Making Us Sick.* New York: John Wiley and Sons, Inc.; 2002.

Bowcock A.M., Kidd J.R., Mountain J.L., *et al.* Drift, admixture, and selection in human evolution: a study with DNA polymorphisms. *Proc Natl Acad Sci USA* 1991;88:839-843.

Bowcock A.M., Ruiz-Linares A., Tomfohrde J., Minch E., Kidd J.R., Cavalli-Sforza L.L. High resolution of human evolutionary tress with polymorphic microsatellites. *Nature* 1994;368:455-457.

Britt R.P., Harper C., Spray G.H. Megaloblastic anaemia among Indians in Britain. *Q J Med* 1971;160:499-520.

Broderick J.P., Adams H.P., Barson W., *et al.* Guidelines for the management of spontaneous intracerebral hemorrhage. A statement for healthcare professionals from a special writing group of the Stroke Council, American Heart Association. *Stroke* 1999;30:905-915.

Burchard E.G., Ziv E., Coyle N., *et al.* The importance of race and ethnic background in biomedical research and clinical practice. *N Eng J Med* 2003;348:1170-1175.

Cann R.L., Stoneking M., Wilson A.C. Mitochondrial DNA and human evolution. *Nature* 1987;325:31-36.

Caplan L.R., Gorelick P.B., Hier D.B. Race, sex and occlusive cerebrovascular disease: A review. *Stroke* 1986;17:648-655.

Carrol S.B. Genetics and the making of *Homo sapiens*. *Nature* 2003;422:849-857.

Cartwright F.F., Biddiss M. *Disease and History*. London: Sutton Publishing; 2004.

Cavalli-Sforza L.L., Menozzi P., Piazza A. *The History and Geography of Human Genes.* Princeton: Princeton University Press; 1994.

Chakravarthy M.V., Booth F.W. Eating, exercise, and "thrifty" genotypes: connecting the dots toward an evolutionary understanding of modern chronic diseases. *J Appl Physiol* 2004;96:3-10.

Cheung R.T.F., Mak W., Chan K.H. Circadian variation of stroke onset in Hong Kong Chinese: A hospital-based study. *Cerebrovascular Diseases* 2001;12:1-6.

Cooper R.S., Kaufman J.S., Ward R. Race and genomics. *N Eng J Med* 2003;348:1166-1170.

Daniel M., Rowley K.G., McDermott R., Mylvaganam A., O'Dea K. Diabetes incidence in an Australian aboriginal population. *Diabetes Care* 1999;22:1993-1998.

Dean M., Stephens J.C., Winkler C., *et al.* Polymorphic admixture typing in human ethnic populations. *Am J Hum Genet* 1994;55:788-808.

Diamond J. *The Third Chimpanzee. The evolution and Future of the Human Animal.* New York: HarperCollins Publishers; 1992.

Douglas J.G., Bakris G.L., Epstein M., *et al.* Management of high blodd pressire in African Americans. Consensus statement of the Hypertension in African Americans Working Group of the International Society on Hypertension in Blacks. *Arch Intern Med* 2003;163:525-541.

Downs J.R., Clearfield M., Weis S., *et al.* Primary prevention of acute coronary events with lovastatin in men and women with average cholesterol levels: results of AFCAPS/TexCAPS. Air Force/Texas Coronary Atherosclerosis Prevention Study. *JAMA* 1998;279:1615-22.

Dyker A.G., Weir C.J., Lees K.R. Influence of cholesterol on survival after stroke: retrospective study. *BMJ* 1997;314:1584-8.

Eastern Stroke and Coronary Heart Disease Collaborative Research Group. Blood pressure, cholesterol, and stroke in eastern Asia. *Lancet* 1998;352:1801-1807.

Eaton S.B., Konner M., Shostak M. Stone Agers in the fast lane: chronic degenerative diseases in evolutionary perspective. *Am J Med* 1988;84:739-749.

Fong P.C., Tam S.C., Tai Y.T., Lau C.P., Lee J., Sha Y.Y. Serum lipid and apolipoprotein distributions in Hong Kong Chinese. *J Epidemiol Community Health* 1994;48:355-359.

Fustinoni O., Biller J. Ethnicity and stroke. Beware of the fallacies. *Stroke* 2000;31:1013-1015.

Gajdusek D.C., Zigas V. Degenerative disease of the central nervous system in New Guinea; the endemic occurrence of kuru in the native population. *N Eng J Med* 1957;257:974-978.

Galvani A.P., Slatkin M. Evaluating plague and smallpox as historical selective pressure for *CCR-Δ32* HIV resistance allele. *Proc Natl Acad Sci USA* 2003;100:15276-15279.

Gamble C. *The Palaeolithic Societies of Europe.* Cambridge: Cambridge University Press; 1999.

Gerber L.M., Crews D.E. Evolutionary perspectives on chronic degenerative diseases. In: Trevathan W.R., editor. *Evolutionary Medicine.* New York: Oxford University Press; 1999; 443-470.

Gonzalez E., Bamshad M., Sato N., *et al.* Race-specific HIV-1 disease-modifying effects associated with *CCR5* haplotypes. *Proc Natl Acad Sci USA* 1999;96:12004-12009.

Gupta A.K., Damji A., Uppaluri A. Vitamin B12 deficiency. Prevalence among South Asians at a Toronto clinic. *Can Fam Physician* 2004;50:743-747.

Hales C.N., Barker D.J. Type 2 (non-insulin-dependent) diabetes mellitus: the thrifty phenotype hypothesis. *Diabetologia* 1992;35:595-601.

Huang C.Y., Chan F.L., Yu Y.L., Woo E., Chin D. Cerebrovascuolar disease in Hong Kong Chinese. *Stroke* 1990;21:230-235.

Ingman M., Kaessmann H., Pääbo S., Gyllensten U. Mitochondrial genome variation and the origin of modern humans. *Nature* 2000;408:708-713.

Ioannidis J.P.A., Rosenberg P.S., Goedert J.J., *et al*, for the International Meta-Analysis of HIV Host Genetics. Effects of *CCR-Δ32*, *CCR2-641*, and *SDF-1 3'A* alleles on HIV-1 disease progression: an international meta-analysis of individual-patient data. *Ann Intern Med* 2001;135:782-795.

Iribarren C., Jacobs D.R., Sadler M., Claxton A.J., Sidney S. Low total serum cholesterol and intra-cerebral hemorrhagic stroke: is the association confined to elderly men? The Kaiser Permanente Medical Care Program. *Stroke* 1996;27:1993-8.

Iso H., Jacobs D.R., Wentworth D., Neaton J.D., Cohen J.D. Serum cholesterol levels and six-year mortality from stroke in 350,977 men screened for the Multiple Risk Factor Intervention Trial. *N Eng J Med* 1989;320:904-10.

Iso H., Stampfer M.J., Manson J.E., *et al*. Prospective study of fat and protein intake and risk of intra-parenchymal hemorrhage in women. *Circulation* 2001;103:856-863.

Kagan A., Popper J.S., Rhoads G.G., Yano K. Dietary and other risk factors for stroke in Hawaiian Japanese men. *Stroke* 1985;16:390-396.

Kay R., Woo J., Kreel L., Wong H.Y., Teoh R., Nicholas M.G. Stroke subtypes among Chinese living in Hong Kong: The Shatin Stroke Registry. *Neurology* 1992;42:985-987.

Klawans H. *Strange Behavior. Tales of Evolutionary Neurology.* New York: W.W. Norton and Company; 2000.

Knowler W.C., Pettitt D.J., Saad M.F., Bennett P.H. Diabetes mellitus in the Pima Indians: incidence, risk factors and pathogenesis. *Diab Metab Rev* 1990;6:1-27.

Krings M., Stone A., Schmitz R.W., Krainitzki H., Stoneking M., Pääbo S. Neandertal DNA sequences and the origin of modern humans. *Cell* 1997;90:19-30.

Libert F., Cochaux P., Beckman G., *et al*. The Δccr5 mutation conferring protection against HIV-1 in Caucasian populations has a single and recent origin in Northeastern Europe. *Hum Mol Genet* 1998;7:399-406.

Lucotte G. Frequencies of 32 base pair deletion of the (*Δ32*) allele of the *CCR5* HIV-1 co-receptor gene in Caucasians: a comparative analysis. *Infect Genet Evol* 2002;1:201-205.

Mayr E. *Animal Species and Evolution.* Cambridge, Mass.: Belknap Press of Harvard University Press; 1963.

Mayr E. *Selected Essays: Evolution and the Diversity of Life.* Cambridge, Mass.: Belknap Press of Harvard University Press; 1976.

Menotti A., Keys A., Blackburn H., *et al*. Twenty-year stroke mortality and prediction in twelve cohorts of the Seven Country Study. *Int J Epidemiol* 1990;19:309-315.

Menotti A., Keys A., Kromhout D., *et al*. Inter-cohort differences in coronary heart disease mortality in the 25-year follow-up of the seven countries study. *Eur J Epidemiol* 1993;9:527-536.

Meyer U.A. Medically relevant genetic variation of drug effects. In: Stearns S.C., editor. *Evolution in Health and Disease.* Oxford: Oxford University Press; 1999; 41-49.

Mithen S. The Mesolithic Age. In: Cunliffe B. (ed). *The Oxford Illustrated History of Prehistoric Europe.* Oxford: Oxford University Press; 1994; 79-135.

Motulsky A.G. Jewish diseases and origin. *Nat Genet* 1995;9:99-101.

Mountain J.L., Cavalli-Sforaza L.L. Multilocus genotypes, a tree of individuals, and human evolutionary history. *Am J Hum Genet* 1997;61:705-718.

Mulherin S.A., O'Brien T.R., Ioannidis J.P.A., *et al*., for the International Meta-Analysis of HIV Host Genetics. Effects of *CCR-Δ32* and *CCR2-64I* alleles on HIV-1 disease progression: the protection varies with duration of infection. *AIDS* 2003;17:377-387.

Multiple Risk Factor Intervention Trial Research Group. Multiple Risk Factor Intervention Trial. Risk factor changes and mortality results. *JAMA* 1982;248:1465-77.

Nakayama T., Date C., Yokoyama T., Yoshiike N., Yamaguchi M., Tanaka H. A 15.5-year follow-up study of stroke in a Japanese provincial city. The Shibata Study. *Stroke* 1997;28:45-52.

Neaton J.D., Blackburn H., Jacobs D., *et al*. Serum cholesterol level and mortality findings for men screened in the Multiple Risk Factor Intervention Trial. *Arch Intern Med* 1992;152:1490-500.

Neel J.V. Diabetes Mellitus: A "thrifty" genotype rendered detrimental by "progress"? *Am J Hum Genet* 1962;14:353-362.

Nesse R.M., Williams G.C. *Why We Get Sick: The New Science of Darwinian Medicine*. New York: Times Books; 1995.

Olson S. *Mapping Human History. Genes, Race, and our Common Origins*. Boston: Mariner Books; 2002.

Richards M., Côrte-Real H, Forster P., *et al*. Paleolithic and Neolithic lineages in the European mitochondrial gene pool. *Am J Hum Genet* 1996;59:185-203.

Richards M., Macaulay V.A., Bandelt H.J., Sykes B.C. Phylogeography of mitochondrial DNA in western Europe. *Ann Hum Genet* 1998;62:241-260.

Richards M., Macaulay V., Hickey E., *et al*. Tracing European founder lineages in the Near Eastern mtDNA Pool. *Am J Hum Genet* 2000;67:1251-1276.

Roquer J., Rodríguez Campello A., Gomis M., Ois A., Munteis E., Böhm P. Serum lipid levels and in-hospital mortality in patients with intracerebral hemorrhage. *Neurology* 2005;65:1198-1202.

Rosenberg N.A., Pritchard J.K., Weber J.L., *et al*. Genetic structure of human populations. *Science* 2002;298:2381-2385.

Rosenberg N.A., Li L.M., Ward R., Pritchard J.K. Informativeness of genetic markers for inference of ancestry. *Am J Hum Genet* 2003;73:1402-1422.

Rubinstein W.S. Hereditary breast cancer in Jews. *Fam Cancer* 2004;3:249-257.

Salem A.H. Distribution of HIV resistance CCR-Δ32 allele among Egyptians. *Suez Canal Univ Med J* 2003;6:61-69.

Saunders E. Hypertension in African-Americans. In: Cardiovascular diseases and stroke in African-Americans and other racial minorities in the United States. A statement for health professionals. *Circulation* 1991;83:1462-1480.

Sauvaget C., Nagano J., Allen N., Grant E.J., Beral V. Intake of animal products and stroke mortality in the Hiroshima/Nagasaki Life Span Study. *Int J Epidemiol* 2003;32:536-543.

Sauvaget C., Nagano J., Hayashi M., Yamada M. Animal protein, animal fat, and cholesterol intakes and risk of cerebral infarction mortality in the Adult Health Study. *Stroke* 2004;35:1531-1537.

Schliekelman P., Garner C., Slatkin M. Natural selection and resistance to HIV. A genotype that lowers susceptibility to HIV extends survival at a time of peak fertility. *Nature* 2001;411:545-546.

Segal A.Z., Chiu R.I., Eggleston-Sexton P.M., Beiser A., Greenberg S.M. Low cholesterol as a risk factor for primary intracerebral hemorrhage: A case-control study. *Neuroepidemiology* 1999;18:185-193.

Semino O., Passarino G., Oefner P.J., *et al*. The genetic legacy of Paleolithic *Homo sapiens sapiens* in extant Europeans: a Y chromosome perspective. *Science* 2000;290:1155-1159.

Shah M.V., Biller J. Medical and surgical management of intracerebral hemorrhage. *Semin Neurol* 1998;18:513-519.

Shen P., Lavi T., Kivisild T., *et al.* Reconstruction of patrilineages and matrilineages of Samaritans and other Israeli populations from Y-chromosome and mitochondrial DNA sequence variation. *Hum Mutat* 2004;24:248-260.

Shimamoto T., Komachi Y., Inada H., *et al.* Trends for coronary heart disease and stroke and their risk factors in Japan. *Circulation* 1989;79:503-515.

Solomon T., Ni H., Beasley D.W.C., Ekkelenkamp M., Cardosa M.J., Barrett A.D.T. Origin and evolution of Japanese encephalitis virus in Southeast Asia. *J Virol* 2003;77:3091-3098.

Solomon T. Flavivirus encephalitis. *N Eng J Med* 2004;351:370-380.

Stearns S.C. Introducing evolutionary thinking. In: Stearns S.C., editor. *Evolution in Health and Disease.* Oxford: Oxford University Press; 1999; 3-15.

Stephens J.B., Reich D.E., Goldstein D.B., *et al.* Dating the origin of the *CCR- Δ32* AIDS-resistance allele by the coalescence of haplotypes. *Am J Hum Genet* 1998;62:1507-1515.

Strassmann B.I., Dunbar R.I.M. Human evolution and disease: putting the Stone Age in perspective. In: Stearns S.C., editor. *Evolution in Health and Disease.* Oxford: Oxford University Press; 1999; 91-101.

Takeya Y., Popper J.S., Shimizu Y., *et al.* Epidemiologic studies of coronary heart disease and stroke in Japanese men living in Japan, Hawaii and California: Incidence of stroke in Japan and Hawaii. *Stroke* 1984;15:15-23.

Tanaka H., Tanaka Y, Hiayashi M, *et al.* Secular trends of mortality for cerebrovascular diseases in Japan, 1960 to 1979. *Stroke* 1982;13:574-581.

Tattersall I., Schwartz J. *Extinct Humans.* Boulder: Westview Press; 2001.

The National Institute of Neurological Disorders and Stroke rt-PA Stroke Study Group. Tissue plasminogen activator for acute ischemic stroke. *N Eng J Med* 1995;333:1581-1587.

Underhill P.A., Shen P., Lin A.A., *et al.* Y chromosome sequence variation and the history of human populations. *Nat Genet* 2000;26:358-361.

Underhill P.A., Passarino G., Lin A.A., *et al.* The phylogeography of Y chromosome binary haplotypes and the origins of modern human populations. *Ann Hum Genet* 2001;65:43-62.

Veith I. *The Yellow Emperor's Classic of Internal Medicine.* Berkeley and Los Angeles: University of California Press; 2002.

Vigilant L., Stoneking M., Harpending H., Hawkes K., Wilson A.C. African populations and the evolution of human mitochondrial DNA. *Science* 1991;253:1503-1507.

Weaver S.C., Barrett A.D.T. Transmission cycles, host range, evolution and emergence of arboviral disease. *Nat Rev Microbiol* 2004;2:789-801.

Wen B., Li H., Lu D., *et al.* Genetic evidence supports demic diffusion of Han culture. *Nature* 2004;431:302-305.

Williams G.C., Nesse R.M. The dawn of Darwinian medicine. *Q Rev Biol* 1991;66:1-22.

Williams B., Poulter N.R., Brown M.J., *et al.* British Hypertension Society guidelines. Guidelines for management of hypertension: report of the fourth working party of the British Hypertension Society, 2004 – BHS IV. *J Hum Hypertens* 2004;18:139-185.

Wilson T.W., Grim C.E. Biohistory of slavery and blood pressure differences in blacks today: a hypothesis. *Hypertension* 1991;17(Suppl I):I122-128.

Wood A.J.J. Racial differences in the response to drugs – pointers to genetic differences. *N Eng J Med* 2001;344:1393-1396.

Xie H.G., Kim R.B., Wood A.J.J., Stein C.M. Molecular basis of ethnic differences in drug disposition and response. *Ann Rev Pharmacol Toxicol* 2001;41:815-850.

Yancy C.W., Fowler M.B., Colucci W.S., *et al*. Race and the response to adrenergic blockade with carvedilol in patients with chronic heart failure. *N Eng J Med* 2001;344:1358-1365.

Yano K., Reed D.M., MacLean C.J.. Serum cholesterol and hemorrhagic stroke in the Honolulu Heart Study. *Stroke* 1989;20:1460-1465.

Yatsu F.M. Stroke in Asians and Pacific-Islanders, Hispanics, and Native Americans. In: Cardiovascular diseases and stroke in African-Americans and other racial minorities in the United States. A statement for health professionals. *Circulation* 1991;83:1462-1480.

Yu T.S.I., Tse L.A., Wong T.W., Wong S.I. Recent trends of stroke mortality in Hong Kong: age, period, cohort analyses and the implications. *Neuroepidemiology* 2000;19:265-274.

Zhou H.H., Richard P.K., Silnerstein D.J., Wilkinson G.R., Wood A.J.J. Racial differences in drug response. Altered sensitivity to and clearance of propranolol in men of Chinese descent as compared with American whites. *N Engl J Med* 1989;320:565-570.

Zimmet P., Thomas C.R. Genotype, obesity and cardiovascular disease – has technical and social advancement outstripped evolution? *J Intern Med* 2003;254:114-125.

In: Racial and Ethnic Disparities in Health and Health Care   ISBN 1-60021-268-9
Editor: Elene V. Metrosa, pp. 101-130   © 2006 Nova Science Publishers, Inc.

Chapter 5

RACIAL DIFFERENCES IN DEVELOPMENTAL RISK AND PROTECTIVE FACTORS FOR CIGARETTE SMOKING

*Helene Raskin White**
Center of Alcohol Studies, Rutgers University, New Jersey, United States
Lisa Metzger
School of Social Work, University of Washington, Washington, United States
Magda Stouthamer-Loeber
Western Psychiatric Institute and Clinic, University of Pittsburgh,
Pennsylvania, United States
Nancy Violette
Center of Alcohol Studies, Rutgers University, New Jersey, United States
Daniel Nagin
H. J. Heinz III School of Public Policy and Management, Carnegie Mellon University,
Pennsylvania, United States

ABSTRACT

The purpose of this study was to examine racial differences in the risk and protective factors for the initiation and maintenance of cigarette smoking during varying developmental periods from childhood through late adolescence. We used data from a sample of 503 males who were first recruited in the first grade and followed annually for 14 years. Trajectory analyses identified three trajectory groups for African Americans and whites: nonsmokers, light smokers, and regular smokers. The following domains of risk and protective factors were included in the analyses: individual [hyperactivity/impulsivity/attention problem (HIA), depression, attitudes toward substance use, school performance, delinquency frequency, and religiosity], family

---

* Correspondence to: Helene Raskin White, Rutgers Center of Alcohol Studies, 607 Allison Road, Piscataway, New Jersey, 08854-8001; hewhite@rci.rutgers.edu

(parental smoking and relationship with parents), peer (peer delinquency), and environmental [socioeconomic status (SES) and neighborhood quality]. First analyses were conducted separately by race to determine which factors represented risk and which represented protection. Then hierarchical logistic regression analyses were conducted to determine how these factors differentiated among the three trajectory groups and whether race interacted with these factors. Many of the variables were both risk and protective factors across different developmental periods. School performance and religiosity were only significantly related to smoking for African Americans and SES was only related for whites. For both races HIA, depression, delinquency, and peer delinquency were significantly related to smoking. In the multivariate analyses, race, SES, and delinquency were related to smoking at younger ages and delinquent peers was related to smoking at all ages. Only four interactions with race were significant for smoking. Good school performance was protective for African Americans at ages 7-9, but not whites. Having many delinquent peers was a stronger risk factor for African Americans at ages 13-16, but having many at ages 17-19 was a risk factor only for whites. Being low in delinquency was a stronger protective factor for whites at ages 13-16. Depression was related to regular smoking only for African Americans and attitudes toward substance use, parental smoking, and neighborhood quality were related only for whites. For both races HIA, school performance, delinquency, and peer delinquency were related to regular smoking. In the multivariate analyses, being African American protected against regular smoking at all ages. Only one interaction was significant; low depression was a protective factor for African American but not white regular smoking. Overall, the fact that there were few significant interactions of risk and protective factors with race suggests that the same factors can be targeted for both whites and African Americans in cigarette prevention programs.

Key Words: race, African Americans, cigarettes, smoking, risk factors, protective factors

INTRODUCTION

Smoking initiation and maintenance are serious public health concerns. In fact, smoking is the number one preventable cause of death in developed countries (Baker, Brandon, and Chassin, 2004). Despite the known health risks, large proportions of young people establish regular smoking habits (Johnston, O'Malley, and Bachman, 2003). Although there have been declines in smoking among adolescents since the mid-1990s, the rate of decline has been decelerating during the past several years. Data from the 2005 Monitoring the Future Study indicate that 50% of high school seniors had tried cigarette smoking, 23% had smoked within the last 30 days, and 14% had smoked daily (www.monitoringthefuture.org).

Racial differences in developmental patterns of cigarette smoking have been identified in numerous studies. Whites compared to African Americans begin smoking earlier and reach higher levels of use into their mid 20s (Griesler and Kandel, 1998; Williams and Covington, 1997). Racial differences in adolescent smoking hold across community and school samples even when bioassays are used to validate self report (Baker et al., 2004). At some point during early adulthood the prevalence of smoking for African Americans increases dramatically (Kandel, Chen, Warner, Kessler, and Grant, 1997; US Department of Health and Human Services, 1998; Williams and Covington, 1997). In fact, recent data indicate that current smoking prevalence rates are similar for white (24%) and African American (22%) adults (National Center for Chronic Disease Prevention and Health Promotion, 2004). White,

Nagin, Repologle, and Stouthamer-Loeber (2004) examined racial differences in developmental trajectories of smoking from late childhood into young adulthood. They identified the same three trajectory groups for African Americans and whites: nonsmokers, light smokers, and regular smokers. For each group, the African American and white trajectories followed similar shapes over time, but for the two smoker groups (light and regular), white trajectory levels were higher than African-American levels. That is, white regular smokers smoked more cigarettes per day than African American regular smokers at each assessment and the same was true for light smokers. In addition, there were differences in the timing and rapidity of development of for regular smokers with whites starting earlier and increasing more rapidly (see below).

Given that the development and patterns of smoking vary by race, it would be expected that the precursors of smoking would also vary by race and, in fact, some studies have found different predictors of smoking for whites and African Americans (e.g., Flint, Yamanda, and Novotny, 1998; Landrine, Richardson, Klonoff, and Flay, 1994; Robinson, Klesges, Zbikowski, and Glaser, 1997). However, other studies have found that similar variables predict smoking for both African Americans and whites (e.g., Gritz, Prokhorov, Hudmon, Chamberlain, Taylor, DiClemente et al., 1998; Kandel, Kiros, Schaffran, and Mei-Chen, 2004). Furthermore, it is possible that risk factors vary at different ages, although few studies have examined this possibility in a single sample. Thus, more research is needed to delineate the common and unique risk and protective factors for transitional stages in smoking behavior in order to develop racially appropriate prevention programs (Flint et al, 1998; Gritz et al., 1998; Gottfredson and Koper, 1996; Landrine et al. 1994). Studying these differences at different age periods can help inform the development of more effective prevention programs, which target adolescents when they are most vulnerable to specific risks. This study examines both risk and protective factors for the initiation of smoking and regular smoking among African Americans and whites at various developmental periods from childhood through late adolescence.

RISK AND PROTECTIVE FACTORS

Over the last few decades, studies of protective (or promotive) and risk (or vulnerability) factors have used alternative conceptualizations to define positive and negative predictors of problem and adaptive behaviors (for a review, see Stouthamer-Loeber, Wei, Loeber, and Masten, 2004). Some researchers view risk and protective factors as opposite ends of a continuum. Others conceptualize protective factors as moderators that buffer the effects of risk factors or as factors that reduce the likelihood that risk factors will occur (Schulenberg and Maggs, 2002, p. 57). In many cases it is not clear whether negative conditions should be viewed as risk factors or whether the absence of such conditions should be viewed as protective factors. Stouthamer-Loeber and colleagues (Stouthamer-Loeber, Loeber, Farrington, Zhang, van Kammen, and Maguin, 1993; Stouthamer-Loeber, Loeber, Wei, Farrington, and Wilkstrom, 2002) have argued that the positive and negative ends of protective/risk factors may have differential significance for varying dependent variables. In other words, they argue that there may be a nonlinear association between protective/risk ends of variables and subsequent outcomes. Furthermore, the positive or negative end of a variable may have differential effects during different developmental periods. In this paper, we examine both the positive and negative end of factors presumed to influence cigarette smoking among youth. We use the term protective factor to refer to the positive end and the term risk factor to refer to the negative end. We examine whether risk and protective factors differ by race across different developmental periods from childhood to late adolescence. We do not, however, examine racial differences in the magnitude of risk and protection (see Wallace and Muroff, 2002).

Current theories of substance use emphasize multiple risk and protective factors across several domains including individual factors and social contexts (Schulenberg, Wadsworth, O'Malley, Bachman, and Johnston, 1996). Multiple factors affect smoking, and their relative impacts vary across the developmental phases of smoking (Baker et al., 2004). In a recent review, Mayhew, Flay, and Mott (2000) identified numerous risk factors, including male gender, white race, positive attitudes and belief about smoking, concerns with body weight, affect regulation, perception of smoking as a relaxation tool, perceptions of cigarette accessibility, number of cigarette offers, intentions to smoke in the future, other drug use, minimization of smoking risks, tolerance for deviance, anti-social behaviors, low academic expectations, less educational achievement, lower expectations for school achievement, and working part time, tobacco use among parents and siblings, parental approval of smoking, adolescent perception of parents' permissiveness toward smoking, parental involvement, and having friends who smoke (for an additional review, see also Baker et al., 2004). After reviewing the literature, Mayhew et al. (2000) and Baker et al. (2004) both concluded that there were more common than unique predictors of smoking among African Americans and whites.

On the other hand, Gardiner (2001) suggested that there were factors related to smoking that were unique for African Americans. He enumerated several protective factors for African Americans that may account for their lower rates of cigarette smoking, including: 1) the cost of cigarettes, 2) sports participation, 3) body-type preferences (i.e., African Americans are less likely to smoke for weight loss); 4) peer and parental smoking status (i.e., having fewer peers and parents who smoke), 5) marijuana use (which often takes the place of tobacco as a gateway drug), and 6) ethical and religious concerns. He also noted several factors that may increase risk for cigarette smoking among African Americans, including: 1) tobacco industry marketing directly to African American teens and sponsorship of African American events, 2) adoption of smoking by segments of the hip-hop culture, 3) greater access to tobacco, and 4) racial discrimination and poverty.

We have selected a set of risk and protective factors across multiple domains, which have been demonstrated to influence the initiation and / or the maintenance of cigarette smoking for whites, African Americans, or both and were available within our data set (Baker et al., 2004; Mayhew et al., 2004). The risk and protective factors that we selected come from four domains: 1) individual (hyperactivity/impulsivity/attention problems, depression, attitudes toward substance use, school performance, delinquency frequency, and religiosity), 2) family (parental smoking and relationship with parents), 3) peer (peer delinquency), and 4) environmental (SES and neighborhood quality). Below, we briefly summarize the literature that supports our choice of these factors and whether racial differences have previously been found.

Negative affect and temperament have been associated with smoking behavior in several studies. There is a relatively strong link between impulsivity, hyperactivity, and attention problems and cigarette use, although studies have not examined racial differences (Baker et al., 2004; Burke, Loeber, and Lahey, 2001). In community samples, higher levels of depression have been found to predict smoking behavior (Glassman, Helzer, Covey, Cottler, Stetner, Tipp et al., 1990; Kandel and Davies, 1986; Newcomb McCarthy, and Bentler, 1989; Patton, Hibbert, Rosier, Carlin, Caust, and Bowes, 1996), although the findings have been inconsistent across studies (e.g., Breslau, Kilbey, and Andreski, 1991; White, Pandina, and Chen, 2002; Winefield, Winefield, and Tiggemann, 1992). In some studies, depression has not been linked to smoking among African Americans (e.g., Juon, Ensminger, and Sydnor, 2002; Lloyd-Richardson, Papandonatos, Kazura, Stanton, and Niaura, 2002).

Beliefs and attitudes concerning substance use have also been shown to be important determinants of smoking behavior (Baker et al., 2004; Chassin, Presson, Rose and Sherman, 1996; Flay, Hu, Siddiqui, Day, Hedeker, Petraitis et al., 1994). African Americans hold less positive attitudes about smoking than whites (Robinson et al., 1997), which might account for African Americans' lower rates of use. Positive attitudes towards smoking are also significant predictors of smoking behavior for whites (Flay et al., 1994). In our analysis, we used attitudes toward substance use (i.e., alcohol and illicit drugs) as a proxy measure because we did not have a measure of attitudes toward tobacco use.

Religiosity is another factor that may differentially protect against smoking initiation for African Americans and whites (Wallace, Brown, Bachman, and Laveist, 2003). Wallace and colleagues (2003) contend that the protective aspects of religiosity for African American youth may be due to the important cultural and social functions offered by church life. Juon and colleagues (2002) found that familial religiosity, as well as church attendance, was a significant protective factor for African American smoking. Other studies have shown that only attitudes towards religion are related to smoking behavior among whites (Griesler and Kandel, 1998).

Studies have consistently found that smoking is related to other deviant behaviors and inversely related to conventional behaviors (Baker et al., 2004; Newcomb et al., 1989). High academic achievement and school attachment appear to be protective factors for both races (Hestick, Perrino, Rhodes, and Sydnor, 2001; Kandel et al., 2004; Lloyd-Richardson et al., 2002). However, Griesler and Kandel (1998) reported that positive attitudes toward school were associated with less smoking for whites, but were not related to smoking for African Americans. In a recent study, Kandel and colleagues (2004) found that a positive scholastic attitude reduced the risk for smoking initiation for whites but not for African Americans. In contrast, they found that a positive scholastic attitude reduced the risk of daily smoking for African Americans but not for whites. Delinquency has been strongly associated with cigarette use (Breslau, Kilbey and Andreski, 1993; Chassin, Presson, Sherman, Montello, and McGrew, 1986; Diem, McKay, and Jamieson, 1994) and this association appears to hold for both races (Derzon and Lipsey, 1999; Kandel et al., 2004; Griesler and Kandel, 1998).

The effects of family smoking are differentially related to smoking by whites and African Americans. Having a parent who currently smokes has a strong predictive effect on adolescent regular smoking behavior and on lower cessation rates for whites (Chassin et al., 1996; Griesler and Kandel, 1998), but has only been shown to be significant for African American cigarette experimentation (Robinson et al., 1997; Hestick et al., 2001). Flay and colleagues (1994) found that parental smoking only had indirect effects on smoking initiation and escalation for both African Americans and whites. Furthermore, for both races, the effects of peer smoking were much stronger than the effects of parent smoking. High quality of parent-child interaction (e.g., closeness and monitoring) has been demonstrated to reduce the likelihood of lifetime smoking among African Americans, but has not had as strong an effect for whites (Griesler and Kandel, 1998). Kandel and colleagues (2004) found that stronger parent-child connectedness protected against daily smoking for both African Americans and whites. In addition, African American parents more closely monitor their children, which can reduce smoking, as well as influence peer group selection (Wallace and Muroff, 2002).

Peer cigarette use has been shown to be one of the strongest predictors of adolescent smoking initiation and maintenance for both whites and African Americans (Botvin, Baker, Botvin, Dusenbury, Cardwell, and Diaz, 1993; Gardiner, 2001; Grtiz et al., 1998; Kandel et al., 2004). We did not have a measure of peer smoking, so we used a measure of peer delinquency as a proxy. Affiliation with delinquent peers has also been shown to predict cigarette use (Baker et al., 2004).

Socioeconomic and neighborhood differences between African Americans and whites may account for differential access to cigarettes. Chaloupka (2003) argued that the high price of cigarettes serves as a deterrent for some youths by limiting access. On the other hand, Wallace and Muroff (2002) have noted that, regardless of race, youngsters of lower SES are more likely to smoke. Yet, family SES appears to have a stronger influence for whites than for African Americans (Griesler and Kandel, 1998). Wallace and Muroff (2002) argued that, because African American teens are more likely to live in poorer neighborhoods with greater availability of both licit and illicit drugs, they are at greater overall risk.

CURRENT STUDY

Although several studies have examined racial differences in the predictors of cigarette use, these studies have had limitations, which weaken their ability to inform and improve prevention programs. Some studies have been cross-sectional, which limits their ability to establish directionality and examine patterns of smoking over time. Many of the longitudinal studies have had high attrition rates, posing generalization and validity issues, especially because dropouts tend to exhibit higher rates of smoking (Chassin, Presson, Sherman, and Kim, 2002). Many studies have not differentiated between different types of smoking (i.e., experimentation and regular use), which prevents them from addressing differences in transitions between levels of use. When smoking levels are taken into account, studies have used different operational definitions, which lead to contradictory findings across studies, as well as the inability to compare results (for greater detail see White et al., 2002). Most studies contain either racially homogeneous samples or heterogeneous samples that tend to have a much greater numbers of whites than African Americans. Furthermore, most studies of racial differences in predictors of smoking have included limited numbers of variables and have not examined multiple domains and predictors at varying age periods. Finally, few studies have empirically differentiated between risk and protection.

The present study attempts to fill a gap in the literature by examining racial differences in risk and protective factors for smoking at different developmental periods from childhood to late adolescence. We address the limitations of previous research by using a community sample with a large proportion of both African Americans and whites, using annually-collected, longitudinal data spanning childhood until late adolescence with low attrition, empirically defining smoking trajectory groups, and including multiple domains of variables and multiple sources of data. In addition, we examine both risk and protective factors for smoking and use a new empirical method for determining risk and protection. We examine these risk and protective factors at various developmental periods marking childhood (ages 7-9), early adolescence (ages 10-12), middle adolescence (ages 13-16) and late adolescence (ages 17-19). Although we have continuous annual data from approximate age 7 to age 19, we divided the ages into these developmental periods to determine if there were developmentally distinct risk and protective factors. Because the risk and protective factors were measured at various developmental periods from ages 7 to 19 and the outcome variable was based on smoking trajectories from ages 10 through 19, only the childhood risk and protective factors precede the trajectory group measurement and represent potential predictors of trajectory group membership. The other risk and protective factors were measured concurrently with smoking behavior and, thus, causal inferences cannot be assumed. Nevertheless, we believe that it is important to examine those variables that are associated with risk and protection of smoking behavior over time. This study will contribute to the literature by exploring risk and protective factors for smoking initiation and regular smoking in the context of specified age ranges. The results should have implications for the design of culturally and age appropriate prevention programs for cigarette smoking.

METHOD

Design and Sample

The data come from the Pittsburgh Youth Study (PYS), a prospective, multiple cohort, longitudinal study of the development of delinquency, substance use, and mental health problems (Loeber, Farrington, Stouthamer-Loeber, and Van Kammen, 1998). In 1987-88, random samples of first, fourth, and seventh grade boys enrolled in the City of Pittsburgh public schools were selected. Approximately 850 boys in each grade (85% of the target sample) were screened. Families were paid for their participation, and informed written consent was obtained from both the participants and their legal guardians. The 15% nonparticipation rate did not result in sample bias, at least in regard to achievement test results and racial distribution, which were the only two variables that could be compared from school records (Loeber et al., 1998).

About 500 boys in each grade (the 30% who scored highest on a risk assessment for later antisocial behavior and another 30% randomly selected from the remainder) were selected for the first follow up 6 months later; therefore, approximately half of each cohort was selected for potential high risk and half was not. There was no significant difference in the percent high risk by race. The present analyses will focus on the youngest cohort (from approximately age 7 through age 19).[1] After the first follow up, the members of the youngest cohort were subsequently followed up at 6-month intervals for six additional assessments and then at

---

[1] We chose to focus on the youngest cohort because they had data spanning childhood through late adolescence. There were no data on childhood precursors for the oldest cohort because they were first sampled at approximately age 12. Follow up of the middle sample stopped after age 13 not allowing for the investigation of the development of subsequent smoking behavior.

yearly intervals for a total of 14 years. Attrition has remained relatively low and the completion rate has averaged above 90% across 14 years of data collection (for more information about recruitment and retention see Stouthamer-Loeber and Van Kammen, 1995). The youngest cohort is 56% African American, 42% white and 2% other or mixed. Over one third of the boys' families received public assistance or food stamps. (For greater detail on design and sample see Loeber et al., 1998.)

Measures

The data come from self reports from the youth, their primary caretaker (usually a mother), and their teacher. The youth and his primary caretaker were interviewed separately, usually in their own home. Teachers completed mailed questionnaires. We combined the early 6-month assessments to create annual measures for each year. The measures were assessed in the same manner at each assessment, unless stated so below.

Race. Youths reported on their *race/ethnicity* at screening. For these analyses, we eliminated the other and mixed groups and included only the African Americans (N=281; coded 2) and whites (N=208; coded 1).

Cigarette use. At screening the respondents were asked if they had ever used tobacco (cigarettes, cigars/pipes and smokeless tobacco) and, if yes, at what age they first used. Subsequent to that, they were asked whether or not they smoked in the last year (last 6-months in the first few assessments). The response to this question was used to indicate annual *prevalence* each year. The first time the respondent reported using tobacco was coded as their *age of onset*. Those who smoked were asked how many cigarettes they smoke per day, which provided a *quantity* measure. Smoking trajectories were based on the number of cigarettes smoked per day.

Risk and protective factors. For the present analyses, we divided the risk and protective factors into four developmental periods representing childhood (ages 7-9), early adolescence (10-12), middle adolescence (ages 13-16), and late adolescence (ages 17-19). Developmental period scores were derived by calculating the mean of all the ages within the period for which data were available.

Hyperactivity/impulsivity/attention (HIA) problems represented 14 descriptors (e.g., "can't concentrate," "can't sit still," "is impulsive") related to hyperactivity, impulsivity, and attention problems. The descriptors were measured by 12 items from the primary caretaker on the Child Behavior Checklist (Extended CBCL; Achenbach and Edelbrock, 1979) and 13 items from the teacher on the Teacher Report Form (Extended TRF; Edelbrock and Achenbach, 1984). If either informant said that a descriptor was true for the boy sometimes or often, the youth received a positive score for that descriptor. The descriptors were then counted to create the final construct. This variable was assessed at all age periods except 17-19 (average alpha across developmental periods = .89).

Depression was the sum of 13 items on the Recent Mood and Feelings Questionnaire (Costello and Angold, 1988) responded to by the youth. The 13 questions covered the symptoms (during the previous 2 weeks) necessary for making a diagnosis of major depression according to the DSM-III-R criteria (American Psychiatric Association, 1987). This variable was assessed at all age periods (average alpha = .84).

Attitude toward substance use was based on the youth's judgment, on a 5-point scale, of the acceptability of behaviors related to drug use. At ages 7-10, it was made from three items about attitudes toward drinking alcohol, smoking marijuana, and sniffing glue. For the later ages, it was made from four items including attitudes about drinking alcohol, smoking marijuana, using hard drugs, and selling hard drugs (average alpha = 80).

Religiosity was measured by two questions asked of the youth: "Do you like going to religious services?" and "If you had to choose between going to a religious service or doing something else, which would you do?" Scores ranged from 0 to 2 with 2 being the least religious (did not attend services) (average alpha = .74). It was measured at all ages except 17-19.

Delinquency was the frequency of youth self-reported delinquency covering theft, violence, vandalism, and fraud but not status offenses (e.g., truancy or running away). It was measured at all ages.

School performance was the sum of the standardized scores for the Academic Achievement and School Motivation scales (average alpha = .86). Academic Achievement combined the caretakers', teachers', and youths' evaluations of the youth's performance in reading, math, writing, and spelling; caretakers and youths also evaluated up to three other academic subjects. Performance was rated on a 4-point scale, ranging from failing (highest score) to above average (lowest score). The ratings of all academic subjects by all informants were averaged to create the construct. School Motivation was based on the teachers' rating, on a 7-point scale, of how hard the youth was working in school. This measure was available at all ages except 17-19.

Parental smoking was a dichotomous measure of whether the male or female caretaker smoked as reported by the primary caretaker when the youth was approximately age 13 and reported by the youth when he was age 17. If either caretaker smoked, then it was coded as 1 and if neither smoked, then it was coded as 0.

Relationship with parents was the sum of the standardized scores for three constructs: Caretaker Positive Parenting, Caretaker/Child Communication, and Relationship with Primary Caretaker (average alpha = .83). Caretaker Positive Parenting combined 9 items from the caretakers' and 7 items from the youths' reports of the frequency of the caretaker's positive behaviors toward the youth (e.g., giving special privileges or compliments). Relationship with Primary Caretaker combined 13 items from the youths' and 16 items from the caretakers' perceptions of the quality of their relationship (e.g., how often the caretaker bugs the youth and how often the caretaker thinks that the youth is a good child). Caretaker/Child Communication summarized 30 items from the caretaker and 28 from the youth regarding everyday communication between caretaker and youth in terms of emotions, disagreements, and problems (e.g., how often they discuss the youth's personal problems together, whether the caretaker could interpret the youth's emotional state without asking). This scale was measured at all ages except 17-19.

Peer delinquency was a construct that summarized the proportion of friends who engaged in various delinquent activities, such as stealing and vandalism, based on the self report of the youth. It was measured at all age periods (average alpha = .83).

Socioeconomic status (SES) was measured using the Hollingshead (1975) index of social status based on data collected from the primary caretaker. It was equal to the highest score attained between the two caretakers or to the score attained by the single caretaker. Scores were reverse coded so that a higher score equals lower SES. It was measured at all age periods except 17-19.

Neighborhood quality was the caretaker's assessment of the neighborhood in which the family lived at the time of the interview. It included 17 items reflecting level of neighborhood safety/stability (e.g., the prevalence of abandoned buildings, unemployment, racial tension, and various criminal activities) (*alpha* = .95). It was measured at all age periods except 17-19.

Analyses

Smoking trajectories.In a previous study (White et al., 2004), we developed smoking trajectories based on the number of cigarettes smoked per day using group-based trajectory modeling (Jones, Nagin, and Roeder, 2001; Nagin, 1999, 2005). This method identifies groups of individuals following distinctive developmental trajectories. As described in Nagin and Tremblay (1999, 2001) and Nagin and Land (1993), the trajectory groups are designed to trace out complex forms of population heterogeneity in developmental patterns using a statistical technique called finite mixture modeling. These unique trajectories not only reveal differences in the level of behavior at a given time, but also identify differences in the development of the particular behavior over time (Nagin and Tremblay, 1999). Model estimation used a SAS-based procedure, called Proc Traj, described in Jones et al. (2001). For the trajectory analyses, the youngest and oldest cohorts were combined and separate trajectory analyses were conducted by race from age 10 through age 25 years.

A key issue in the application of a group-based model is making a determination of how many groups define the best fitting model. We followed the lead of D'Unger, Land, McCall, and Nagin (1998) and used the Bayesian Information Criterion (BIC) as a basis for selecting the optimal model (see Raftery, 1995). They recommend selection of the model with the maximum BIC. We tested four sequential models each adding another group. Based on the BIC criteria, a three-group model fit the data best for each race. These three trajectories groups were: nonsmokers, light smokers, and regular smokers (see results below for greater detail). Individuals in the estimation sample were then assigned to the group to which they most likely belonged based on a statistic called the posterior probability of group membership (PPGM) (see Nagin, 1999, 2005). The PPGM measures the probability that the individual belongs to that trajectory group. Ideally, the PPGM for an individual for his/her assigned group is 1; when the mean classification probability for individuals assigned to each of the respective trajectory groups exceeds .7, conventional normal-based hypothesis tests of differences across trajectory groups are little affected by classification error (Roeder, Lynch, and Nagin, 1999; Nagin, 2005). For these models the average PPGM for all individuals assigned to each group was .97 and above for both whites and African Americans (for greater details on the analytic technique and the creation of the trajectory groups see White et al., 2004). For some of the analyses below, the trajectory groups were dichotomized to reflect smoking (nonsmokers vs. light and regular smokers) and regular smoking (light vs. regular smokers).

Risk and protective factors. We used an empirical method developed by Stouthamer-Loeber et al. (2004) to identify whether a variable's relation to cigarette smoking was determined by the protective and / or the risk end. All variables were coded so that the higher score reflected potentially greater risk for cigarette smoking. We first tested each variable to see whether it had a significant protective association, a significant risk association, or both. To do this, each variable was trichotomized separately for whites and African Americans into the bottom 25%, the middle 50%, and the top 25%, which served to isolate the 25% of the youth at the potentially protective end, the 50% neutral, and the 25% at the potentially risk end, respectively. We then cross-tabulated the protective end (bottom 25%) with the 50% neutral (excluding those at the risk end) and cross-tabulated the risk end (top 25%) with the 50% neutral (excluding those at the protective end) by the smoking (nonsmokers vs. light and regular smoker) and regular smoking (light vs. regular smokers) dichotomies to determine whether the independent variable had a risk or protective association for each race.

After determining the protective and / or risk association of each variable for each race, the variable was then dichotomized 25%/75% (either the 25% protective vs. the rest or the 25% risk vs. the rest) so that all youth were included in the analyses. Chi-square analyses (2 X 2) and odds ratios were calculated for each protective and / or risk factor by the two dichotomized measures of smoking trajectory group membership described above separately by race. Parental smoking was treated as a dichotomy throughout the analyses to reflect the presence or absence of the risk factor.

Those protective and risk factors that were significantly associated ($p<.05$) with smoking initiation or regular smoking in the second set of cross-tabulations were then included in hierarchical logistic regression analyses for the age period and trajectory dichotomy for which they were significant. None of the independent variables were multicollinear within models. For the present analyses we conducted two sets of logistic regressions as suggested by Cohen, Cohen, West, and Aiken (2003). In the first set examining risk and protective factors for smoking initiation, we compared nonsmokers to light and regular smokers. In the second set examining risk and protective factors for regular smoking, we compared light to regular smokers. In the first step of the hierarchical logistic regression analyses, we entered each of the significant risk and protective factors and race; in the second step, we added the interactions between race and each of the risk and protective factors simultaneously. The models were tested separately at four points in time: childhood (ages 7-9), early adolescence (ages 10-12), middle adolescence (ages 13-16), and late adolescence (ages 17-19).

RESULTS

Descriptive Results

Whites (mean=12.6 years) began smoking significantly earlier than African Americans (mean=13.6 years) by about one year (t= -2.20, p=.029). By age 19 significantly more whites (67.0%) than African Americans (47.6%) had ever smoked a cigarette (chi square= 27.56, df=1, p<.001).

The average number of cigarettes smoked per day over time for each trajectory group is shown in Figure 1 for whites and Figure 2 for African Americans. Group membership differed significantly by race (chi square = 7.23, df=2, p<.03). There were more African Americans (56.6%) than whites (48.6%) in the nonsmoker group and more whites (28.4%) than African Americans (18.1%) in the regular smoker group. There were similar proportions of whites (23.1%) and African Americans (25.3%) in the light smoker group. Within both the light and regular smoker groups, whites began smoking earlier and smoked more cigarettes per day than African Americans at all ages (for greater detail see White et al., 2004).

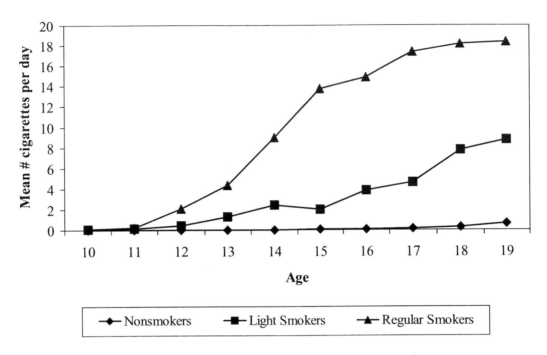

Figure 1. Observed Mean Number of Cigarettes Smoked for White Trajectory Groups

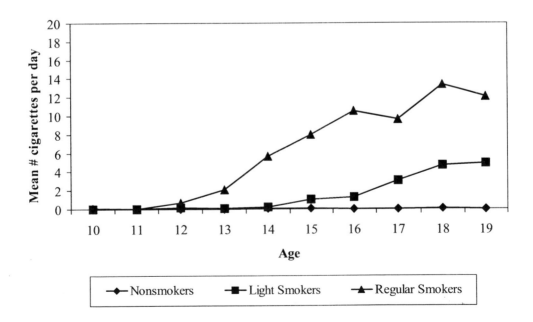

Figure 2. Observed Mean Number of Cigarettes Smoked for African American Trajectory Groups

Racial Differences in Risk and Protective Factors for Smoking

Table 1 shows the risk and protective factors significantly related to smoking based on the chi square analyses for the total sample conducted separately for whites and African Americans. We did not control for the number of chi square analyses that were conducted because we were first trying to classify all variables into risk or protection. The later multivariate analyses helped to isolate those variables that were most strongly related to smoking. Depression, delinquency, school performance, peer delinquency, and attitude toward substance use acted as both risk and protective factors for smoking either at the same age period or at different age periods. In other words, these variables had both positive and negative ends. Within each age period, those variables that had only a risk effect are listed first, followed by those that had only a protective effect, and then those that had both protective and risk effects. Only variables that were significant in the chi square analyses are listed.

For whites at ages 7-9, having many delinquent peers was a risk factor and having few was a protective factor. As an example of how to read Table 1, 39% of the nonsmokers compared to 16.8% of the smokers had few delinquent peers and having few delinquent peers reduced the risk of smoking by about one-third [Odds Ratio (OR) = .32]. Also, 35.5% of the smokers compared to 13% of the nonsmokers had many delinquent peers and having many delinquent peers increased the risk of smoking almost four-fold [Odds Ratio (OR) = 3.69]. In addition, being high in delinquency was a risk factor and being low in depression and coming from a high SES family were protective factors. At ages 10-12, being high in HIA was a risk factor and having few delinquent peers and coming from a high SES family were protective factors. At ages 13-16, school performance, delinquent peers, and attitudes toward substance use had both protective and risk associations with smoking. In addition, low depression, low delinquency, and good relationships with parents were protective factors. At ages 17-19 having a parent who smoked and many delinquent peers were risk factors, whereas having negative attitudes toward substance use was a protective factor.

Many of the same risk and protective factors for smoking were identified for African Americans, although not necessarily at the same ages as whites. At ages 7-9, high HIA, depression, and delinquency were risk factors for African Americans, whereas doing well in school, good relationships with parents, and having few delinquent peers were protective factors. At ages 10-12 high HIA and poor school performance were risk factors and low delinquency and few delinquent peers were protective factors for smoking among African Americans. At ages 13-16, having many delinquent peers was a risk factor and having few was a protective factor for smoking. In addition, having high HIA, positive attitudes toward substance use, and a parent who smoked were risk factors and being high in religiosity and doing well in school were protective factors. At ages 17-19, none of the variables were risk factors, but having negative attitudes toward substance use and low depression were protective factors.

In summary, all of the factors except neighborhood quality were significantly related to smoking for at least one race at one or more developmental period. School performance (as a risk and protective factor) and religiosity (as a protective factor) were significant only for African Americans. SES (as a protective factor) was related only for whites. The variables most frequently related to smoking for both races were HIA (only as a risk factor), depression (mostly as a protective factor), delinquency (as both a risk and protective factor), and peer delinquency (more often as a protective factor than a risk factor).

Table 1. Significant Risk and Protective Factors for Cigarette Smoking by Race and Developmental Period

	White			African American		
	Nonsmoker %	Smoker %	OR (95% CI)	Nonsmoker %	Smoker %	OR (95% CI)
Ages 7-9						
Risk Factors						
High HIA				18.9	32.0	2.02 (1.17-3.50)
High Delinquency	11.0	38.3	5.03 (2.40-10.51)	15.1	32.0	2.64 (1.48-4.71)
Protective Factors						
Good School Performance				34.0	13.9	.32(.17-.58)
Good Relationship with Parents				30.2	19.7	.57 (.32-.99)
High SES	33.3	16.8	.40 (.21-.78)			
Both Risk and Protective Factors						
High Depression				18.2	31.2	2.03 (1.16-3.54)
Low Depression	38.0	13.1	.25 (.12-.49)			
Many Delinquent Peers	13.0	35.5	3.69 (1.82-7.46)			
Few Delinquent Peers	39.0	16.8	.32 (.17-.60)	33.3	13.9	.32 (.18-.60)
Ages 10-12						
Risk Factors						
High HIA	17.5	29.5	1.97 (1.01-3.86)	18.4	33.3	2.21 (1.27-3.87)
Poor School Performance				17.8	34.2	2.40 (1.37-4.21)
Protective Factors						
Low Delinquency				47.0	30.0	.48 (.29-.80)
Few Delinquent Peers	35.1	13.3	.29 (.14-.57)	28.8	14.2	.41 (.22-.76)
High SES	34.0	16.2	.37 (.19-.73)			
Ages 13-16						
Risk Factors						
High HIA				17.8	33.9	2.37 (1.34-4.19)
Parental Smoking				54.6	69.8	1.93 (1.15-3.23)
Protective Factors						
Low Depression	31.9	16.4	.42 (.21-.82)			
High Religiosity				30.8	17.0	.46 (.25-.83)
Low Delinquency	68.1	30.8	.21 (.11-.38)			
Good Relationship with Parents	34.7	16.4	.37 (.19-.72)			
Both Risk and Protective Factors						
Positive Attitude to Substance Use	16.0	34.6	2.79 (1.41-5.53)	16.4	36.4	2.91(1.64-5.19)
Negative Attitude to Substance Use	28.7	12.5	.36 (.17-.74)			
Many Delinquent Peers	12.8	34.6	3.62 (1.75-7.49)	11.0	39.0	5.19 (2.74-9.82)
Few Delinquent Peers	37.2	14.4	.28 (.14-.57)	34.9	14.4	.31 (.17-.58)
Poor School Performance	11.6	37.5	4.58 (2.18-9.64)			
Good School Performance	37.9	13.5	.26 (.13-.51)	37.7	9.3	.17 (.08-.34)
Ages 17-19						
Risk Factors						
Parental Smoking	35.6	55.3	2.24 (1.24-4.06)			
Many Delinquent Peers	12.4	35.6	3.92 (1.85-8.27)			
Protective Factors						
Low Depression				33.1	20.4	.52 (.29-.93)
Negative Attitude To Substance Use	33.7	14.4	.33 (.16-.67)	34.6	15.0	.34 (.18-.63)

Table 2. Hierarchical Logistic Regression Results for Smoking[a]

	Model I	Model II
Ages 7-9 (N= 487)		
High HIA	1.15 (0.72-1.84)	0.89 (0.17-4.76)
Low Depression	0.55 (0.34-0.88)*	0.13 (0.03-0.67)
High Delinquency	2.46 (1.53-3.96)*	6.21 (1.10-35.15)
Good School Performance	0.64 (0.40-1.03)	3.93 (0.75-20.66)
Good Relationship with Parents	0.79 (0.50-1.24)	0.84 (0.18-3.97)
Few Delinquent Peers	0.47 (0.29-0.75)*	0.51 (0.11-2.40)
High SES	0.66 (0.42-1.04)	0.21 (0.04-1.05)
Race	0.66 (0.45-0.98)*	0.66 (0.32-1.37)
Race x HIA		1.20 (0.45-3.25)
Race x Depression		2.52 (0.95-6.70)
Race x Delinquency		0.57 (0.21-1.57)
Race x School Performance		0.32 (0.12-0.89)*
Race x Relationship with Parents		0.96 (0.37-2.46)
Race x Delinquent Peers		0.96 (0.36-2.51)
Race x SES		2.04 (0.78-5.34)
Likelihood Ratio χ^2	68.87***	80.33***
Ages 10 – 12 (N=466)		
High HIA	1.59 (0.97-2.60)	2.20 (0.32-15.28)
Low Delinquency	0.59 (0.39-0.91)*	0.39 (0.10-1.59)
Poor School Performance	1.53 (0.94-2.48)	0.38 (0.06-2.39)
Few Delinquent Peers	0.49 (0.29-0.82)*	0.28 (0.05-1.47)
High SES	0.52 (0.32-0.83)*	0.22 (0.05-1.08)
Race	0.64 (0.43-0.96)*	0.39 (0.19-0.78)
Race x HIA		0.87 (0.29-2.63)
Race x Delinquency		1.30 (0.55-3.10)
Race x School Performance		2.32 (0.80-6.69)
Race x Delinquent Peers		1.42 (0.50-4.00)
Race x SES		1.71 (0.66-4.47)
Likelihood Ratio χ^2	49.76***	54.59***
Ages 13 – 16 (N=414)		
High HIA	1.61 (0.95-2.72)	2.63 (0.42-16.61)
Low Depression	1.03 (0.60-1.76)	0.69 (0.11-4.43)
Positive Attitude to Substance Use	1.65 (0.97-2.83)	2.07 (0.32-13.52)
High Religiosity	0.77 (0.45-1.33)	2.13 (0.30-15.27)
Low Delinquency	0.73 (0.44-1.20)	0.07 (0.01-0.38)
Good School Performance	0.34 (0.19-0.60)*	1.66 (0.25-10.93)
Parental Smoking	1.64 (1.04-2.58)*	0.83 (0.17-4.01)
Good Relationship with Parents	0.88 (0.51-1.52)	0.61 (0.09-4.31)
Many Delinquent Peers	2.48 (1.36-4.51)*	0.30 (0.04-2.39)
High SES	0.74 (0.43-1.27)	0.40 (0.06-2.56)

Table 2. Hierarchical Logistic Regression Results for Smoking (Continued)

	Model I	Model II
Race	0.68 (0.44-1.06)	0.26 (0.08-0.81)
Race x HIA		0.75 (0.25-2.25)
Race x Depression		1.33 (0.43-4.08)
Race x Attitude to Substance Use		0.86 (0.28-2.66)
Race x Religiosity		0.56 (0.18-1.81)
Race x Delinquency		4.53 (1.59-12.87)[*]
Race x School Performance		0.35 (0.11-1.16)
Race x Parental Smoking		1.61 (0.62-4.23)
Race x Relationship with Parents		1.15 (0.36-3.68)
Race x Delinquent Peers		3.76 (1.06-13.27)[*]
Race x SES		1.40 (0.44-4.41)
Likelihood Ratio χ^2	84.07[***]	97.62[***]
Ages 17 – 19 (N=405)		
Low Depression	0.92 (0.57-1.49)	2.12 (0.43-10.37)
Negative Attitude to Substance Use	0.30 (0.18-0.51)[*]	0.20 (0.03-1.21)
Parental Smoking	1.74 (1.14-2.66)[*]	2.91 (0.67-12.62)
Many Delinquent Peers	1.80 (1.09-2.97)[*]	13.93 (2.33-83.19)
High SES	0.51 (0.30-0.86)[*]	0.91 (0.16-5.17)
Race	0.75 (0.49-1.13)	1.37 (0.62-3.03)
Race x Depression		0.59 (0.22-1.56)
Race x Attitude to Substance Use		1.30 (0.44-3.85)
Race x Parental Smoking		0.73 (0.30-1.75)
Race x Delinquent Peers		0.28 (0.10-0.80)[*]
Race x SES		0.71 (0.24-2.09)
Likelihood Ratio χ^2	50.12[***]	57.23[***]

[a] Odds Ratio presented; 95% Confidence Intervals in parentheses.
* $p < .05$; ** $p < .01$; *** $p < .001$

We selected all of the risk and protective factors that were significant at each developmental age period for either race and included them in multivariate hierarchical logistic regression analyses with smoking trajectory group as the dependent variable (light or regular smokers versus nonsmokers). In the previous analysis, we found that high SES was a protective factor in the two younger age periods (7-9 and 10-12) for whites. We decided to include SES as a protective factor in all of the models because of the need to control for SES when examining race differences (Rose, Chassin, Presson, and Sherman, 1996). In the 17-19 age period, we used the SES measure from ages 13-16 because family SES was not available at ages 17-19. If a variable had both a risk and protective effect for one race, but a clear risk or protective effect for the other race, then we went with the clear effect. Otherwise, if a variable had both a risk and a protective effect, then we included the effect with the best odds ratio from the cross-tabular analyses reported above. The analyses were conducted separately for each developmental period. We first tested the main effects of the risk and protective factors and race. Then we added the interactions of race with each of the risk factors simultaneously. The results are presented in Table 2.

In the main effects model, at ages 7-9, depression, delinquency, peer delinquency, and race were all significant predictors of smoking. Being low in depression, having few delinquent peers, and being African American protected against smoking; frequently engaging in delinquent activities increased the risk for smoking. In the second model that included the interactions, only the interaction between race and school performance was significant. A probe of that interaction showed that high school performance protected against smoking for African Americans (OR = .32, CI = .18-.60, p<.001), but was not a protective factor for whites (OR= .82, CI= .44-1.55, p>.05).

At ages 10-12 delinquency, peer delinquency, family SES, and race were significantly related to smoking. Being non-delinquent, having few delinquent peers, coming from a high SES family, and being African American were protective factors for smoking. None of the interactions was significant.

In middle adolescence (ages 13-16), school performance, parental smoking, and peer delinquency were significantly related to smoking. Having a parent who smoked and having many delinquent peers increased the risk of smoking, whereas good school performance decreased the risk. In the second model, low delinquency and many delinquent peers interacted with race. Probes of these interactions indicated that being low in delinquency was a stronger protective factor for whites (OR = .21, CI = .11-.38, p<.001) than for African Americans (OR = .48, CI = .29-.81, p<.01). On the other hand, having many delinquent peers was a somewhat stronger risk factor for African Americans (OR = 5.19, CI = 2.74-9.82, p<.001) than whites (OR = 3.62, CI = 1.75-7.49, p<.001).

There were several factors in late adolescence (ages 17-19) that were significantly related to smoking in the multivariate analyses, including attitude toward substance use, parental smoking, peer delinquency, and family SES. At ages 17-19, those young men who had a parent who smoked and many delinquent peers were at increased risk for smoking. On the other hand, those who came from a higher SES family and held negative attitudes toward substance use were less likely to smoke. The interaction between race and delinquent peers was significant. Having many delinquent peers at ages 17-19 was a risk factor for whites (OR = 3.92, CI = 1.85-8.27, p<.001), but not for African Americans (OR = 1.76, CI = .99-3.15, p>.05)

Racial Differences in Risk and Protective Factors for Regular Smoking

Table 3 shows the significant risk and protective factors for regular smoking for whites and African Americans. At each age period, fewer significant risk and protective factors were identified for regular smoking than for smoking, possibly due to less power (i.e., eliminating the nonsmokers from the analyses).

For whites at ages 7-9, poor school performance was a risk factor for regular smoking and living in a good neighborhood was a protective factor. At ages 10-12, no risk factors were identified, but good school performance was a protective factor. At ages 13-16, positive attitudes towards substance use, high delinquency, having many delinquent peers, and having a parent who smoked were risk factors, whereas low HIA and doing well in school were protective factors. At ages 17-19, having a parent who smoked was the only factor related to regular smoking for whites.

Table 3. Significant Risk and Protective Factors for Regular Cigarette Smoking by Race and Developmental Period

	White			African American		
	Light Smoker %	Regular Smoker %	OR (95%CI)	Light Smoker %	Regular Smoker %	OR (95%CI)
Ages 7-9						
Risk and Factors						
Poor School Performance	16.7	37.3	2.97(1.18-7.49)			
Protective Factors						
Low HIA				29.6	11.8	.32 (.12-.86)
Good Neighborhood	14.6	35.7	3.24 (1.16-9.02)			
Ages 10-12						
Protective Factors						
Low Depression				25.7	6.0	.18 (.05-.67)
Low Delinquency				38.6	18.0	.35 (.15-.83)
Good School Performance	36.2	13.8	.28 (.11-.73)			
Ages 13-16						
Risk Factors						
Positive Attitude to Substance Use	21.7	44.8	2.93 (1.20-6.99)			
High Delinquency	21.7	50.0	3.60 (1.51-8.59)	19.1	52.0	4.58 (2.02-0.41)
Parental Smoking	46.7	72.2	2.97 (1.29-6.85)			
Many Delinquent Peers	19.6	46.6	3.58 (1.47-8.74)			
Protective Factors						
Low HIA	30.4	8.8	.22 (.07-.67)	26.5	6.0	.18 (.05-.64)
Risk and Protective Factors						
Poor School Performance				23.5	48.0	3.0 (1.36-6.60)
Good School Performance	28.3	1.7	.04 (.01-.36)			
Ages 17-19						
Risk Factors						
Parental Smoking	39.0	67.9	3.3 (1.41-7.76)			
Protective Factors						
Few Delinquent Peers				11.6	27.3	2.86 (1.06-7.71)

For African Americans, low HIA protected against regular smoking at ages 7-9 and low depression and low delinquency protected at ages 10-12. At ages 13-16, high delinquency and poor school performance were risk factors, and low HIA was a protective factor. Having few delinquent peers at ages 17-19 was a risk factor for regular smoking rather than a protective factor as would be expected.

In sum, all of the variables except religiosity and SES were related to regular smoking across developmental periods for at least one race. Depression (as a protective factor) was related to regular smoking for African Americans only and attitudes toward substance use (protective), parental smoking (risk), and neighborhood quality (protective) were related for whites only. The variables related to smoking for both races were HIA (only protective), school performance (both risk and protective), delinquency (risk and protective), and peer delinquency (only protective).

As was done before for the smoking analyses, for each developmental period, the significant risk and protective factors were included in hierarchical logistic regression analyses. Now regular smoking was the dependent variable (i.e., the regular smoker group vs.

the light smoker group). (Nonsmokers were not included in these analyses.) The same criteria as above were used to determine whether the risk or protective end would be used in the regression analyses. For these analyses, we also controlled for high SES. The results are presented in Table 4.

Table 4. Hierarchical Logistic Regression Results for Regular Smoking[a]

	Model I	Model II
Ages 7-9 (N=208)		
Low HIA	0.53 (0.24-1.17)	2.34 (0.18-30.97)
Poor School Performance	1.36 (0.72-2.58)	11.99 (1.15-125.06)
High SES	0.63 (0.29-1.34)	0.26 (0.02-3.51)
Good Neighborhood	1.90 (1.00-3.61)	6.54 (0.66-64.69)
Race	0.49 (0.28-0.87)[*]	0.97 (0.40-2.38)
Race x HIA		0.39 (0.08-2.01)
Race x School Performance		0.25 (0.06-1.01)
Race x SES		1.68 (0.35-8.15)
Race x Neighborhood		0.44 (0.11-1.71)
Likelihood Ratio χ^2	16.16[***]	22.45[***]
Ages 10-12 (N=224)		
Low Depression	0.60 (0.28-1.26)	10.81 (0.78-150.18)
Low Delinquency	0.73 (0.40-1.32)	3.31 (0.47-23.57)
Good School Performance	0.42 (0.20-0.89)[*]	0.13 (0.01-1.39)
High SES	0.81 (0.39-1.72)	0.74 (0.06-8.66)
Race	0.49 (0.28-0.87)[*]	0.86 (0.40-1.88)
Race x Depression		0.14 (0.02-0.77)[*]
Race x Delinquency		0.35 (0.10-1.22)
Race x School Performance		1.97 (0.41-9.30)
Race x SES		0.99 (0.21-4.60)
Likelihood Ratio χ^2	15.75[***]	26.53[***]
Ages 13-16 (N=193)		
Low HIA	0.30 (0.11-0.78)[*]	0.19 (0.01-4.49)
Positive Attitude to Substance Use	1.13 (0.56-2.28)	3.69 (0.27-50.44)
High Delinquency	2.58 (1.21-5.53)[*]	0.88 (0.06-13.08)
Good School Performance	0.19 (0.05-0.74)[*]	0.01 (<0.01-1.00)
Parental Smoking	2.13 (1.04-4.36)[*]	4.17 (0.37-47.07)
Many Delinquent Peers	1.32 (0.61-2.85)	1.31 (0.09-18.57)
High SES	1.38 (0.56-3.42)	0.12 (0.01-2.86)
Race	0.44 (0.23-0.84)[*]	0.38 (0.09-1.66)
Race x HIA		1.23 (0.17-9.18)
Race x Attitude to Substance Use		0.55 (0.12-2.59)
Race x Delinquency		2.05 (0.41-10.33)
Race x School Performance		9.38 (0.55-160.10)
Race x Parental Smoking		0.64 (0.14-2.89)
Race x Delinquent Peers		0.95 (0.19-4.73)
Race x SES		4.98 (0.75-33.28)
Likelihood Ratio χ^2	45.67[***]	53.48[***]

Table 4. Hierarchical Logistic Regression Results for Regular Smoking[a] (Continued)

	Model I	Model II
Ages 17-19 (N=193)		
Parental Smoking	1.57 (0.87-2.83)	8.77 (1.23-62.76)
Few Delinquent Peers	1.26 (0.57-2.81)	0.25 (0.02-3.66)
High SES	0.74 (0.33-1.69)	0.16 (0.01-2.21)
Race	0.48 (0.27-0.86)[*]	0.62 (0.24-1.65)
Race x Parental Smoking		0.31 (0.09-1.04)
Race x Delinquent Peers		2.95 (0.58-15.10)
Race x SES		3.03 (0.58-15.99)
Likelihood Ratio χ^2	9.71[*]	17.88[*]

[a] Odds Ratio presented; 95% Confidence Intervals in parentheses

* $p < .05$; ** $p < .01$; *** $p < .001$

None of the predictors at ages 7-9, except race, was significantly related to regular smoking. African Americans were less likely to become regular smokers than whites. None of the interactions was significant.

At ages 10-12, school performance and race were significantly related to regular smoking. Those who did well in school compared to those who did worse were less likely to be regular smokers and African Americans were less likely to be regular smokers than whites. In the second model, there was a significant interaction of race with depression. Being low on depression protected against regular smoking for African Americans (OR = .18, CI= .05-.67, p<.01), but not for whites (OR = .99, CI= .37-2.63, p>.05).

In middle adolescence (ages 13-16), HIA, delinquency, school performance, parental smoking, and race were significantly related to regular smoking. Those who had a parent who smoked and were high in delinquency had an increased risk for regular smoking. Being low in HIA, having good school performance, and being African American protected against regular smoking. None of the interactions was significant.

Finally, in late adolescence (ages 17-19) only race was related to regular smoking. African Americans were more likely to be regular smokers than whites. None of the interactions with race was significant.

CONCLUSION

In this chapter we examined risk and protective factors for smoking and regular smoking among African Americans and whites across multiple domains. We had expected to find differential risk and protective factors for African Americans and whites. Instead we found that, for the most part, similar variables were related to smoking and regular smoking for both races. Our findings are consistent with those of Kandel and colleagues (2004), who also found that the same variables predicted smoking initiation and regular smoking for whites and African American youth. In addition, some variables acted as protective factors, others acted as risk factors, and many acted as both. We also found that similar variables acted as risk and / or protective factors across different development periods.

In accord with other research (Baker et al., 2004; Griesler and Kandel, 1998; Hestick et al., 2001; Lloyd-Richardson et al., 2002), we found that school performance was related to smoking; however it appears to be more consistently related to regular smoking than to smoking initiation. It was significantly associated (as a protective factor) with smoking only for African Americans and with regular smoking (as both a risk and protective factor) for both races. Regardless of its risk or protective association, the implications for prevention are clear. Smoking prevention programs should be targeted to students doing poorly in school and those with low school motivation (see also Kandel et al., 2004). Helping such students to improve their academic skills and motivation may also reduce smoking (see Storr, Ialongo, Kellam, and Anthony, 2002). Targeting students with poor school performance could also be preventative for other substance use, as well as problem behaviors such as delinquency, given the reciprocal nature of these relationships (Baker et al., 2004). Because the temporal order between smoking and school performance was not assessed at each developmental period, it is also possible that smoking may have led to declines in academic achievement and motivation over time (e.g., through associations with deviant peers). Nevertheless, childhood good school performance protected against smoking for African Americans highlighting the importance of early school performance as a target for smoking prevention.

Having or not having delinquent peers and being high or low on delinquency were also consistently related to smoking and regular smoking for both races. Deviant adolescents are more likely to affiliate with deviant and substance using peers due both to socialization and selection effects (Baker et al., 2004; Gorman and White, 1995). In this study, we did not have a measure of peer cigarette smoking and we used delinquent peers as a proxy measure. The findings indicate that affiliation with delinquent peers is related to cigarette smoking regardless of peer cigarette use. However, given the association between delinquency and cigarette smoking (Baker et al., 2004), it is reasonable to assume that many of the delinquent peers were also cigarette smokers, who could have influenced smoking by modeling smoking behavior, increasing perceptions that smoking is normative, and / or providing opportunities for use (Baker et al., 2004). Previous research examining the association between an adolescent's cigarette use and his or her friends' use has found that the effect of peers is stronger for whites than African Americans (Baker et al., 2004; Unger, Rohrbach, Cruz, Baezconde-Garbanati, Palmer, and Johnson, 2001). Our results suggest that when other types of deviance are included in the peer measure, the associations between smoking and peer behaviors in childhood and adolescence are equally strong for both races, although the effects varied at different periods of development. In late adolescence, having few compared to many delinquent peers was a risk rather than protective factor for regular smoking among African Americans. The reasons for this finding are unclear, but perhaps the negative influence of peers diminishes over time for African Americans. Nevertheless, the overall results suggest that smoking prevention programs need to target delinquent youth. It should be noted that peer delinquency was reported by the youth and thus reflects perceptions of peer behavior rather than peer actual behavior. Other studies have shown that the effects of peers may be overestimated because youth are likely to attribute their own behavior to those of peers (e.g., Bauman and Ennett, 1994).

As found in previous research, parental smoking was a risk factor for smoking (Chassin et al., 1996; Griesler and Kandel, 1998; Hestick et al., 2001; Robinson et al., 1997). Among African Americans it was related to smoking and for whites it was related to regular smoking. These findings are consistent with those of other studies that found that parental smoking was related to initiation for African Americans, but not to regular use (Hestick et al., 2001; Robinson et al., 1997). Parental smoking retained its significance in three of the four multivariate analyses in which it was included. This strong association between a youth's smoking and his parent's smoking may reflect modeling or effects or heredity (i.e., heritable individual differences in the pharmacological effects of tobacco or personality characteristics) (Baker et al., 2004, p. 470). In this study we could not disentangle such effects.

High HIA was consistently a risk factor for smoking over time, especially for African Americans. In contrast low HIA was a protective factor for regular smoking for both races. However, HIA was only significant in one of the multivariate models (age 13-16 for regular smoking). It is possible that the inclusion of other variables, such as delinquency, in the models may have mediated the effects of HIA. That is, attention deficit/hyperactivity disorder has not been found to predict adolescent substance use when co-occurring conduct disorder is included in the model (Baker et al., 2004). Our measure of HIA did not separate out the effects of attention problems from hyperactivity problems, and some studies have found that these differential components have varying effects on tobacco use (Burke et al., 2001). Nevertheless, the results suggest that boys high in HIA during childhood may be an important risk group for early cigarette prevention.

Low depression was primarily a protective factor for smoking for both races, however, it did not maintain significance in the multivariate analyses. There was one significant interaction with depression indicating that low depression was protective for African Americans, but not whites (at ages 10-12). Our failure to find a stronger association between depression and cigarette smoking is consistent with some of the previous research (Baker et al., 2004; White et al., 2002) and may reflect the fact that we did not have a diagnostic measure of depression nor of cigarette dependence. We expected that depression would be especially important for regular smoking inasmuch as cigarettes are often used for negative affect regulation (Baker et al., 2004). Overall, our findings are consistent with the literature in that externalizing factors were more strongly related to smoking than were internalizing factors (see Baker et al., 2004).

In middle and late adolescence, attitudes toward substance use were related to smoking for both races and, in middle adolescence, attitudes were related to regular smoking by whites. However, attitudes were only significant in one multivariate model. Our measure did not include attitudes towards cigarettes, which might explain the absence of a stronger effect. Nevertheless, the fact that the attitude variable was significant at all suggests that negative attitudes about substance use generalize across substances. Therefore, prevention programs need to reinforce negative attitudes and counter positive attitudes toward substance use among youth.

High religiosity was protective only at one age period (13-16) for smoking for African Americans and at no age periods for regular smoking for either race. Furthermore, in the multivariate models, religiosity did not emerge as a protective factor in contrast to what has been found in other studies, especially of African Americans (e.g., Juon et al., 2002). However, our measure was quite weak and may not have captured religiosity as used in other research.

High SES was protective against smoking in childhood and early adolescence for whites, but not for African Americans at any age and SES was not related to regular smoking for either race. Similarly, neighborhood quality was not related to smoking for either race and was only related to regular smoking at one age period for whites. These findings are in contrast to claims that low SES and disadvantaged neighborhoods increase the risk of smoking for African Americans (Gardiner, 2001). In the presence of behavioral variables (i.e., delinquency and school performance), SES and neighborhood may not be important. It is possible, however, that SES has an indirect impact on smoking behavior through its impact on school performance, delinquency, and peer delinquency. Future research should test such mediation models.

The fact that we found mostly similar risk and protective factors for both races may have had to do with the way we defined our factors. That is, we identified the risk and protective end cutoffs separately by race. Therefore, African Americans and whites may have differed in terms of absolute levels of risk and protective factors but not in terms of relative effects (see Wallace and Muroff, 2002). For example, the means for delinquency frequency were higher for African Americans than whites (not shown), however, for both races being in the highest 25% in terms of delinquency frequency for one's race was a significant risk factor for smoking. In contrast, Griesler and Kandel (1998) found that although African Americans experienced a disproportionate number of risk factors for smoking compared to whites, these factors were more often associated with smoking for whites than for African Americans. They found few consistent predictors across race except for behavior problems. Most of our common risk factors were also related to behavior (i.e., school performance, delinquency, peer delinquency, and HIA). In the presence of other risk and protective factors, being African American was a protective factor for smoking in childhood and early adolescence and for regular smoking from childhood through late adolescence.

The results of the present study should be considered within the limitations of the data. The present study was limited to one geographical location. However, lifetime prevalence rates for the whites and African-Americans at age 17 were very close to their racial counterparts of male (and female) high school seniors in the 2000 and 2001 Monitoring the Future studies (Johnston et al., 2003). We only included males, and the findings may not be generalizable to females. Because the PYS study oversampled boys who were at risk for antisocial behavior, it is possible that the significant associations may not generalize to other samples. However, the association between race and whether the boy was originally in the high antisocial risk group was not statistically significant and, therefore, racial differences identified in this study do not appear to be influenced by the high-risk nature of the sample.

For the present study, we relied on self reports and did not confirm our smoking measures with bioassays. However, other studies have found that self-reports of smoking behavior are valid (e.g., Chassin, Presson, Rose, and Sherman, 1990; Patrick, Cheadle, Thompson, Diehr, Koepsell, and Kinne, 1994). In addition, not all independent variables were measured at each age period. Therefore, analyses within age periods relied on different sets of risk and protective factors, which could have influenced the number of significant associations found. In addition, the meaning of certain variables may differ over time, and certain measures may have better validity in childhood than adolescence or vice versa. Also, we did not measure the pharmacological effects of nicotine nor individual's motivations for smoking. These types of measures are especially important for understanding why individuals transition from experimental to regular smoking (Baker et al., 2004). In addition, we did not have a measure of nicotine dependence within the data set and our group of regular smokers was based solely on their quantity of cigarettes over time. Therefore, we could not address potential racial differences in the use of cigarettes for negative affect control or in the development of dependence.

Many of the risk and protective factors were measured at the same time as the smoking behaviors. Therefore, as discussed in the Introduction, we were not able to assess the temporal associations between the adolescent risk and protective factors and smoking behavior. We could, however, identify those factors that were significantly associated with different smoking trajectories during adolescence. In addition, we could identify those childhood risk and protective factors that predicted later smoking trajectory group membership.

In addition, there are contextual influences, which we did not measure, that can play an important role in the onset of smoking. It is important to consider the influence of the community, racial discrimination, pricing, media access, school policies, and smoke-free air laws, and how these differentially affect African Americans compared to other ethnic/racial groups (Chaloupka, 2003; Gardiner, 2001; Wilcox, 2003). Kandel and colleagues (2004) found that individual factors were better predictors of smoking initiation and daily smoking than were contextual factors. In their multivariate analyses, the only significant contextual predictor of smoking initiation was state-level bans on cigarette vending machines. Given that our sample all came from the same state, and, in fact, the same city, this variable would not have had any variance in this study. In addition, in the Kandel et al. (2004) study, the racial composition of the school predicted daily smoking for both African Americans and whites. Unfortunately, we did not measure this variable. We did include a measure of neighborhood quality, which included characteristics, such as racial tension. Also, we did not have measures of cultural or ethnic/racial identity, although this factor has been shown to affect racial and ethnic differences in cigarette smoking (Nichter, 2003). Other cultural factors may also account for increased smoking among African Americans, such as the commercial hip-hop culture which has adopted cigarette, cigar, and marijuana smoking, and the tobacco industry's increased sponsorship of African American community events and aggressive marketing to African American youth (Gardiner, 2001). We could not assess these influences within our data set, and, thus, more research is needed to examine cultural influences (Nichter, 2003).

Despite these limitations, this study had several strengths. It used prospective data and followed African American and white youth at least annually for 14 years. We utilized a new technique for examining both risk and protection. Our measures were collected from multiple sources and covered multiple domains across varying developmental periods. The findings, as well as those of previous studies, indicate that there are multiple factors that are related to the development of smoking behaviors including individual, family, and peer factors (Baker et al., 2004). Nevertheless, in this study we have identified several factors that were related to both the initiation and maintenance of cigarette smoking for African American and white youths and very few that were unique to either race. African American and white young men with low academic achievement and motivation, who are delinquent, who belong to delinquent peer groups, and / or who are high in hyperactivity, inattention, and impulsivity appear to be key targets for smoking prevention efforts in childhood and adolescence. For the most part, it appears that the same types of school-based smoking prevention programs (see Sussman, Dent, Stacy, Burton, and Flay, 1995) can be used with whites and African Americans in middle school and high school.

ACKNOWLEDGEMENTS

This research was supported, in part, by grants from the Robert Wood Johnson Foundation (043747), the National Institute on Drug Abuse (DA 17552; DA 411018), the Office of Juvenile Justice and Delinquency Prevention (96-MU-FX-0012), and the National Institute of Mental Health (MH 050778). Points of view in this document are those of the authors and do not necessarily represent the official position or policies of the U.S. Department of Justice. We acknowledge Rebecca Stallings for assistance in preparing the data files and Adam Thacker for his help with manuscript preparation. An earlier version of this paper was presented at the Society of Prevention Research annual meeting, May 28, 2004, Quebec City, Canada.

REFERENCES

Achenbach, T.M., and Edelbrock, C.S. (1979). The child behavior profile: II. Boys ages 12-16 and girls ages 6-11 and 12-16. *Journal of Consulting and Clinical Psychology, 47,* 223-233.

American Psychiatric Association (1987). *Diagnostic and statistical manual of mental disorders.* Washington, DC: American Psychiatric Association.

Baker, T.B., Brandon, T.H., and Chassin, L. (2004). Motivational influences on cigarette smoking. *Annual Review of Psychology, 55,* 463-491.

Bauman K.E. and Ennett, S.T. (1994). Peer influence on adolescent drug use. *American Psychologist, 49,* 820-822.

Botvin, G.J., Baker, E., Botvin, E.M., Dusenbury, L., Cardwell, J., and Diaz, T. (1993). Factors promoting cigarette smoking among black youth: A casual modeling approach. *Addictive Behaviors, 18,* 397-405.

Breslau, N., Kilbey, M., and Andreski, P. (1991). Nicotine dependence, major depression, and anxiety in young adults. *Archives of General Psychiatry, 48,* 1069-1074.

Breslau, N., Kilbey, M., and Andreski, P. (1993). Nicotine dependence and major depression: New evidence from a prospective investigation. *Archives of General Psychiatry, 50,* 31-35.

Burke, J.D., Loeber, R., and Lahey, B.B. (2001). Which aspects of ADHD are associated with substance use in early adolescence? *Journal of Child Psychology and Psychiatry, 42,* 493-502.

Chaloupka, F.J. (2003). Contextual factors and youth tobacco use: Policy linkages. *Addiction, 98,* 147-149.

Chassin, L., Presson, C.C., Rose, J.S., and Sherman, S.J. (1996). The natural history of cigarette smoking from adolescence to adulthood: Demographic predictors of continuity and change. *Health Psychology, 15,* 478-484.

Chassin, L., Presson C.C., and Sherman S.J. (1990). Social psychological contributions to the understanding and prevention of adolescent cigarette smoking. *Personality and Social Psychology Bulletin, 16,* 133-151.

Chassin, L., Presson C.C., Sherman S.J., and Kim, K. (2002). Long-term psychological sequelae of smoking cessation and relapse. *Health Psychology, 21,* 438-443.

Chassin, L., Presson, C.C., Sherman, S.J., Montello, D., and McGrew, J. (1986). Changes in peer and parent influence during adolescence: Longitudinal versus cross-sectional perspectives on smoking initiation. *Developmental Psychology, 22,* 327-334.

Cohen, J., Cohen, P., West, S.G., and Aiken, L.S. (2003). *Applied multiple regression/correlation analysis for the behavioral sciences* (3rd ed.). Mahwah, NJ: Erlbaum.

Costello, E.J., and Angold, A. (1988). Scales to assess child and adolescent depression-Checklists, screens and nets. *Journal of the American Academy of Child and Adolescent Psychiatry, 27,* 726-737.

Derzon, J.H., and Lipsey, M.W. (1999). Predicting tobacco use to age 18: A synthesis of longitudinal research. *Addiction, 94,* 995-1006.

Diem, E.C., McKay, L.C., and Jamieson, J.L. (1994). Female adolescent alcohol, cigarette, and marijuana use: Similarities and differences in patterns of use. *The International Journal of the Addictions, 29,* 987-997.

D'Unger, A.V., Land, K.C., McCall, P.L., and Nagin, D.S. (1998). How many latent classes of delinquent/criminal careers? Results from mixed Poison regression analyses. *American Journal of Sociology, 103,* 1593-1630.

Edelbrock, C.S., and Achenbach, T.M. (1984). The teacher version of the Child Behavior Profile: I. Boys ages 6-11. *Journal of Consulting and Clinical Psychology, 52,* 207-217.

Flay, B., Hu, F.B., Siddiqui, O., Day, L.E., Hedeker, D., Petraitsi, J., Richardson, J., and Sussan, S. (1994). Differential influence of parental smoking and friends' smoking on adolescent initiation and escalation of smoking. *Journal of Health and Social Behavior, 35,* 248-265.

Flint, A.J., Yamanda, E.G., and Novotny, T.E. (1998). Black-white differences in cigarette smoking uptake: Progression from adolescent experimentation to regular use. *Preventive Medicine, 27,* 358-364.

Gardiner, P. (2001). African American teen cigarette smoking: A review. In D. Burns (Ed.), *Changing adolescent smoking prevalence: Where is it and why.* Tobacco Control Monograph 14 (pp. 213-226) (NIH Pub. No. 02-5086). Bethesda, MD: National Cancer Institute.

Glassman, A.H., Helzer, J.E., Covey, L.S., Cottler, L.B., Stetner, F., Tipp, J.E., and Johnson, J. (1990). Smoking, smoking cessation, and major depression. *Journal of the American Medical Association, 264,* 1546-1549.

Gorman, D., and White, H.R. (1995). You can choose your friends, but do they choose your crime? Differential association theories for crime prevention policy. In H. Barlow (Ed.), Criminology and public policy: Putting theory to work, pp. 131-155. Boulder, CO: Westview Press.

Gottfredson, D.C., and Koper, C.S. (1996). Race and sex differences in the prediction of drug use. *Journal of Consulting and Clinical Psychology, 64,* 305-313.

Griesler, P.C., and Kandel, D.B. (1998). Ethnic differences in correlates of adolescent smoking. *Journal of Adolescent Health, 23,* 167-180.

Gritz, E.R., Prokhorov, A.V., Hudmon, K.S., Chamberlain, R.M., Taylor, W.C., DiClemente, C.C., Johnston, D.A., Hu, S., Jones, L.A., Jones, M.M., Rosenblum, C.K., Ayars, C.L., and Amos, C. (1998). Cigarette smoking in a multiethnic population of youth: Methods and baseline findings. *Preventive Medicine, 27,* 365-384.

Hestick, H., Perrino, S.C., Rhodes, W.A., and Sydnor, K.D. (2001). Trial and lifetime smoking risks among African American college students. *Journal of American College Health, 49,* 213-219.

Hollingshead, A.B. (1975). *Four factor index of social status.* Unpublished manuscript. Department of Sociology at Yale University, MA.

Johnston, L.D., O'Malley, P.M., and Bachman, J.G. (2003). *Monitoring the Future: National survey results on drug use from the Monitoring the Future Study, 1975-2001. Vol. I, Secondary school students.* Bethesda. National Institute on Drug Abuse.

Jones, B.L., Nagin, D.S., and Roeder, K. (2001). A SAS procedure based on mixture models for estimating developmental trajectories. *Sociological Methods and Research, 29,* 374-393.

Juon, H.S., Ensminger, M.E., and Sydnor, K.D. (2002). A longitudinal study of developmental trajectories to young adult cigarette smoking. *Drug and Alcohol Dependency, 66,* 303-314.

Kandel, D.B., Chen, K., Warner, L.A., Kessler, R.C., and Grant, B. (1997). Prevalence and demographic correlates of symptoms of last year dependence on alcohol, nicotine, marijuana, and cocaine in the US population. *Drug and Alcohol Dependence, 44,* 11-29.

Kandel, D.B., and Davies, M. (1986). Adult sequelae of adolescent depressive symptoms. *Archives of General Psychiatry, 43,* 255-262.

Kandel, D.B., Kiros, G.-E., Schaffran, C., and Hu, M.-C. (2004). Racial/ethnic differences in cigarettes smoking initiation and progression to daily smoking: A multilevel analysis. *American Journal of Public Health, 94,* 128-135.

Landrine, H., Richardson, J.L., Klonoff, E.A., and Flay, B. (1994). Cultural diversity in the predictors of adolescent cigarette smoking: The relative influence of peers. *Journal of Behavioral Medicine, 17,* 331-346.

Lloyd-Richardson, E.E., Papandonatos, G., Kazura, A., Stanton, C., and Niaura, R. (2002). Differentiating stages of smoking intensity among adolescents: Stage-specific psychological and social influences. *Journal of Consulting and Clinical Psychology, 70,* 998-1009.

Loeber, R., Farrington, D.P., Stouthamer-Loeber, M., and Van Kammen, W.B. (1998). *Antisocial behavior and mental health problems: Explanatory factors in childhood and adolescence.* Mahwah, NJ: Lawrence Erlbaum Associates.

Mayhew, K.P., Flay, B.R. and Mott, J.A. (2000). Stages in the development of adolescent smoking. *Drug and Alcohol Dependence, 59,* s-61-s81.

Nagin, D.S. (1999). Analyzing developmental trajectories: A semiparametric, group-based approach. *Psychological Methods, 4,* 139-157.

Nagin, D.S. (2005). *Group-based modeling of development.* Cambridge, MA: Harvard University Press.

Nagin, D.S., and Land, K.C. (1993). Age, criminal career, and population heterogeneity: Specification and estimation of a nonparametic mixed Poisson model. *Criminology, 31,* 327-362.

Nagin, D.S., and Tremblay, R.E. (1999). Trajectories of boy's physical aggression, opposition, and hyperactivity on the path to physically violent and non-violent juvenile delinquency. *Child Development, 7,* 1181-1196.

Nagin, D.S., and Tremblay, R.E. (2001). Analyzing developmental trajectories of distinct but related behaviors: A group-based method. *Psychological Methods, 6,* 18-34.

National Center for Chronic Disease Prevention and Health Promotion. (2004). Adult cigarette smoking in the united states: Current estimates. Fact Sheet, May 2004 obtained on-line http://www.cdc.gov/tobacco/factsheets/AdultCigaretteSmoking_FactSheet.htm)

Newcomb, M.D., McCarthy, W.J., and Bentler, P.M. (1989). Cigarette smoking, academic lifestyle, and social impact efficacy: An eight-year study from early adolescence to young adulthood. *Journal of Applied Social Psychology, 19*, 251-281.

Nichter, M. (2003). Smoking: What does culture have to do with it? *Addiction, 98*, 139-145.

Patrick, D.L., Cheadle, A., Thompson, D.C., Diehr, P., Koepsell, T., and Kinne, S. (1994). The validity of self-reported smoking: A review and meta-analysis. *American Journal of Public Health, 84*, 1086-1093.

Patton, G.C., Hibbert, M., Rosier, M.J., Carlin, J.B., Caust, J., and Bowes, G. (1996). Is smoking associated with depression and anxiety in teenagers? *American Journal of Public Health, 86*, 225-230.

Raftery, A.E. (1995). Bayesian model selection in social research. *Sociological Methodology, 25*, 111-164.

Robinson, L.A., Klesges, R.C., Zbikowski, S.M., and Glaser, R. (1997). Predictors of risk for different stages of adolescent smoking in a biracial sample. *Journal of Consulting and Clinical Psychology, 65*, 653-662.

Roeder, K., Lynch, K.G., and Nagin, D.S. (1999). Modeling uncertainty in latent class membership: A case study in criminology. *Journal of the American Statistical Association, 94,* 766-776.

Rose, J., Chassin, L., Presson, C. C., and Sherman, S. J. (1996). Demographic factors in adult smoking status: Mediating and moderating influences. *Psychology of Addictive Behaviors, 10*, 28-37.

Schulenburg, J.E., and Maggs, J.L. (2002) A developmental perspective on alcohol use and heavy drinking during adolescence and the transition to young adulthood. *Journal of Studies on Alcohol, Supplement No. 14*, 54-70.

Schulenberg, J., Wadsworth, K.N., O'Malley, P.M., Bachman, J.G., and Johnston, L.D. (1996). Adolescent risk factors for binge drinking during the transition to young adulthood: Variable-and pattern-centered approaches to change. *Developmental Psychology, 32*, 659-674.

Storr, C.L., Ialongo, N.S., Kellam, S.G., Anthony, J.C. (2002). A randomized controlled trial of two primary intervention strategies to prevent early onset of tobacco smoking. *Drug and Alcohol Dependence, 66*, 51-60.

Stouthamer-Loeber, M., Loeber, R., Farrington, D.P., Zhang, Q., van Kammen, W., and Maguin, E. (1993). The double edge of protective and risk factors for delinquency: Interrelations and developmental patterns. *Development and Psychopathology, 5*, 683-701.

Stouthamer-Loeber, M., Loeber, R., Wei, E., Farrington, D.P., and Wilkstrom, P-O. (2002). Risk and promotive effects in the explanation of persistent serious delinquency in boys. *Journal of Consulting and Clinical Psychology, 70*, 111-123.

Stouthamer-Loeber, M., Wei, E., Loeber, R., and Masten, A.S. (2004). Desistance from persistent serious delinquency in the transition to adulthood. *Development and Psychopathology, 16,* 897-918.

Stouthamer-Loeber, M. and Van Kammen, W. (1995). Stouthamer-Loeber, M., and Van Kammen,

W. B. (1995). Data collection and management: A practical guide. Newbury Park, CA.: Sage.

Sussman, S., Dent, C.W., Stacy, A.W. Burton, D., and Flay, B.R. (1995). Developing school-based tobacco use prevention and cessation programs. Thousand Oaks, CA: Sage Publications, Inc., 1995.

Unger, J.B., Rohrbach, L.A., Cruz, T.B., Baezconde-Garbanati, L., Howard, K.A. Palmer, P.H., and Johnson, C.A. (2001). Ethnic variation in peer influence on adolescent smoking. *Nicotine and Tobacco Research, 3*, 167-176.

US Department of Health and Human Services (1998). *Tobacco use among US racial/ethnic minority groups: A report of the surgeon general.* Atlanta, Georgia: USDHHS, CSC.

Wallace, J.M. and Muroff, J.R. (2002). Preventing substance abuse among African American children and youth: Race differences in risk factor exposure and vulnerability. *The Journal of Primary Prevention, 22*, 235-261.

White, H.R., Nagin, D., Replogle, E., and Stouthamer-Loeber, M. (2004). Racial differences in trajectories of cigarette use. *Drug and Alcohol Dependence, 76*, 219-227.

White, H.R., Pandina, R.J., and Chen, P-H. (2002). Developmental trajectories of cigarette smoking from adolescence to young adulthood. *Drug and Alcohol Dependence, 65*, 167-178.

Wilcox, P. (2003). An ecological approach to understanding youth smoking trajectories: Problems and prospects. *Addiction, 98*, 57-78.

Williams, J.G., and Covington, C.J. (1997). Predictors of cigarette smoking among adolescents. *Psychological Reports, 80*, 481-482.

Winefield, H.R., Winefield, A.H., and Tiggemann, M. (1992). Psychological attributes of young adult smokers. *Psychological Reports, 70*, 675-681.

www.monitoringthefuture.org. The Monitoring the Future Study, the University of Michigan.

In: Racial and Ethnic Disparities in Health and Health Care
Editor: Elene V. Metrosa, pp. 131-147

ISBN 1-60021-268-9
© 2006 Nova Science Publishers, Inc.

Chapter 6

Addressing Mental Health Disparities: A Preliminary Test of the Multicultural Assessment Intervention Process (MAIP) Model

Glenn Gamst, * *Richard Rogers and Aghop Der-Karabetian*
University of La Verne, La Verne, CA
Richard H. Dana
Regional Research Institute, Portland State University

Abstract

Racial and ethnic disparities in American health and healthcare are becoming increasingly apparent and are garnering a growing body of research attention (e.g., La Viest, 2005). These disparities are particularly problematic regarding mental health service delivery to multicultural populations (Snowden and Yamada, 2005; U.S. Department of Health and Human Services, 2001). The present study explores a variety of key parameters associated with the Multicultural Assessment Intervention Process (MAIP) model proposed by Dana (1993, 1998, 2000) and Dana, Aragon, and Kramer, (2002). This model provides a mental health agency and its practitioners with the necessary conceptual scaffolding and theoretical clarity to address service delivery disparities by positing that mental health consumers are best served when factors such as (1) consumer-provider ethnic/racial match, (2) consumer acculturation status and/or ethnic/racial identity, and (3) provider cultural competence are assessed and factored into the treatment process and clinical outcome. Toward this end, a sample of 123 university counseling center consumers was measured on the 4 previous independent variables (i.e., ethnic/racial match, acculturation status, ethnic identity, and staff cultural competence). Five clinical outcome dependent measures were assessed including Global Assessment of Function (GAF) pre and post treatment differences, and 4 subscales of the Brief

---

* Correspondence concerning this chapter should be addressed to Glenn Gamst, Department of Psychology, University of La Verne, 1950 Third Street, La Verne, CA 91750 (e-mail: gamstg@ulv.edu).

Psychiatric Rating Scale (BPRS): Thinking Disturbance, Withdrawal/Retardation, Hostile-Suspicious, and Anxious-Depression, all of which served as dependent variables. A 2 x 2 x 2 x 2 factorial between-subjects multivariate analysis of covariance (MANCOVA) indicated a statistically significant multivariate interaction effect between Ethnic Match x Client Acculturation x Client Ethnic Identity for the BPRS-thinking disturbance measure. Implications for the MAIP model with this college student population are discussed.

INTRODUCTION

The issue of health disparities or inequality in the United States is receiving more attention from researchers, practitioners, and politicians. The National Institutes of Health (cited by LaViest, 2005, p. 108) operationalize the concept of health disparities as "differences in the incidence, prevalence, mortality and burden of diseases and other adverse health conditions that exist among specific population groups in the United States".

A recent groundbreaking monograph by the Institute of Medicine (2002) titled *Unequal treatment: Confronting Racial and Ethnic Disparities in Health Care*, documented a considerable body of evidence demonstrating that White Americans receive better quality of health care than do people of color. This report aptly contextualized the poor clinical outcomes, underutilization of services, and low levels of service satisfaction that racial/ethnic minorities experience as part of the historical legacy of racism and discrimination people of color continue to cope with.

In the realm of mental health, these same concerns regarding disparities were echoed in the 2001 U.S. Surgeon General's supplemental report titled *Mental Health: A Report of the Surgeon General* (U.S. Department of Health and Human Services, 2001). In this report, it is argued that the U.S. mental health system may be ill prepared to meet the mental health needs of racial/ethnic groups due to deficiencies in the level of cultural competence among service providers of all types (e.g., psychiatrists, therapists, case managers) (see also, Gamst, et al., 2004). Cultural competence deficiencies are exacerbated by the unique cultural differences displayed by racial/ethnic groups with regard to coping styles, utilization of services, help-seeking attitudes and behaviors, and the use of family and community as resources (U.S. Department of Health and Human Services, 2001).

RACIAL /ETHNIC GROUP RISK FACTORS

While not meant to be a comprehensive compilation, below is a brief overview of some significant and unique mental health challenges and needs of the four underserved racial/ethnic groups in the United States.

African Americans

Evidence indicates that African Americans may be at a higher risk of mental disorders than White Americans due to socioeconomic differences (Reiger, et al.,1993) and perceived racism (Dana, 2002). African Americans tend to be underrepresented in outpatient treatment, yet overrepresented in inpatient treatment facilities at the rate of twice that for White Americans (Snowden and Cheung, 1990; Snowden, 1999). Additionally, African Americans are more likely to utilize emergency room services for mental health problems than White Americans (Snowden, 1999).

Native American Indians

A genuine paucity of epidemiological survey research exists currently on the incidence of mental disorders or the mental health needs of this population. High levels of poverty, poor general health and mental health are disproportionately associated with Native Americans (Manson, 2000). Depression and alcohol abuse continue to be a significant problem for many Native American Indians, along with increasing suicide rates (see Novins, Duclos, Martin, Jewett, and Manson, 1999).

Asian Americans/Pacific Islanders

It is difficult to assess this population's mental illness prevalence rates due to methodological challenges such as lack of adequate population sub-sampling. In general, Asian Americans/Pacific Islanders tend to not seek help for mental health problems (Leong and Lau, 2001), and underutilize both outpatient and inpatient treatment because of perceived stigma, and language barriers (Leong, 2001).

Latino Americans

The Epidemiologic Catchment Area Study (ECA) (Robins and Reiger, 1991) found similar rates of psychiatric disorders between Mexican Americans and White Americans, however, higher rates of depression and phobias were reported among acculturated Latino Americans in comparison to White Americans. Differential needs among Latino subgroups have been identified (U.S. Department of Health and Human Services, 2001). Specifically, Central American immigrants who have experienced trauma in their country of origin may have the greatest mental health needs. Exacerbating these problems is the fact that over one-third of Latino Americans have no health insurance (National Center for Health Statistics, 2003).

Clearly, the mental health needs and challenges of these racial and ethnic minority groups is real, immediate, and growing. To address these needs, the U.S. Surgeon General's Supplemental Report has encouraged the development and evaluation of culturally responsive evidence-based mental health treatment services. For example, this report notes that "culture and language affect the perception, utilization, and potentially, the outcomes of mental health services. Therefore, the provision of culturally and linguistically appropriate mental health services is a key ingredient for any programming design to meet the needs of diverse racial and ethnic populations" (U.S. Department of Health and Human Services, 2001, p. 166). The development of the Multicultural Assessment Intervention Process (MAIP) model is one attempt to address mental health disparities within a comprehensive system.

THE MULTICULTURAL ASSESSMENT INTERVENTION PROCESS (MAIP) FRAMEWORK

The MAIP has its roots in a multicultural historical trichotomy that includes issues of social justice, multicultural training and assessment, and large-scale mental health systems of care models. Persistent public sector mental health services disparities are addressed with the MAIP by routinely probing client preference for ethnic, gender, or linguistic match with their provider, using culturally appropriate social etiquette and service delivery styles, with culturally competent mental health providers, evaluating client acculturation status and ethnic identity, and determining the beneficial application of cultural formulations and ethnic-specific services.

The MAIP developed essentially as a multiculturally sensitive assessment model for mental health consumer populations (Dana, 1993, 1998, 2000), and was one of six models recently reviewed by Ponterotto, Gretchen, and Chauhan, (2000). The most recent iteration of the MAIP (see, Dana, Aragon, and Kramer, 2002) and its component parts can be seen in Figure 1.

In its bare essence, The MAIP can be construed as a funnel that routes a diverse mental health consumer clientele to a limited amount of agency resources. As can be seen in Figure 1, this is accomplished in a seven-step process. First, clients are screened, presenting problems and personal history are evaluated, client matching preferences are noted, preliminary diagnosis, Global Assessment of Function (GAF), and other initial clinical outcome and cultural assessments are made. Second, cultural, linguistic, and gender client preferences and needs are addressed, with the overall aim of achieving a balance between the client goals and the available agency human resources. Recent evidence indicates that client requests for specific ethnic/cultural matches range between one-fourth and one-third of community mental health populations. For example, Gamst et al. (2003) reported that 24.2% of their Asian American sample requested a cultural match. Similarly, Gamst et al. (2002) reported 32.9% of their Latino Americans requested a cultural match. Third, determining acculturation status of ethnic/racial minority clients through standard classification procedures (e.g., acculturated, bicultural, marginal, traditional) and assessing ethnic identity status of all clients (e.g., high or low ethnic identity) provides crucial information in the treatment planning and service delivery process. Fourth, to this point the model has focused on the mental health consumer. However, the MAIP also postulates that we scrutinize the cultural competence of the mental health provider. Due to differences in training and clinical experience, providers vary in their cultural knowledge, skills, and abilities (Gamst et al., 2004). Hence, cultural competence of all mental health providers must be routinely assessed and the results of that assessment incorporated into the client disposition or resource allocation process. Fifth, these differences in staff cultural competencies will drive the allocation of multicultural training resources (Dana et al., 2006). Sixth, based on the previous steps, a determination is made as to the viability and usefulness of providing the client with a culture/ethnic-specific clinical intervention. Most clients neither seek nor desire ethnic-specific services. The key question then becomes which clients would benefit from these ethnic-specific services and which clients might be engaged alternatively with more standard culture-general treatment interventions? The MAIP model weighs in on this fundamental resource allocation question by suggesting that traditional (unacculturated) clients may need to be linguistically and ethnically matched with culturally competent providers using specialized cultural formulations and interventions. Conversely, many acculturated clients do not expect or require mental health services from an ethnically matched provider or a culture-specific intervention. However, the MAIP model does prescribe that all mental health consumers be treated with dignity and respect, including provider service delivery styles and social etiquette that acknowledge and embrace such consideration. The seventh and final step of the MAIP model is the client/provider completion of a variety of posttest outcome measures of the client's functioning at the end of treatment or at annual review. Consumer service satisfaction measures would also be completed at this juncture.

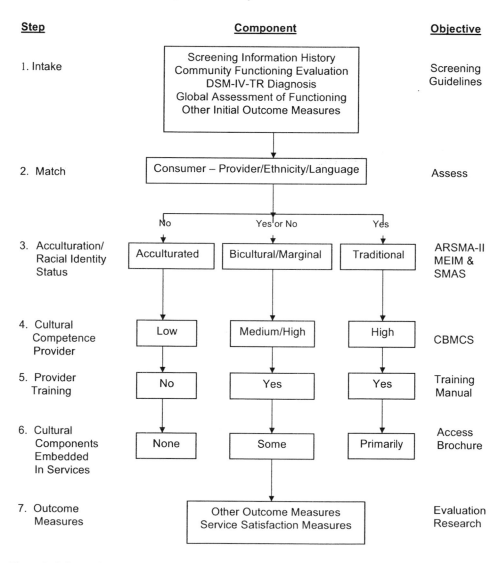

Figure1. Schematic Flow Chart of MAIP Model Components.

Clearly, the MAIP model as depicted in Figure 1 proscribes or argues against the typical community mental health practice of connecting a mental health consumer to the first available mental health provider resource. Rather, this model encourages a thoughtful and careful evaluation of the client as a cultural being in a multicultural milieu. By injecting a multicultural focus and formulation into the therapeutic process, the MAIP should increase consumer satisfaction and attitudes toward the counseling process. These beneficial attitudes should, in turn, reduce the client "churn" or dropout rate after the first session, thereby, reducing mental health disparities.

Present Study

The present study examined key parameters of the MAIP (e.g., client-provider ethnic match, client acculturation, client ethnic identity, and provider cultural competence) on the clinical outcome of a sample of college students seeking mental health services at a university counseling center. The basic question under study is to what extent do the MAIP variables interact with each other, and contribute to clinical outcome?

Method

The population under study included all students who received mental health services at a southern California, private university counseling center between September 2004 and May 2005. The process of assigning students to mental health providers was a random process, driven primarily by staff caseloads and occasionally the special needs or preferences of the student. Client and provider ethnicity were based on self-report. The racial composition of the sample data reflect a complete census of university students who received mental health services at an university counseling center during the course of Academic Year 2004-2005. Twenty clients were eliminated from the present study (8 African American, 6 bi-racial, 4 Asian American, 2 other) due to small sub-sample sizes. The final total sample of 123 clients included 66 (53.7%) White American and 57 (46.3%) Latino American clients.

Clients received culture-general services from nine mental health providers, 8 of whom were female. The ethnic breakdown of the providers was 4 White Americans, 3 Latino Americans, 1 Asian American, and 1 bi-racial provider. Provider degree status was as follows: 1 Psy.D, 4 Psy.D 3rd year graduate students, 2 Psy.D 2nd year graduate students, and 2 Marriage and Family Counseling 2nd year graduate students. Clients received a variety of outpatient services including individual therapy, group therapy, and case management.

Variables

Four main independent variables were used in this study: client ethnicity, client-provider ethnic match, client ethnic identity, and client acculturation status. Two additional variables served as covariates to adjust the dependent variables: client-provider gender match, and provider cultural competence. Client ethnicity was dichotomized as White American, and Latino American (coded 1, or 0, respectively).

Client-provider ethnic match was dichotomized as match or no match (coded as 1, or 0, respectively) and followed the operationalization offered by Gamst, Dana, Der-Karabetian, and Kramer, (2004), who considered that an ethnic match existed when the provider who made the admission evaluation of functioning had the same ethnicity as the client.

Client ethnic identity was dichotomized as either high or low (coded as 1, or 0, respectively), and was based on the 12-item Multigroup Ethnic Identity Measure (MEIM) (Phinney, 1992; Roberts et al., 1999). This measure is composed of two subscales (ethnic identity search, and affirmation, belonging, and commitment). Internal consistency as measured by Cronbach's alpha was computed on all clients who completed the MEIM. High reliability was observed for both subscales: Ethnic identity search (alpha = .79) and affirmation, belonging, and commitment (alpha = .92). Because the present study found strong positive correlation ($r = .52$) between the two MEIM subscales, only one (affirmation, belonging, and commitment) was used as a measure of ethnic identity.

Likewise, client acculturation was measured using the 32-item Stephenson Multigroup Acculturation Scale (SMAS) (see, Stephenson, 2000). This measure is composed of two subscales (ethnic society immersion, and dominant society immersion). Internal consistency as measured by Cronbach's alpha was again high for both subscales: Ethnic society immersion (alpha = .82) and dominant society immersion (alpha = .86). Again, the present study discovered strong positive correlation between the two SMAS subscales ($r = .79$) indicating considerable conceptual and empirical overlap, thus only one of the subscales (dominant society immersion) was used as our measure of client acculturation status. This measure was dichotomized as high or low (coded as 1, or 0, respectively) and was based on a median split of the dominant society immersion subscale of the SMAS. The correlation observed between the composite SMAS and MEIM scales was $r = -.32$, indicating that the two scales were measuring separate constructs.

Two dichotomous covariates were used to adjust the dependent variables. Gender match between client and provider was defined as either gender match or no gender match (coded as 1, or 0, respectively). Provider cultural competence was based on the California Brief Multicultural Competence Scale (CBMCS) developed by Gamst et al. (2004). This 21-item scale is composed of four subscales that include multicultural knowledge, awareness of cultural barriers, sensitivity and responsiveness to consumers, and sociocultural diversities. For purposes of the present study, a median split was computed on the entire 21-item scale which classified providers as being either high or low in overall cultural competence (coded as 1, or 0, respectively).

Clinical Outcome Variables

Five dependent variables were used in the present study. One dependent measure was the Global Assessment of Functioning (GAF) Axis V rating of the *Diagnostic and Statistical Manual of Mental Disorders*, fourth edition (DSM-IV; American Psychiatric Association, 1994). The GAF was completed by the mental health provider at intake, and again at termination, and a computed difference score examined all phases of the treatment process. GAF scale values can range from 1 (severe impairment) to 100 (good general functioning). GAF-difference scores were computed for each client by means of subtraction (e.g., GAF at time 2 minus GAF at time 1). A positive GAF-difference score indicated a more positive clinical assessment by the counselor at termination; conversely, a negative GAF-difference score indicated a more pessimistic clinical assessment by the mental health provider at termination. Adequate reliability and validity have been reported using this subjective measure (e.g., Jones, Thornicroft, Coffey, and Dunn, 1995).

Four additional dependent measures were developed from the 18-item Brief Psychiatric Rating Scale (BPRS; Overall and Gorham, 1988). Following the factor analytic work with this scale by Hedlund and Vieweg, (1980), four subscales were computed by summing the individual items comprising the subscale. These subscales (dependent measures) included: Thinking disturbance (three items, alpha = .44), withdrawl/retardation (two items, alpha = .32), hostile/suspiciousness (three items, alpha = .55), and anxious/depression (three items, alpha = .72). Clients were evaluated on the BPRS at intake and at termination. A difference score was computed on the sums of each BPRS subscale (i.e., time 2 minus time 1). A negative subscale value indicates improvement in client functioning. A positive value indicates a more pessimistic appraisal of the client by the mental health provider at termination. The relatively weak internal consistency of several of the BPRS subscales is possibly due to the paucity of items making up each individual subscale, and also may indicate a lack of sensitivity among these BPRS subscales in discriminating client functioning among college students seeking mental health services.

Sample Characteristics

A breakdown of sample characteristics by client ethnicity can be seen in Table 1. Of the 123 students who received mental health services, 57 (46.3%) were Latino Americans and 66 (53.7%) were White Americans. The mean age of the clients was 24 years and nearly three-fourths were female. Over eight of ten of the clients were single, never married. Roughly, four of ten clients were ethnically matched with a mental health provider. Gender matches occurred for about seven of ten clients, primarily for the females. High ethnic identity was found in half of the Latino Americans and in about four of ten White Americans. High acculturation was twice the level for Latino Americans (70.2%) as for White Americans (35.6%).

Analysis Strategy

Two sets of statistical analyses were computed with several independent and dependent variables. First inter-item correlations were computed among all independent, dependent, and covariate measures in this study. Second, one four-way between-subjects multivariate analysis of covariance (MANCOVA) was conducted using client ethnicity (2 levels), ethnic match (2 levels), client acculturation (2 levels), and client ethnic identity (2 levels) as independent variables and GAF-difference, and four BPRS subscales (thinking disturbance, withdrawl/retardation, hostile/suspiciousness, anxious/depression) served as dependent measures. Two covariates were used to adjust the five dependent variables in the MANCOVA model. These covariates were gender match and provider cultural competence. The first covariate has been found in previous research (see, Gamst et al., 2000; 2001; 2003) to provide significant adjustment.

Table 1. Sample Characteristics by Client Ethnicity

	Total	Latino American	White American
Sample size	123	57	66
Mean age	24.0	23.8	24.2
Percentage female	74.0	77.2	71.2
Percentage single marital status	84.6	86.0	83.3
Percentage ethnic match	43.9	35.1	51.5
Percentage gender match	69.9	71.9	68.2
Percentage high ethnic identity	45.3	50.9	40.0
Percentage high acculturation	52.6	70.2$_a$	35.6$_b$

Note. Tests of statistical significance of difference between proportions is used for variables summarized by percentages. Variables represented by means are evaluated with analysis of variance. Percentages or means in the same row with subscripts that differ are statistically significantly different at the .01 level of significance. The ethnic identity measure is based on a median split of the affirmation, belongingness, and commitment subscale of the MEIM. The acculturation measure is based on a median split of the dominant society immersion subscale of the SMAS.

RESULTS

As can be seen in Table 2, Pearson correlations among the covariates and independent and dependent variables in the study generated low to moderate correlation. Specifically, client ethnicity was negatively correlated with client acculturation. Ethnic match produced a low negative correlation with the BPRS- thinking-disturbance measure. The GAF-difference measure was found to be negatively correlated with the BPRS thinking disturbance and anxious/depression measures.

Table 2. Pearson Correlations Among Independent and Dependent Variables and Covariates

Variables	1	2	3	4	5	6	7	8	9	10	11
1. Ethnic match	--	.17	-.17	-.13	.01	.08	.05	-.23*	.03	-.09	.11
2. Client ethnicity		--	-.35*	-.11	.06	-.04	.05	-.14	.17	-.12	.13
3. Client acculturation			--	-.14	.07	.04	.01	.02	-.15	.08	-.25*
4. Client ethnic identity				--	-.03	-.14	-.05	.14	.15	.15	-.18
5. Provider cultural competence					--	.15	.12	-.13	-.17	21*	.01
6. Gender match						--	-.07	-.12	-.19	-.12	-.05
7. GAF-difference							--	-.29*	-.19	-.07	-.37*
8. BPRS-TD								--	.14	.20*	.10
9. BPRS-WR									--	.29*	.32*
10. BPRS-HS										--	-.05
11. BPRS-AD											--

N=123

*p<.01

BPRS-TD=Brief Psychiatric Rating Scale-Thinking Disturbance, BPRS-WR=Brief Psychiatric Rating Scale-Withdrawal/Retardation, BPRS-HS=Brief Psychiatric Rating Scale-Hostile/Suspiciousness, BPRS-AD=Brief Psychiatric Rating Scale-Anxious/Depression.

Multivariate Analysis of Covariance Model

A 2 x 2 x 2 x 2 between-subjects multivariate analysis of covariance (MANCOVA) was performed on five dependent measures associated with client outcomes: GAF-difference, BPRS-thinking disturbance, BPRS-withdrawl/retardation, BPRS-hostile/suspiciousness, BPRS-anxious/depression. Adjustment was made for two covariates: gender match and provider cultural competence. Independent variables were client ethnicity (White American, Latino American), ethnic match (match, no match), client acculturation (high, low), and client ethnic identity (high, low).

SPSS General Linear Model: Multivariate was used for this analysis. Total $N = 123$ cases with no cases eliminated due to missing data. There were no univariate or multivariate within-cell outliers at $\alpha = .01$. Evaluation of cases for multivariate assumptions was satisfactory, and covariates were considered reliable for covariate analysis.

Due to a statistically significant Box's M Test of equality of covariance matrices ($p < .001$), Pillai's Trace was used as the multivariate test statistic (see, Meyers, Gamst, and Guarino, 2006). Using Pillai's criterion, the combined dependent variables were statistically significantly related to ethnic match $F (5, 75) = 2.24$, $p < .05$, partial $\eta^2 = .13$, client acculturation $F (5, 75) = 2.69$, $p < .03$, partial $\eta^2 = .15$, and the multivariate interaction effects of, Ethnic Match x Client Acculturation $F (5, 75) = 2.41$. $p < .04$, partial $\eta^2 = .14$, Ethnic Match x Client Ethnicity $F (5, 75) = 3.08$, $p < .01$, partial $\eta^2 = .17$, and Ethnic Match x Client Acculturation x Client Ethnic Identity $F (5, 75) = 3.04$, $p < .01$, partial $\eta^2 = .17$.

Neither covariate (gender match or provider cultural competence) significantly adjusted the dependent measures ($p > .05$). While five multivariate main and interaction effects were found in the present study, we will focus on interpreting the multivariate triple interaction of Ethnic Match x Client Acculturation x Client Ethnic Identity, since it takes interpretive precedence over the other statistically significant effects.

Table 3. Adjusted Means and Standard Errors for BPRS-Thinking Disturbance by Ethnic Match, Client Acculturation, and Client Ethnic Identity.

Ethnic Match	Acculturation	Ethnic Identity	M	SE
Match	Low	Low	-.27	.34
		High	-.04	.27
	High	Low	-.04	.25
		High	-.57	.54
No Match	Low	Low	1.86	.47
		High	-.01	.26
	High	Low	-.18	.20
		High	.44	.25

Note. A Negative BPRS-Thinking Disturbance Mean indicates an improvement in client functioning between intake and termination as assessed by the mental health provider. A positive value indicates a more pessimistic appraisal between Time 1 and Time 2.

Univariate three-way between-subjects analyses of covariance (ANCOVAs), followed by simple-simple effects analyses, were conducted on each dependent measure separately to determine the locus of the statistically significant multivariate triple interaction effect. Only the BPRS-thinking disturbance dependent variable reached statistical significance, $F(1, 79) = 11.34$, $p < .001$, partial $\eta^2 = .13$. Table 3 displays the means for the BPRS-thinking disturbance triple interaction effect.

Due to the fact that after adjusting for differences on the covariates, only the univariate Ethnic Match x Client Acculturation x Client Ethnic Identity interaction effect was found to be statistically significant, a simple-simple effects analysis (see Levine, 1991) collapsed across each level of ethnic match and client acculturation was conducted ($p < .05$). No statistically significant differences were observed among the ethnic match treatment conditions ($p > .05$). However, clients in the no match, low acculturation, and low ethnic identity conditions ($M = 1.86$, $SE = .47$) garnered more pessimistic appraisals from their mental health providers than did their no match, low acculturation, and high ethnic identity counterparts ($M = -.01$, $SE = .26$). This result produced the multivariate triple interaction effect for the BPRS-thinking disturbance measure.

DISCUSSION

The present study examined relationships among client ethnicity, client-provider ethnic match, client acculturation, and client ethnic identity on five types of clinical outcome, while controlling for client-provider gender match and provider cultural competence with college student clients. Results, adjusted for the effects of the covariates, indicated a statistically significant multivariate triple interaction effect among the client-provider ethnic match, client acculturation, and client ethnic identity variables. Subsequent univariate analyses indicated the locus of the multivariate effect to be with the BPRS-thinking disturbance dependent measure. Specifically, this dependent measure indicated poorer outcome or lack of clinical progress (between initial intake and termination of services) among clients who were not ethnically matched, and were unacculturated, and indicated low ethnic identity. This finding provides limited support for the MAIP model in that poorer clinical outcomes are predicted among college student clients who are culturally marginalized, have low ethnic identity, and who do not experience mental health services from providers who are culturally similar to them.

Surprisingly, the independent variables produced a statistically significant impact on only one of the five dependent measures (BPRS-thinking disturbance). This finding suggests that the GAF-difference and other three BPRS subscales may not be sensitive enough to capture variability for this particular college student population.

This study underscores the importance of including salient independent variables (e.g., matching, acculturation, ethnic identity, cultural competence), identified by the MAIP model during the course of mental health assessment and intervention.

Recent reviews of the ethnic/racial matching literature (e.g., Karlsson, 2005; Maramba and Hall, 2002; Shin et al., 2005) indicate the importance of client-provider matching in the context of the other MAIP variables. Additional empirical evidence demonstrating the importance of ethnic matching to clinical outcome, and analogous to the present findings, can be found with adult African American, Latino American, and White American community mental health consumers (e.g., Gamst, Dana, Der-Karabetian, and Kramer, 2000), Adult Asian American community mental health consumers (Gamst et al., 2003; Gamst, Dana, Der-

Karabetian, and Kramer, 2001), and African American, Latino American, and White American child and adolescent community mental health consumers (Gamst, Dana, Der-Karabetian, and Kramer, 2004). Some of the variability in the previous match literature may be affected by the unspecified professional identities of public sector mental health providers. An additional source of variability is that match is almost always confounded by provider cultural competence.

The role of acculturation or adaptation of a group to a host culture has garnered a great deal of attention in the theoretical (Dana, 1993; 1998;Van de Vijver, and Phalet, 2004) and empirical (e.g., Marin, Balls Organista, and Chun, 2003) literature. Many acculturation scales are ethnic-specific (e.g., Cuellar, Arnold, and Maldonado, 1995), while some profess to be ethnic-general (e.g., Stephenson, 2000). Currently, a paucity of empirical research exists concerning the use of ethnic-specific versus general acculturation devices with mental health consumer populations. The present study employed the Stephenson (2000) ethnic-general (SMAS) acculturation instrument with good success. One benefit of using this instrument is that it provides the researcher with a cost effective means of measuring acculturation with a diverse client base. Conversely, employment of such a measure may not be sensitive enough to address acculturative stress and transformation issues of each cultural group.

Like acculturation, ethnic and racial identity research is also expanding at a rapid rate (Dana, 1993; Trimble, Helms, and Root, 2003). Identity issues have been successfully explored for specific cultural groups and also in the multigroup domain. The present research successfully employed the Phinney (1992) multigroup measure (MEIM) with this college student population. The finding of an elusive triple interaction of ethnic match, acculturation, and ethnic identity supports the MAIP model contention of both the complexity and value of disentangling these cultural factors in allocating scarce mental health human resources. The present interaction effect parallels somewhat the acculturation and ethnic identity effects found by Gamst et al., (2002) with Latino Americans. This finding underscores the multicultural complexity that identity and acculturation manifest themselves in the real world.

The issue of a mental health provider's cultural competence has also garnered a tremendous amount of historical (e.g., Sue et al., 1982; Sue, Arredondo, and McDavis, 1992) and recent (e.g., Pope-Davis, Coleman, Liu, and Toporek, 2003) attention in the literature. Currently, six instruments have been developed that purport to measure aspects of the original 11 and later 31 specific competencies identified in the Sue et al. (1982; 1992) publications. These instruments included the Cross-Cultural Counseling Inventory-Revised (CCCI-R; LaFromboise et al., 1991), the Multicultural Awareness, Knowledge, Skills Survey (MAKSS; D'Andrea et al., 1991), the Multicultural Counseling Knowledge and Awareness Scale (MCKAS; Ponterotto, and Potere, 2003), the Multicultural Counseling Inventory (MCI; Sodowski, Kuo-Jackson, Richardson, and Corey, 1998), the Multicultural Competency and Training Survey (MCCTS; Holcomb-McCoy, 2000), and the California Brief Multicultural Competence Scale (CBMCS; Gamst et al., 2004). The present study employed the CBMCS, an amalgamation of four of the above instruments, due to its brevity and good reliability and validity among a large number of mental health practitioners. The dichotomized CBMCS variable was used as a covariate in the present study and not an independent variable due to the small number (9) of providers who rendered mental health services to our sample. While this covariate (as well as the gender match covariate) failed to statistically significantly adjust the dependent measures, we believe its measurement is crucial in implementing human resource allocations governed by the MAIP model. Specifically, mental health providers' scores on the CBMCS four subscales can demarcate essential staff multicultural training needs and future training interventions (e.g., Dana et al., 2006).

Some obvious limitations to the present study should be noted. First, due to the relatively small sample size, an examination of the present independent variables' *simultaneous* impact on the dependent measures (e.g., through structural equation modeling) was not conducted in the present study. Recent structural equation modeling of MAIP variables with a large adult community mental health sample has supported many of the MAIP postulates (e.g., Gamst, Dana, Der-Karabetian, Meyers, and Guarino, 2006). Second, this study is based on a relatively small sample of college students who sought help for mental health issues, and thus, may not be generalizable to the adult mental health consumer (non-student) population. Third, clients and providers were paired on the basis of availability, rather than a deliberate allocation process based on the MAIP model. Fourth, for the most part, all clients received culture-general clinical intervention, which may have impacted the clinical outcomes used in this study. Fifth, clients' responses to some of the BPRS subscales achieved relatively low reliability, and may not have been sensitive enough to detect any group differences.

CONCLUSION

The MAIP model affords a community mental health agency, or as in the present case, a university counseling center, with opportunities to integrate culturally responsive and evidence-based treatments and outcomes. The MAIP helps focus management attention on the critical question of who should provide what services to whom? The answer to this query is multifaceted and constrained by organizational human resource limitations and shaped ultimately by an organization's cultural competence.

The strength of the MAIP model lies in its empirical basis and flexibility in conducting culturally sensitive client assessments, clinical interventions, client outcome evaluation, and the targeting of provider multicultural competence in-service training needs. The MAIP premise of examining client ethnic identity and acculturation status provides researchers and practitioners with empirical tools for pondering consumer within-group differences. Such scrutiny, by MAIP model proponents should provide exciting and practical mental health payoffs over time for agencies providing services to diverse communities.

Future research with the MAIP would be enhanced by examining, simultaneously, MAIP variables in a variety of mental health contexts (e.g., university counseling center consumers, adult community mental health consumers, child/adolescent community mental health consumers, etc.). Systematic assessment of the most cost-effective instruments for measuring cultural identity needs to be undertaken. Ways of engaging MAIP methodology (see, Gamst and Dana, 2006) in the context of public-sector managed systems of care will surely garner increasing attention from researchers, practitioners, and mental health care and university counseling center administrators.

ACKNOWLEDGEMENTS

The authors acknowledge the helpful comments of Chris Liang (Department of Psychology, University of La Verne) on an earlier draft of this chapter.

REFERENCES

American Psychiatric Association. (1994). *Diagnostic and statistical manual of mental disorders* (4th ed.). Washington, DC: Author.

Cuellar, I., Arnold, B., and Maldonado, R. (1995). The Acculturation Rating Scale for Mexican Americans-II (ARSMA-II): A revision of the original ARSMA scale. *Hispanic Journal of Behavioral Sciences, 17(3)*, 275-304.

Dana, R. H. (2002). Mental health services for African Americans: A cultural/racial perspective. *Cultural Diversity and Ethnic Minority Psychology, 8 (1)*, 3-18.

Dana, R. H. (Ed.). (2000). An assessment-intervention model for research and practice with multicultural populations. In R.H. Dana (Ed.), *Handbook of cross-cultural and multicultural personality assessment* (pp. 6-16). Mahwah, NJ: Erlbaum.

Dana, R. H. (1998). *Understanding cultural identity in intervention and assessment.* Thousand Oaks, CA: Sage Publications.

Dana, R. H. (1993). *Multicultural assessment perspectives for professional psychology.* Needham Heights, MA: Allyn and Bacon.

Dana, R. H., Aragon, M., and Kramer, T. (2002). Public sector mental health services for multicultural populations: Bridging the gap from research to clinical practice. In M. N. Smyth (Ed.), *Health care in transition* (Vol. 1, pp.1-13). Hauppauge, NY: Nova Science Publishers.

Dana, R. H., Gamst, G., and Der-Karabetian, A., (2006). *The California Brief Multicultural Training Program: A manual for trainers.* La Verne, CA: University of La Verne Press.

D'Andrea, M., Daniels, J., and Heck, R. (1991). Evaluating the impact of multicultural counseling training. *Journal of Counseling and Development, 70,* 143-150.

Gamst, G. and Dana, R. H. (2006). Testing the MAIP model: A proposed method for assessing culturally sensitive mental health service delivery for adults and children. Unpublished manuscript, University of La Verne.

Gamst, G., Dana, R. H., Der-Karabetian, A., and Kramer, T. (2004). Ethnic match and treatment outcomes for child and adolescent mental health center clients. *Journal of Counseling and Development, 82,* 457-465.

Gamst, G., Dana, R. H., Der-Karabetian, A., Aragon, M., Arellano, L., Morrow, G., and Martenson, L. (2004). Cultural competency revised: The California Brief Multicultural Competence Scale. *Measurement and Evaluation in Counseling and Development, 37,* 163-183.

Gamst, G., Aguilar-Kitibutr, A., Herdina, A., Hibbs, S., Krishtal, E., Lee, R., Roberg, R., Ryan, E., Stephens, H., and Martenson, L. (2003). Effects of racial match on Asian American mental health consumer satisfaction. *Mental Health Services Research, 5,* 197-208.

Gamst, G., Dana, R. H., Der-Karabetian, A., Aragon, M., Arellano, L., and Kramer, T. (2002). Effects of Latino acculturation and ethnic identity on mental health outcomes. *Hispanic Journal of Behavioral Sciences, 24,* 479-505.

Gamst, G., Dana, R. H., Der-Karabetian, A., and Kramer, T. (2001). Asian American mental health clients: Effects of ethnic match and age on global assessment and visitation. *Journal of Mental Health Counseling, 23 (1),* 57-71.

Gamst, G., Dana, R. H., Der-Karabetian, A., and Kramer, T. (2000). Ethnic match and client ethnicity effects on global assessment and visitation. *Journal of Community Psychology, 28 (5),* 547-564.

Gamst, G., Dana, R. H. , Der-Karabetian, A., Meyers, L. S., and Guarino, A. J. (2006, May). Assessing the validity of the Multicultural Assessment Intervention Process (MAIP) model for mental health consumers. Poster presented at the Western Psychological Association Meeting, Palm Springs, CA.

Hedlund, J. L., and Vieweg, B. W. (1980). The Brief Psychiatric Rating Scale (BPRS): A comprehensive review. *Journal of Operational Psychiatry, 11,* 48-65.

Holcomb-McCoy, C. C. (2000). Multicultural counseling competencies: An exploratory factor analysis. *Journal of Multicultural Counseling and Development, 28,* 83-97.

Institute of Medicine. (2002). *Unequal treatment: Confronting racial and ethnic disparities of health care.* Washington, DC: National Academies Press.

Jones, S. H., Thornicroft, G., Coffey, M., and Dunn, G. (1995). A brief mental health outcome scale: Reliability and validity of the global assessment of functioning. *British Journal of Psychiatry, 166,* 654-659.

Karlsson, R. (2005). Ethnic matching between therapist and patient in psychotherapy: An overview of findings, together with methodological and conceptual issues. *Cultural Diversity and Ethnic Minority Psychology, 11,* 113-129.

LaFromboise, T. D., Coleman, H. L. K., and Hernandez, A. (1991). Development and factor structure of the Cross-Cultural Counseling Inventory-Revised. *Professional Psychology: Research and Practice, 22,* 380-388.

LaVeist, T. A. (2005). *Minority populations and health: An introduction to health disparities in the United States.* San Francisco, CA: Jossey-Bass.

Leong, F. T. L. (2001). Guest editor's introduction to the special issue: Barriers to providing effective mental health services to racial and ethnic minorities. *Mental Health Services Research, 3,* 179-180.

Leong, F. T. L. and Lau, A. S. L. (2001). Barriers to providing effective mental Health services to Asian Americans. *Mental Health Services Research, 3,* 201-211.

Levine, G. (1991). *A guide to SPSS for analysis of variance.* Hillsdale, NJ: Lawrence Erlbaum Associates, Publishers.

Manson, S. M. (2000). Mental health services for American Indians: Need, use, and barriers to effective care. *Canadian Journal of Psychiatry, 45,* 617-626.

Maramba, G. G., and Hall, G. C. N. (2002). Meta-analyses of ethnic match as a predictor of dropout, utilization, and level of functioning. *Cultural Diversity and Ethnic Minority Psychology, 8 (3),* 290-297.

Marin, G., Balls Organista, P., and Chun, K. M. (2003). Acculturation research: Current issues and findings. In G. Bernal, J. E. Trimble, A. K. Burlew, and F. T. L. Leong (Eds.), *Handbook of racial and ethnic minority psychology* (pp. 208-219). Thousand Oaks, CA: Sage Publications.

Meyers, L. S., Gamst, G., and Guarino, A. (2006). *Applied multivariate design and interpretation.* Thousand Oaks, CA: Sage Publications.

National Center for Health Statistics. (2003). *Health, United States, 2003.* Hyattsville, MD: Author, Centers for Disease Control and Prevention, U.S. Department of Health and Human Services.

Novins, D. K. , Duclos, C. W., Martin, C., Jewett, C. S., and Manson, S. M. (1999). Utilization of alcohol, drug, and mental health treatment services among American Indian adolescent detainees. *Journal of the American Academy of Child and Adolescent Psychiatry, 38,* 1102-1108.

Overall, J. E., and Gorham, D. R. (1988). The Brief Psychiatric Rating Scale (BPRS): Recent developments in ascertainment and scaling *Psychopharmocology Bulletin, 24,* 97-99.

Phinney, J. S. (1992). The Multigroup Ethnic Identity Measure: A new scale for use with diverse groups. *Journal of Adolescent Research, 7,* 156-176.

Ponterotto, J. G., and Potere, J. C. (2003). The Multicultural Counseling Knowledge and Awareness Scale (MCKAS): Validity, reliability, and user guidelines. In D. B. Pope-Davis, H. L. K. Coleman, W. Ming Liu, and R. L. Toporek (Eds.), *Handbook of multicultural competencies in counseling and psychology.* Thousand Oaks, CA: Sage Publications.

Ponterotto, J. G., Gretchen, D., and Chauhan, R. V. (2000). Cultural identity and multicultural assessment: Quantitative and qualitative tools for the clinician. In L. A. Suzuki, J. G. Ponterotto, and P. J. Meller, (Eds.), *Handbook of multicultural assessment: Clinical, psychological, and educational applications* (2nd ed., pp. 67-100). San Francisco, CA: Jossey-Bass.

Pope-Davis, D. B., Coleman, H. L. K., Liu, W. M., and Toporek, R. L. (Eds.) (2003). *Handbook of multicultural competencies in counseling and psychology.* Thousand Oaks, CA: Sage Publications.

Reiger, D. A., Narrow, W. E., Rae, D. S., Manderscheid, R. W., Locke, B. Z., and Goodwin, F. K. (1993). The de facto U.S. mental and addictive disorders service system. Epidemiologic Catchment Area prospective 1-year prevalence rates of disorders and services. *Archives of General Psychiatry, 50,* 85-94.

Roberts, R., Phinney J., Masse, L., Chen, Y., Roberts, C., and Romero, A. (1999). The structure of ethnic identity in young adolescents from diverse ethnocultural groups. *Journal of Early Adolescence, 19,* 301-322.

Robins, L., and Reiger, D. A. (1991). *Psychiatric disorders in America: The Epidemiologic Catchment Area Study.* New York: The Free Press.

Shin, S.-M., Chow, C., Camacho-Gonsalves, Levy, R. J., Allen, I., E., and Leff, H. S. (2005). A meta-analytic review of racial-ethnic matching for African American and Caucasian American clients and clinicians. *Journal of Counseling Psychology, 52,* 45-56.

Snowden, L. R. (1999). African American service use for mental health problems. *Journal of Community Psychology, 27,* 303-313.

Snowden, L. R., and Yamada, A.-M. (2005). Cultural differences in access to care. *Annual Review of Clinical Psychology, 1,* 143-166.

Snowden, L. R., and Cheung, F. K. (1990). Use of inpatient mental health services by members of ethnic minority groups. *American Psychologist, 45,* 347-355.

Sodowsky, G. R., Kuo-Jackson, P. Y., Richardson, M. F., and Corey, A. T. (1998). Correlates of self-reported multicultural competencies: Counselor multicultural social desirability, race, social inadequacy, locus of control, racial ideology, and multicultural training. *Journal of Counseling Psychology, 45,* 256-264.

Stephenson, M. (2000). Development and validation of the Stephenson Multigroup Acculturation Scale (SMAS). *Psychological Assessment, 12,* 77-88.

Sue, D. W., Arredondo, P., and McDavis, R. J. (1992). Multicultural counseling competencies: A call to the profession. *Journal of Multicultural Counseling and Development, 20,* 64-88.

Sue, D. W., Bernier, J. E., Durran, A., Feinberg, L., Pedersen, P., Smith, E. J., et al. (1982). Position paper: Cross-cultural counseling competencies. *The Counseling Psychologist, 10,* 45-52.

Trimble, J. E., Helms, J. E., and Root, M. P. P. (2003). Social and psychological perspectives on ethnic and racial identity. In G. Bernal, J. E. Trimble, A. K. Burlew, F. T. L. and Leong (Eds.), *Handbook of racial and ethnic minority psychology* (pp.239-275). Thousand Oaks, CA: Sage Publications.

U.S. Department of Health and Human Services. (2001). *Mental health: Culture, race, and ethnicity—a supplement to mental health: A report of the Surgeon General.* Rockville, MD: Author.

Van de Vijver, F. J. R., and Phalet, K. (2004). Assessment in multicultural groups: The role of acculturation. *Applied Psychology: An International* Review, 53 (2), 215-236.

In: Racial and Ethnic Disparities in Health and Health Care   ISBN 1-60021-268-9
Editor: Elene V. Metrosa, pp. 149-204   © 2006 Nova Science Publishers, Inc.

Chapter 7

RACIAL AND ETHNIC DISPARITIES IN MENTAL HEALTH CARE FOR YOUTH

Judy Ho, June Liang, Jonathan Martinez, Cindy Huang and May Yeh*

San Diego State University/University of California San Diego Joint Doctoral Program
in Clinical Psychology, Child and Adolescent Services Research Center,
Children's Hospital San Diego, San Diego, CA

ABSTRACT

The continuing racial and ethnic diversification of the youth population in the United States necessitates greater understanding of issues related to the delivery of appropriate youth mental health services. There is a dire need for greater research in this area, and recent studies have begun to form a strong foundation of knowledge regarding mental health service delivery for various racial and ethnic groups. This chapter will review the empirical literature on racial and ethnic disparities in mental health care use, treatment retention, and outcomes for youth across a variety of service types (e.g., inpatient services, outpatient services, school-based services, clinical trials). Barriers that may explain racial and ethnic disparities in mental health care will be reviewed, and a model illustrating the influence of barriers in creating and sustaining disparities in the mental health treatment process will be introduced. Recent public policy documents highlighting the nation's priority upon addressing racial/ethnic disparities in mental health care for youth will be identified, and recommendations for future directions in research and clinical practice will be discussed.

---

* phone 858-966-7703).

INTRODUCTION

Approximately 20% of all children and adolescents in the U. S. have diagnosable mental health disorders with at least a minimum level of functional impairment (United States Department of Health and Human Services [USDHHS], 1999), yet only 20% of these children in need are receiving any type of mental health care (United States Public Health Service, 2000). It is estimated that 7.5 million U. S. children have unmet mental health needs (Kataoka, Zhang, and Wells, 2002), and within this underserved population of youth, minorities are of particular concern. Recent research suggests that African American, Asian/Pacific Islander, and Latino youth have an even higher level of unmet mental health need than do non-Hispanic White youth (Hough et al., 2002; Kataoka et al., 2002); one study of an at-risk sample found unmet need rates of 48% for African Americans, 72% for Asian/Pacific Islanders, and 47% for Latinos as compared to 31% for non-Hispanic Whites (Yeh, McCabe, Hough, Dupuis, and Hazen, 2003). These disparities are troublesome because research suggests that minorities have similar community rates of mental health problems compared to non-Hispanic Whites (USDHHS, 2001). Adding to the urgency of addressing these needs is the rapid diversification of the U. S. population. Minority youth will continue to experience more rapid growth than non-minority youth (U. S. Department of Commerce, 1999), and it is estimated that in approximately 20 years, 48% of children will be from racial and ethnic minority backgrounds (USDHHS, 2001). This population growth is even higher for very young children; minority children ages 5 and under are projected to exceed non-minority children in the next 25 years (U. S. Department of Commerce, 1999).

National task forces have recognized the need to address racial/ethnic disparities in current mental health care and improve services for ethnic minorities. The Surgeon General's report *Mental Health: Culture, Race, and Ethnicity* (USDHHS, 2001) recommends that the nation place studying and understanding minority mental health and mental health care as a top priority. The Surgeon General also released *Healthy People 2010*, urging the Nation to address disparities in health care access and outcomes by encouraging the field to strive toward the highest quality of care and health outcomes across all groups. In addition, the National Institute of Health (NIH) introduced mandatory guidelines in the NIH Revitalization Act of 1993, which required all NIH-supported research projects to include women and ethnic minority groups in all human subject research and in phase III clinical trials. The President's New Freedom Commission on Mental Health recommends that empirical research should be conducted in order to monitor racial and ethnic disparities in access, availability, quality, and outcomes of mental health services, and that this knowledge should be incorporated into Comprehensive State Mental Health Plans (The President's New Freedom Commission on Mental Health, 2003). These guidelines from national agencies help to promote the examination of mental health services and outcomes across different cultural groups (Hohmann and Parron, 1996).

In line with these national initiatives, this chapter aims to provide a deeper understanding of current mental health care for minority youth. We will provide a synthesis of current literature on minority youth mental health care, identify existing racial/ethnic disparities and examine inconsistencies and gaps in the evidence base, discuss barriers that account for current disparities, provide suggestions for future research directions and offer recommendations for improving mental health care for ethnic minority youth.

THE CURRENT STATE OF MENTAL HEALTH CARE
FOR MINORITY YOUTH

Disparities in Service Utilization

Disparities exist for minority youth in mental health services, and youth in different cultural groups exhibit differential patterns of mental health service use compared to non-Hispanic Whites (USDHHS, 2001). Our discussion of utilization disparities will be organized by the same racial/ethnic categories described by the Surgeon General in *Mental Health: Culture, Race, and Ethnicity* (USDHHS, 2001): African Americans, Hispanic Americans/Latinos, Asian and Pacific Islanders, American Indian and Alaska Natives, and non-Hispanic Whites.

African Americans

Studies with African American youths have produced mixed results, with evidence of overrepresentation in mental health services as well as both higher and lower rates of use compared to non-Hispanic White youth. African American youth have been found to be overrepresented in the mental health sector (Bui and Takeuchi, 1992; McCabe et. al., 1999) and in school-based services for children with severe emotional disturbance (SED, now called ED) compared to their representation in the local population (McCabe et al., 1999). In a survey of SED classrooms nationwide, African American youth were found to be overrepresented (21% of SED classrooms) compared to their representation in the U. S. census (14%; U. S. Department of Education, 1990). African American youth were overrepresented in community mental health clinics in metropolitan areas (Takeuchi, Bui, and Kim, 1993; Costello and Janiszewski, 1990), and overrepresentation in outpatient mental health services was found even when analyses controlled for other demographic characteristics (i.e., gender, age, and poverty status), diagnosis, and referral choice (Bui and Takeuchi, 1992). Studies examining utilization rates across cultural groups show that African American youth were more likely than non-Hispanic Whites to receive mental health services in the public sector (Stehno, 1982). However, Pumariega, Holzer, and Nguyen (1993) found that African American adolescents used mental health services at lower rates than that of Caucasian Americans in a school sample. Similarly, one study found that African American youth were less likely than non-Hispanic White youth to utilize outpatient mental health services even when analyses controlled for caregiver strain and socioeconomic status (Garland et al., 2005). In a study of service types used by youth who were already enrolled in public mental health services, African American youth were more likely than non-Hispanic White youth to receive outpatient mental health services but were less likely than non-Hispanic White youth to receive school-based mental health services (Yeh et al., 2002).

Beyond inconsistencies in utilization rates compared to non-Hispanic Whites, the current literature consistently suggests that African Americans youth have higher rates of unmet needs, defined as lack of mental health service use when mental health needs (e.g., psychopathology or associated functional impairment) were present (Yeh, McCabe, Hough, Dupuis, and Hazen, 2003; Flisher et al., 1997). In a study of U. S. and Puerto Rico youth, African Americans had higher rates of unmet need compared to Caucasian children in the previous 6 months (Flisher et al., 1997). African American youth were also found to have significantly higher rates of unmet need (47.7%) compared to non-Hispanic White youth (30.7%) in a large at-risk sample in the U. S. (Yeh et al., 2003). Taken together, these findings suggest that greater barriers to mental health service use may exist for African American children compared to non-Hispanic White children.

Hispanic Americans/Latinos

Studies with Latino youth generally show patterns of underutilization in mental health services. Latino youth have been found to be underrepresented in mental health services compared to their representation in the local population (Bui and Takeuchi, 1992), and were underrepresented in school-based services for children with severe emotional disturbance (SED) children in a study of a large urban area (McCabe et al., 1999). Latino youth were also found to be underrepresented in SED classrooms nationwide (4% of SED classrooms) when compared to their proportion in the U. S. census (14%; U. S. Department of Education, 1990). McCabe and colleagues (1999) found that Latino youth were represented in public mental health services at the expected rates compared to their representation in the local population, but were underrepresented when socioeconomic status was taken into account and when compared to their representation in school enrollment data.

Studies examining utilization rates across cultural groups have yielded conflicting results, with evidence of lower and higher use compared to non-Hispanic White youth. In one study, Latino junior high and high school students had lower average rates of outpatient mental health services use than non-Hispanic White youth (Pumariega, Glover, Holzer, and Nguyen, 1998). Another study of at-risk youth also found that Latino youth utilized outpatient mental health services less than did non-Hispanic White youth; however, this result was not significant after caregiver strain and socioeconomic status were accounted for in analyses (Garland et al., 2005). In a study of youth who were already using public mental health services, Latino children were less likely to receive day treatment services and other school-related services than were non-Hispanic Whites, especially when the services required a referral from school personnel, but were more likely than non-Hispanic White children to receive outpatient mental health services (Yeh et al., 2002). These inconsistencies in existing findings may be due to differences in methodologies and study samples (e.g., at-risk sample, community sample, youth already enrolled in services).

Beyond representation rates and cross-ethnic comparisons, there is evidence of higher levels of unmet mental health needs for Latino youth. Latino children were found to have significantly higher rates of unmet need (47.2%) compared to non-Hispanic White children in an at-risk sample (30.7%; Yeh et al., 2003). Another study found that 88% of Latino youth who were in need of mental health services did not receive them, compared to a rate of 75% for all U. S. youth, and that Latino youth had higher unmet needs than non-Hispanic White youth even when socioeconomic and insurance status were accounted in analyses (Kataoka et al., 2002). These findings are particularly troubling given that these youth have higher rates of depressive and anxious symptomatology and higher rates of suicidal thoughts compared to non-Hispanic White youth (Centers for Disease Control and Prevention, 2000). Taken together, representation and unmet needs studies to date suggest that Latino youth may encounter a greater number of barriers in mental health service entry than non-Hispanic White youth.

Asian/Pacific Islanders

Although there is a scarcity of data concerning Asian/Pacific Islander youth, available data shows underrepresentation and lower rates of use of mental health services compared to non-Hispanic Whites. Some studies have found that Asian/Pacific Islander youth are underrepresented in mental health services and in school-based SED services compared to their representation in the local population (Bui and Takeuchi, 1992; McCabe et al., 1999). Studies examining utilization rates across cultural groups show that Asian/Pacific Islander youth underutilize special education services for youths with emotional disturbance compared to non-Hispanic White children (Yeh, Forness, Ho, McCabe, and Hough, 2004). Garland and colleagues found that Asian/Pacific Islander youth have the lowest utilization rates in mental health services compared to African American, Latino, and non-Hispanic White youth, even when analyses controlled for caregiver strain and socioeconomic status (Garland et al., 2005). In addition, Asian/Pacific Islanders are most severe in their symptom presentation at time of initial service use (USDHHS, 2001), which suggests that Asian/Pacific Islander youth may delay services until problems become too difficult to manage without professional help, or until a certain severity of problem is reached.

Beyond representation studies and comparisons with non-Hispanic Whites indicating underutilization, Asian/Pacific Islander youth also demonstrate a high level of unmet mental health need. One study of at-risk youth found that Asian/Pacific Islander youth had the highest rates of unmet need (71.8%) compared to African American, Latino, and non-Hispanic White youth (47.7%, 47.2%, and 30.7%, respectively; Yeh et al., 2003). Literature indicating underutilization and higher levels of unmet needs compared to other cultural groups, coupled with evidence that Asian/Pacific Islander youth delay seeking services until symptoms are very severe, suggest that many challenging barriers to mental health service use exist for this population.

American Indian/Alaskan Natives

Only a handful of studies have examined utilization rates for American Indian and/or Alaskan Native youths. Limited evidence suggests that American Indian and Alaskan Native youth used outpatient mental health services at rates equal to their representation in the U. S. population (Breaux and Ryujin, 1999). However, beyond representation rates, American Indian children have demonstrated higher unmet mental health needs compared to non-Hispanic White youth and compared to American Indian adults. One study showed that only 1 in 7 Cherokee youth with diagnosable psychiatric disorders received mental health treatment in the past 3 months compared to 1 in 4 White youth, even when insurance status was taken into account (Costello, Farmer, Angold, Burns, and Erkanli, 1997). Another study found that only 39% of Plains Indian youth who needed mental health care (as identified by parents and/or teachers) received services, and most were seen through school-provided services instead of services in the specialty mental health sector (Novins, Feming, Beals, and Manson, 2000). Evidence also suggests that American Indian children have higher unmet needs than their adult counterparts; American Indian children make up 32% of the American Indian population, but only receive 10% of the mental health care provided especially for American Indians (LaFromboise and Low, 1989). Unfortunately, no studies to date have examined unmet need for Alaskan Natives. The amount of limited evidence for these populations is problematic, as existing data suggests that American Indian youth suffer a disproportionate burden of mental health problems compared with other racial/ethnic groups

(Beals et al., 1997; USDHHS, 2001). Much work is needed in this area to expand the evidence base for these youths who may experience even more mental health concerns than other Americans.

Disparities in Service Utilization: Summary

Disparities in mental health service utilization for minority youths are well-established. Although literature regarding representation have yielded some inconsistent results for certain cultural groups (e.g., African American, Latinos), there is consistent evidence of higher unmet needs for African American, Latino, Asian/Pacific Islander, and American Indian youth compared to their non-Hispanic White counterparts. These higher rates of unmet need are concerning, particularly because there is limited evidence of racial/ethnic differences in the prevalence of mental health problems for U. S. youth (Achenbach and Edelbrock, 1981); in fact, some minority youths (i.e., Latino, American Indian, Alaskan Native) are thought to suffer a greater number of mental health problems compared to non-Hispanic White youth (USDHHS, 2001). Equally troubling is the finding that some minority groups (e.g., Asian/Pacific Islander youths) may delay service seeking until problems significantly worsen (Center for Disease Prevention and Control, 2000; USDHHS, 2001). Taken together, these disparities provide evidence for the existence of formidable barriers to mental health service use for minority youth that may be greater than those experienced by non-minority youth.

Quality of Services for Minorities

After barriers to initial access have been surmounted, disparities in mental health care may continue to exist for minority youth (Snowden and Yamada, 2005). Existing research largely focuses on examining quality of care for minority adults and suggests a greater likelihood of receiving poorer quality of services as compared to Whites. Although little is known about the quality of services for minority youth, it is possible that disparities in quality of care for minority adults may extend to their younger counterparts. In addition, caregivers and other adult family members are often involved in youth mental health treatment (Morrissey-Kane and Prinz, 1999), and their experience with mental health services may help to determine the experience of services by the child (e.g., parents who feel they are being mistreated in family therapy may opt to stop treatment). Therefore, much can be drawn from the adult literature as it relates to youth, and relevant literature on quality of care for minority adults will be presented in addition to available findings on quality of care for minority youth.

African Americans

Findings suggest that there are disparities in the quality of mental health services received by African Americans adults. African Americans adults were found to be less likely than non-Hispanic Whites to receive appropriate care (defined as care that adheres to guidelines that are based on results of clinical trials) for depression and anxiety (Wang, Burgland, and Kessler., 2000; Young, Klap, Shebourne and Wells (2001). In a separate study, they were also less likely than non-Hispanic Whites to receive an antidepressant when depression was first diagnosed, and were less likely to receive the newer selective serotonin reuptake inhibitor (SSRI) medications, which carry fewer side effects and are more easily tolerated (Melfi,

Croghan, Hanna, and Robinson, 2000). Existing research has not examined racial/ethnic differences specifically for children, and future studies should examine whether these findings in the adult literature extend to youth.

Differential utilization patterns by type of care and service sector may also lead to a lesser likelihood of receiving adequate care. African Americans adults were less likely to receive services in the specialty mental health sector and were more likely to receive care in the general medical setting than were non-Hispanic Whites (USDHHS, 2001; Pingitore, Snowden, Sansome, and Klinkman, 2001). However, primary care providers may not be adequately trained to recognize mental health disorders and may not be equipped to provide the specific services patients need for their mental health problems, especially if they have co-existing physical disorders (Rost et al., 2000). The likelihood of receiving services in the primary care setting, coupled with the finding that minorities are at greatest risk for missed and/or incorrect diagnoses in this setting (Borowsky et al., 2000), raises questions about the quality of care in this sector for African Americans with mental health concerns. Beyond higher enrollment in the primary care setting for mental health problems, findings also suggest that African Americans often enter less desirable and/or more restrictive services. African American adults were more likely than non-Hispanic Whites to receive emergency care for their mental health problems (Hu, Snowden, Jerrell, and Nguyen, 1991) and were more likely to be hospitalized in psychiatric hospitals (Snowden and Cheung, 1990; Breaux and Ryujin, 1999). African Americans with mental health concerns also relied heavily on public sector programs (Swartz et al., 1998), and child welfare authorities often acted as gatekeepers to mental health care for African American youth (Halfon, Berkowitz, and Klee, 1992; Takayama, Bergman, and Connell, 1994). Entering services through less desirable mechanisms, and/or mechanisms that may not be specifically designed to address mental health concerns (e.g., child welfare) may lead to a lesser likelihood of receiving appropriate treatment.

African American adults were also more likely to endorse mistreatment by health providers. Recent studies found that African Americans were more likely than non-Hispanic Whites to feel that a doctor or health provider judged them unfairly or that they were disrespected because of their ethnic background (Brown, Cohen, Johnson, and Smailes, 1999; LaVeist, Diala, and Jarrett, 2000). Clinician bias and stereotyping can also lead to inappropriate treatment or mistreatment; for example, the stereotype that African Americans are more violent than Whites may have contributed to the finding that African American youth were four times more likely than Whites to be restrained, even when both groups acted in similarly aggressive ways (Bond, DiCandia, and Mackinnon, 1988). Findings indicating inadequate specialized care and mistreatment of this group, coupled with attitudes of mistrust toward mental health professionals frequently held by minority individuals (USDHHS, 2001), suggest that the experience of African Americans in mental health services may be significantly compromised.

Hispanic Americans/Latinos

Findings suggest that there are disparities in the quality of mental health services received by Latino adults. For example, in one study, Latinos were less likely than non-Hispanic Whites to receive appropriate care for depression and anxiety (24% and 34% received appropriate care, respectively; Young et al., 2001). Differential utilization patterns by type of care and service sector may also lead to a lesser likelihood of receiving adequate care. Latino adults were less likely to receive services in the specialty mental health sector and were more likely to receive care in the general medical setting than were non-Hispanic Whites (Vega, Kolody, Aguilar-Gaxiola, and Catalano, 1999). As mentioned earlier, these findings are concerning because a greater likelihood of misdiagnoses and inadequate treatment may occur in the primary care setting (Borowsky et al., 2000; USDHHS, 2001); for example, Latino adults were approximately half as likely as Whites to receive a diagnosis of depression or antidepressant medication in a general medical sector (Sclar, Robison, Skaer, and Galin, 1999). Perception of mistreatment has also been endorsed by this group; Latino adults were more likely than non-Hispanic Whites to feel that a doctor or health provider judged them unfairly or that they were disrespected because of their ethnic background (Brown et al., 1999; LaVeist et al., 2002). These findings, coupled with attitudes of mistrust toward mental health professionals frequently held by minority individuals (USDHHS, 2001), suggest that the experience of Latino adults in mental health services may be significantly compromised. Future research should examine whether these findings in the adult literature extend to youth as well.

Asian/Pacific Islanders

There is a dearth of studies examining quality of care for Asian/Pacific Islanders, although evidence suggests that they are less likely to receive evidence-based care (Miranda et al., 2005). The widely held stereotype of Asian Americans as "problem free" may lead to clinicians overlooking their problems and need for treatment (Takeuchi and Uehara, 1996). Borowsky and colleagues (2000) suggested that primary care doctors may not identify depression in their Asian American clients as often as in White clients, although the study sample was too small to draw strong conclusions. Regarding perceptions of treatment, findings indicate that Asian American adult clients reported less satisfaction with outpatient mental health services received than did Whites (Zane, Enomoto, and Chun, 1994). The current knowledge base in this area is significantly lacking and further investigations need to be conducted to evaluate quality of services for this group, although existing research suggests that Asian/Pacific Islanders are more likely to receive compromised mental health care. Future research on quality of care is needed with both Asian/Pacific Islander adults and youth to address these gaps in the evidence base.

American Indian/Alaskan Native

Research examining quality of care for American Indian and Alaskan Natives is severely lacking, although existing findings suggest that American Indians often enter less desirable and/or more restrictive services. An evaluation of federal and non-federal hospitals in the U. S. found that American Indian adults were admitted to state and county hospitals at higher rates than Whites, but were admitted to private psychiatric hospitals at lower rates than Whites (Snowden and Cheung, 1990). Findings that paralleled results in the adult literature were found for American Indian youth; Cherokee children were more likely to receive treatment through the juvenile justice system and inpatient services than were non-Indian children. Thus, the current limited evidence base suggests some inequality in the treatment of American Indian in mental health services, and future research is needed to examine other factors involved in quality of care for both American Indian and Alaskan Native youth.

Summary: Quality of Services for Minorities

Existing literature examining quality of services for minority youth is lacking; however, studies with adults suggest that minorities may receive poorer quality mental health services as compared to Whites. Minorities are less likely to receive state of the art, evidence-based care (Miranda et al., 2005), are more likely to receive inappropriate or inadequate treatment for their mental health concerns, are more likely to receive services in less desirable or more restrictive settings than non-Hispanic Whites, and are more likely to endorse mistreatment by mental health professionals. Taken together, these findings suggest that the current standards for quality of care for minorities need to be strengthened in order to improve the experience in the mental health sector for these cultural groups. Future studies are needed that specifically examine quality of care for minority youth.

Treatment Retention of Minority Youth

Cultural factors, along with the receipt of poorer quality services compared to non-Hispanic Whites, may lead minority families to exit services prematurely before emotional/behavioral problems of the youth are resolved. It is often hypothesized that minority families are more likely to have poorer treatment retention compared to non-Hispanic Whites in mental health services, due to adherence to cultural values, beliefs, attitudes, and behaviors that may be incompatible with Western conceptualizations of mental health treatment (USDHHS, 2001). For example, evidence suggests that there are differential patterns of beliefs regarding the etiology of youth emotional/behavioral problems. Asian/Pacific Islander parents were more likely than non-Hispanic Whites to cite American culture as causes of their child's problems, and both African American parents and Asian/Pacific Islander parents were more likely to endorse prejudice (Yeh, Hough, McCabe, Lau, and Garland, 2004) that may not necessarily lead to service-seeking in the mental health sector. It is possible that these beliefs, which may be incompatible with Western conceptualizations of mental illness, will subsequently reduce treatment retention. Indeed, disparities in treatment retention have been found for minority families in youth mental health services. Although only a handful of studies for minority youth are available, current evidence suggests that minority families exhibit even higher rates of dropout and premature termination than non-minority families (Morrisey-Kane and Prinz, 1999; McCabe, 2002).

Treatment retention is usually measured by dropout (defined as the failure to return for treatment after one session) and/or premature termination (defined as parent or family terminating treatment before completing the recommended number of sessions and when doing so is considered inadvisable and against the advice of the clinician) (Bui and Takeuchi, 1992; O'Sullivan, Peterson, Cox, and Kirkeby, 1989; Sue, Fujino, Hu, and Takeuchi, 1991; Sue and McKinney, 1975; Kazdin, Stolar, and Marciano, 1995; Kazdin, Holland, and Crowley, 1997). Dropping out after one session or terminating services before treatment completion is likely to indicate that the family is dissatisfied with their initial contact with the agency/therapist and/or the services they have received up to the point of termination, although it is possible (albeit less likely) that the family has received the services they wanted, have experienced significant improvement, and/or are satisfied with the outcomes (Bui and Takeuchi, 1992). Usually, however, clients who drop out are not likely to receive the maximum benefits services offer, and may continue to experience significant levels of impairment (Kazdin, Holland, and Crowley, 1994; Larsen, Nguyen, Green, and Attkisson., 1983).

Treatment retention studies with African American families have yielded somewhat inconsistent results. It has been reported that Black families had a higher rate of drop out than White families for treatment on their child's externalizing problems over and above the effects of socio-demographic and clinical variables (Kazdin, Stolar, and Marciano, 1995). Bui and Takeuchi (1992) found that the dropout rates of African American adolescents did not differ from those of White adolescents; however, African American youth had a shorter length of treatment than Whites. Literature comparing drop out rates between Latino and non-Hispanic White youth is lacking; however, McCabe (2002) conducted a study examining factors that predict premature termination among Mexican American families and found that negative attitudes toward mental health services (an attitude more likely held by Latino groups than non-Hispanic Whites) predicted lower treatment retention. This may have some implications regarding differential rates of premature termination between Latino and non-Hispanic White families, although further research is needed to elucidate these effects. There is a dearth of literature examining dropout rates of Asian Pacific Islander youth in mental health services. However, in a study on dropout rates of adolescents in outpatient mental health services, Asian American youth were found to attend more sessions than non-Hispanic Whites (Bui and Takeuchi, 1992). Unfortunately, no studies to date have examined treatment retention for American Indian or Alaskan Native youth.

Summary: Treatment Retention of Minority Youth

In summary, the field is greatly lacking research on treatment retention for different cultural groups and studies comparing dropout and premature termination rates across racial/ethnic groups, especially for school-based services which are often considered the "de facto" source of mental health care for children (Burns et al., 1995). Research is needed to examine treatment retention for minority families in school-based services as well as outpatient services, and to study the relationship between retention and other variables such as barriers experienced by the family and therapy outcomes. Studies show that engaging families in youth mental health services can serve to decrease dropout and premature termination rates for youth services (e.g., McKay et al., 2004). Future research is needed to investigate whether there are differences in the types of engagement strategies that may be more or less effective at achieving treatment retention for different cultural groups.

Outcomes for Minority Children

It is often hypothesized that minority families are more likely to have poorer outcomes in mental health services, due to adherence to cultural values, beliefs, attitudes, and behaviors that may be incompatible with western conceptualizations of mental health treatment (e.g., USDHHS, 2001, Telles et al., 1995; Zane et al., 1994). For example, evidence suggests that there are differential patterns of beliefs regarding the etiology of youth emotional/behavioral problems, such that Asian/Pacific Islander parents were more likely than non-Hispanic Whites to cite American culture as causes of their child's problems, and both African American parents and Asian/Pacific Islander parents were more likely to endorse prejudice (Yeh, Hough et al., 2004). These types of beliefs that may be less consistent with service-seeking in the mental health sector. It is possible that these beliefs, which may be incompatible with Western conceptualizations of mental illness, will subsequently reduce treatment retention, satisfaction, and outcomes. Some recent research efforts have examined treatment outcomes for minority youth. Although only a few studies have been completed in this area to date, existing literature suggests that minorities do benefit from services. However, whether these groups differ in outcomes to non-Hispanic White youth is unclear.

Outcomes of mental health care are obtained through either efficacy or effectiveness studies. Efficacy studies, or mental health clinical trials, are randomized, controlled studies in which considerable control has been exercised by researchers over sample selection criteria (usually recruited samples without comorbid disorders), delivery of intervention (e.g., use of manuals), and conditions under which treatment occurs (e.g., carefully controlled laboratory settings). The goal of efficacy studies is to determine the outcomes of an intervention for specific syndromes. Efficacy studies examining outcomes of mental health care for minorities are rarely available. These studies have usually been conducted in nonminority populations, and even when minorities were included, the small sample sizes did not yield the power necessary to examine outcomes for specific groups. Of 7,670 participants involved in 69 adult efficacy studies for the treatment of bipolar disorder, schizophrenia, and depression, only 558 Black/African American, 40 Hispanic/Latino, 5 Asian American/Pacific Islander, and 0 American Indians/Alaskan Natives were included (USDHHS, 2001). Furthermore, only one of these studies compared outcomes between minorities and nonminorities. Data examining inclusion rates of minority youth in 32 randomized intervention trials (N = 1, 657) for attention-deficit/hyperactivity disorder (ADHD) indicated that only 126 were African American, 55 Hispanic/Latino, 4 Asian/Pacific Islander, and 0 American Indians/Alaskan Natives were included. Although no other data on youth inclusion in clinical trials is currently available, it is likely that similar patterns of minority youth underrepresentation may exist in clinical trials for other disorders.

In contrast, effectiveness studies evaluate outcomes of care in more naturalistic settings. Once an intervention is found to be efficacious, effectiveness studies examine this intervention when implemented with a "real-world" sample that is typically more heterogeneous in nature (e.g., diagnosis, comorbidities, therapist training, etc.). Effectiveness studies to date have not usually included significant numbers of ethnic minorities, and even when minority samples are included, outcomes are rarely examined across cultural groups (USDHHS, 2001). However, a few recent studies (described in the following section) have specifically included a minority sample (Miranda et al., 2005).

Due to lack of inclusion of minority samples in most mental health outcomes research, not much is known in this area. Studies that include adequate samples of minorities provide some evidence of racial/ethnic disparities in mental health outcomes for African American, Latino, and Asian Pacific Islander adults, especially for those who are less acculturated to mainstream American society (USDHHS, 2001). Research focusing on minority youth outcomes is even more lacking than the adult evidence base and have yielded inconsistent findings. In our discussion, we will summarize available data in outcome studies involving minority youth samples, which consists of a greater number of efficacy studies.

African Americans

Studies on outcomes for African American youth show that mental health treatment may be beneficial at reducing emotional/behavioral problems. A study of African American youth demonstrated positive effects from enrollment in multisystemic therapy (Borduin, Mann, Cone. Henggeler, and Fucci, 1995), and another study showed positive outcomes from medication treatment for African American youth with ADHD (Brown and Sexson, 1988). A pilot study examining the efficacy of a culturally-adapted version of Silverman and colleagues' (1999) school-based group cognitive-behavioral intervention demonstrated that African American youth experienced a significant reduction of symptoms posttreatment (Ginsburg and Drake, 2002), and a study evaluating a school-based social skills training program reported that treatment was effective in reducing aggression and peer rejection among African American boys (Lochman, Coie, and Underwood, 1993).

Whether African American youth benefit from services as much as other cultural groups is still under investigation, and current findings support the notion that there are no significant differences in outcomes between African American and non-Hispanic White youth. One study that evaluated the effectiveness of a parenting program found no significant differences in treatment effects between youths of African American and non-Hispanic White mothers (Reid, Webster-Stratton, and Beauchaine, 2001). Another study found Cognitive-Behavioral Therapy to be effective in reducing aggression in African American boys (Hudley and Graham, 1993), and another study found no significant racial/ethnic effect on outcome (Dubow, Huesman, and Eron, 1987). After behavioral and medication treatment, African American youth did not differ significantly from their matched pair non-Hispanic White youth participants on ADHD and ODD symptomatology as reported by teachers, after controlling for socioeconomic disadvantage (MTA Cooperative Group, 1999).

In summary, the limited studies on outcomes have shown that African American youth do benefit from mental health services delivered in clinical trials and in more generalized settings, and that there are no significant differences in outcomes compared to non-Hispanic White youth.

Hispanic Americans/Latinos

Few studies on the response of Latino youth to mental health treatment are available; the existing research mostly involves adults (Comas-Diaz, 1981; Alonso and Val., 1997; Rossello and Bernal, 1999) and findings have been inconsistent. A limited number of studies suggest that Latino youth do experience symptom improvement in mental health services. One study found that a parent management training program was successful at reducing behavioral problems of Latino youth (Pantin et al., 2003), and another study of Latino boys with emotional and behavioral problems reported that structural family therapy improved child functioning posttreatment (Szapocsnik et al., 1989).

Whether Latino youth benefit from services as much as White youth is still under investigation, and current literature offers little basis for conclusions about outcome differences between these populations. Some studies suggest that there are no significant outcome differences between Latino and non-Hispanic White children. A study that evaluated the effectiveness of a parenting program found that youths of Latino mothers exhibited a reduction in behavioral problems after treatment, and that there were no significant differences in treatment effects between youths of Latino and non-Hispanic White mothers. (Reid et al., 2001). After behavioral and medication treatment, Latino youth did not differ significantly from their matched pair non-Hispanic White youth participants on ADHD and ODD symptomatology as reported by teachers, after controlling for socioeconomic disadvantage (MTA Cooperative Group, 1999). Similarly, no significant ethnic differences in outcomes were found between Latino and non-Hispanic White youths with anxiety disorders who received CBT treatment (Silverman et al., 1999). However, a parent training program demonstrated differential effects on outcomes for Latino and non-Hispanic White youths; specifically, that teacher-rated internalizing problems was reduced in the non-Hispanic White sample but not for the Latino sample. This study illustrates the possibility that racial/ethnic disparities in outcomes exist for Latinos, and further research is needed before any generalizations can be made.

In summary, there is evidence that Latino youth do benefit from services delivered in clinical trials and in more generalized settings, but there is inconsistent evidence when comparing their treatment gains with non-Hispanic White youth. It is possible that racial/ethnic disparities in outcomes do exist for Latinos and further research is needed before any generalizations can be made.

Asian/ Pacific Islanders

Research involving Asian/Pacific Islander youth is lacking (USDHHS, 2001), although limited research with Asian American adults suggest that they had poorer short term results than Whites (Zane, Enomoto, and Chun, 1994). One study reported a reduction in behavioral problems for children of Asian American mothers after completing a parent management program, and that there were no significant differences in outcomes between youths of Asian and non-Hispanic White mothers (Reid et al., 2001).

American Indian/Alaskan Native

To date, no studies examining treatment outcomes in mental health services for American Indian or Alaskan Native youth (or adults) have been published (USDHHS, 2001). However, a review of the literature on American Indian youth by Miranda and colleagues (2005) revealed that prevention interventions offered through schools are successful at decreasing depression, hopelessness, and suicidal ideation among American Indian youth.

Outcomes for Minority Children: Summary

Review of the current evidence base suggests that African American and Latino youth experience symptom improvement in mental health services. No significant racial/ethnic differences in outcomes were found for African American youth in the current evidence base, although some inconsistencies exist for Latino youth in currently available studies. Only one study examined an Asian youth sample, and there are no studies examining outcomes for American Indian and Alaskan Native children. Taken together, the extent to which evidence-based mental health services are beneficial for populations other than African American and Latino youths is unknown.

To address these gaps in the outcome literature for minority youth, researchers should make inclusion of minority youth in both efficacy and effectiveness studies a priority. Obtaining adequate samples to enable comparison of outcomes across groups would be most desirable; however, when this is not possible, providing information on racial/ethnic breakdowns of study samples will help to contextualize results and enable the generalizability of findings. Despite these limitations, current trends demonstrate that this evidence base has been growing, especially efficacy studies that include minority youth. This is encouraging because efficacy studies may be considered the first necessary step to building the evidence base for outcomes research, as effectiveness studies focus on the real-world examination of treatments found to be efficacious. To continue bridging the gap between efficacy and effectiveness in research, a focus on effectiveness studies is also needed to examine how efficacious treatments work in real-world delivery settings, and whether culturally adapted efficacious treatments are beneficial for minority youth.

BARRIERS

We have provided a review of research on the current state of minority youth mental health care. To summarize the current findings, racial and ethnic minority youth

- Experience higher levels of unmet mental health need as compared to non-Hispanic Whites
- May experience higher rates of premature termination and dropout than do non-Hispanic Whites
- May receive lower quality care as compared to non-Hispanic Whites, similar to patterns observed in their adult counterparts
- Experience some improvement from therapy
- Are significantly underrepresented in outcome studies

Despite national and local efforts for improving youth mental health care in the U. S., findings in the current evidence base suggest that many obstacles exist in the service utilization pathway for ethnic minority families. Understanding the unique sets of barriers experienced by various racial/ethnic groups is a necessary first step to reducing these documented disparities in minority mental health care; however, few studies have examined specific barriers to mental health care for minority families. Despite the limited number of empirical studies, researchers have hypothesized that numerous contextual and cultural barriers discourage mental health service use and effective care for different cultural groups above and beyond those for non-Hispanic White populations. For youth mental health care, adult caretakers play a critical role in the child's utilization and experience of mental health services, as children are rarely self-referred and adults are usually the key decision-makers (McKay, Pennignton, Lynn, and McCadam, 2001). The experience of obstacles is rarely focused solely on the youth; instead, the experience of barriers by the family (i.e., parent/caregivers) will be pivotal to youth mental health care. As such, we will also summarize applicable findings from the minority adult literature. In the following discussion, we illustrate how contextual factors, client factors, provider factors, and client and provider interactions may act as barriers to minority mental health care.

Contextual Barriers

Contextual barriers in this discussion include social and economic influences present in the immediate environment that may act as barriers to mental health care for minority youths.

These contextual barriers can be presented in three broad classifications: concrete barriers, stressor barriers, and referral barriers.

Concrete Barriers

Concrete obstacles such as inaccessible locations (Baekeland and Lundwall, 1975; Boyd-Franklin, 1993), lack of monies to pay for services and general financial disadvantage (Leong, Wagner, and Tata, 1995; McNeil and Kennedy, 1997; Tolan and McKay, 1996), lack of private insurance (Kataoka et al., 2002; Smedley, Stith, and Nelson, 2003), transportation problems (Koroloff, Elliot, Koren, and Frisen, 1994), lack of time (Tolan and McKay, 1996), and lack of child care (Hahn, 1995; McKay, McCadam, and Gonzales, 1996) have been found to be significant barriers to obtaining mental health care for low-income minority families and low-income families in general. There is evidence that minority groups are overrepresented among the poor (USDHHS, 2001), and low-income minority children are more likely higher-income children to demonstrate increased mental health difficulties. However, these children, compared to higher income or non-minority children, are the least likely to use services (Kazdin, 1993; Regier et al., 1993). These findings suggest that concrete barriers may have implications for service utilization, may impact treatment retention once in therapy, and may play a larger role in impeding effective youth mental health care for minorities with lower socioeconomic status than for other groups.

Stressor Barriers

Stressor barriers such as lack of social support, stress associated with poverty, family dysfunction, and negative life events have been linked with lower initial utilization of services, ongoing engagement of families and treatment retention rates, and eventual outcomes in youth and family intervention studies for various cultural groups including non-Hispanic Whites (Harrison, McKay, and Bannon, 2004; Morrisey-Kane and Prinz, 1999; McKay, Pennington, Lynn, and McCadam, 2001). In one study, mothers' social networks (both in terms of quality and quantity) were important in the service utilization process as parents tended to consult family members and friends for feedback about how to handle their youth's problems (Arcia and Fernadez, 2003). Parents frequently used social support networks to discuss their youth's mental health problems and agreed that using services would be appropriate; parents who attended at least one appointment had spoken to their primary social support person prior to entering services (Harrison et al., 2004), and encouragement from social support networks to seek help was significantly associated with keeping a first appointment at an outpatient mental health program and longer length of stay in services for youth and their families (McKay et al., 2001; Harrison et al., 2004). Therefore, lack of social support systems for families in distress acted as an impediment to receiving needed services. Higher levels of family stress significantly predicted lower attendance at scheduled appointments for youths (McKay et al., 2004) and utilization of mental health services for adults (Abe-Kim, Takeuchi, and Hwang, 2002), suggesting that families in great distress may be unlikely to enter or stay in services. There is some evidence that these stressor barriers may be more prevalent for minority families than for non-Hispanic Whites. Studies indicate that minority families report more stress and experience greater caregiver burden, and that these stressors tend to increase hostile parenting, reduce parental warmth, and decrease the likelihood of recognizing problems and seeking help to address them (Hill and Herman-Stahl, 2002; Pinderhughes, Nix, Foster, Jones, and The Conduct Problems

Prevention Research Group, 2001; Brannan, Helfinger, and Bickman, 1995). It is possible that the increase of hostile parenting may also lead to service referrals to the child welfare system, and there is evidence that suggest African American children have a higher likelihood of receiving treatment in this sector instead of the mental health sector (Halfon et al., 1992; Takayama et al., 1994). These experiences of hardship are also more likely to occur for low-income families, as reported stress and burden often relate to inadequate resources (either financial or social, such as lack of funds to purchase necessities or weak social support systems). In other words, parents experiencing more distress were less likely to enroll and retain their youth in mental health services (Harrison et al., 2004), which is alarming because these families may need more assistance with the youth's emotional/behavioral concerns compared to less distressed families.

Referral Barriers

Children rarely seek services on their own and are often referred by adults (e.g., parents, school personnel, county officials), and there is evidence that barriers exist in the youth service referral process. For example, parents often act as gatekeepers to their child's care, and the receipt of services may be determined by whether the parent recognizes the problem as needing intervention (McMiller and Weisz, 1996; Cauce et al., 2002). Thus, parental recognition of problems and decision to seek services for the youth are important factors, and delays in recognition or decision-making can act as barriers to referral. For children, schools are also a primary gatekeeper to enrollment in mental health services (Forness, 2003). However, there is evidence that school psychologists and educators were "back-loading" most of their efforts, only referring children to needed services long after the diagnosis was fully realized (Hoagwood and Johnson, 2003). For example, Duncan, Forness, and Hartsough (1995) found that average placement in special classrooms for emotional or behavioral disorders was 10.4 years, but parents had recognized some symptomatology at an average age of 3.5 years. Therefore, not "front loading" at the earliest signs of trouble may delay or even prevent treatment for youth. Furthermore, there is evidence that there are differential referral patterns for minority children. For example, Latino children who were using public mental health services were less likely to have received school-based mental health services than were non-Hispanic Whites, especially when the services required a referral from school personnel (Yeh et. al., 2002), and there is evidence that African American youth with mental health problems were more likely to enter services through the child welfare or juvenile justice sector (Halfon et al., 1992; Takayama et al., 1994; USDHHS, 2001).

Research also suggests that misidentification of by referral sources (e.g., schools) was common (Forness, 2003). Fewer than one in four youth identified for special education services was correctly detected as having emotional or behavioral disorders by school personnel (Redden et al., 1999), and instead, these youth were labeled as having only learning or related problems (Redden et al., 1999; Lopez, Forness, MacMillan, Bocian, and Gresham, 1996). Such misidentification of mental health problems may result in a lack of specific treatment for these problems. In the adult literature, there is evidence that misidentification of mental health problems is more common in minority adults by medical professionals (e.g., Sclar et al., 1999). It is possible that these racial/ethnic differences in misidentification rates extend to children by school personnel, and it would be important to determine if such trends exist for children, as well. Future research is needed to elucidate these relationships. Taken together, literature to date suggest that while factors in the referral process may act as barriers to youth mental health service entry for minorities and non-minorities alike, it is likely that referrals are even more problematic for minority children and may act as significant barriers to effective mental health care.

Client Barriers

Client barriers in this discussion include factors that are most attributable to individual characteristics of the youth and family (e.g., beliefs, values, attitudes). These client barriers include perceived and cultural barriers.

Perceived and Cultural Barriers
In addition to concrete barriers, a number of perceived barriers (i.e., perception that there are difficulties to using or staying in services) also seem to greatly impede minority youth service utilization (USDHHS, 2001). Perceived barriers have been found to be significant predictors of higher premature termination of services rates and low adherence to treatment recommendations (McNaughton, 2001), indicating that continuity of care may be severely compromised if the family perceives a high number of barriers to mental health service use.

Minority families tend to perceive greater barriers to using services, and these barriers are often culture-related (USDHHS, 2001). For minority families, cultural factors may act as barriers to youth mental health care, and we adopt Cauce's model (2002) to describe cultural variables identified in the current literature that play key roles in youth mental health care. Cauce states that culture plays a role in three junctions of the service utilization pathway: 1) problem recognition and definition, 2) the decision to seek help, and 3) service selection (Cauce et al., 2002). Although Cauce's model is more specific to service utilization, we also include in our discussion the impact cultural factors may have in treatment retention, quality of services received, and outcomes from therapy. It is also important to note that for youth mental health care, parents' cultural background and experience with barriers may be more important to service utilization, treatment retention, and eventual outcomes from therapy, as children rarely refer themselves for services and parents usually act as gatekeepers to youth mental health care (McMiller and Weisz, 1996). Therefore, we will include relevant discussions of findings from the minority adult evidence base when applicable.

Problem Recognition and Definition
Problem recognition is the first step to help-seeking, and families may be less likely to seek services in the mental health sector if they do not believe their child's emotional/behavioral problems are mental health related. Indeed, there is evidence that cultural groups differ on what is perceived to be a mental health problem (Fabrega, Ulrich, and Mezzich, 1993), and minority parents are more likely to identify their child's emotional/behavioral problems as non-mental health related than non-Hispanic White parents or not identify them as problems at all (USDHHS, 2001). For example, some cultures may be more accepting of certain psychiatric symptoms and have different "distress thresholds," or variations in what is considered undesirable or abnormal (Weisz and Weiss, 1991); Thai parents rated their child's emotional/behavioral problems as less worrisome, less likely to reflect stable traits, and more likely to improve with time compared to American parents

(Weisz, Walter, Chaiyasit, Anderson, 1988). Parents who hold these beliefs may not be likely to seek help of any sort, as they do not view their child's behaviors as problematic or needing intervention.

There are also cultural differences in the explanation of youths' emotional/behavioral problems. African American parents were less likely than White parents to describe their child's ADHD symptoms using medical or mental health labels (Bussing, Schoenberg, Rogers, Zima, and Angus, 1998). African American and Asian/Pacific Islander parents held etiological beliefs about their child's emotional/behavioral problems that were more sociological in nature and less consistent with biopsychosocial explanations compared to non-Hispanic Whites (Yeh, Hough et al., 2004), and parental beliefs about their child's problems helped in part to explain racial/ethnic disparities in the utilization of special education services for youth with emotional disturbance (Yeh, Forness et al., 2004) and specialty mental health service use (Yeh et al., 2005). Evidence suggests that Mexican American parents value parental authority (Rosello and Bernal, 1996) and are more likely to view their child's problems as a matter of ineffective discipline (e.g., requiring more strict discipline) rather than a mental health concern needing to be addressed with psychotherapy (McCabe, 2002). These cultural differences in the problem recognition stage illustrate how minority parents may be less likely to recognize their child's emotional/behavioral problems as needing intervention in the mental health sector or needing intervention of any type.

Adding to the complexity of problem recognition is the developmental course of mental health problems in children. Many psychiatric disorders in their earliest stages are not always recognized as such (Forness, 2003). Parents and professionals may have been concerned about emotional/behavioral problems in children but did not view them as early symptoms of mental illness. The failure to recognize early symptoms of psychopathology may be an important barrier for minority and non-minority youth alike, with important implications in the recognition process and subsequent help-seeking behavior in any sector.

The Decision to Seek Help

Once a mental health problem is recognized as abnormal, undesirable, and/or needing intervention, cultural factors play a key role in whether families actually seek help. Attitudes toward mental health problems and mental health treatment act as very influential barriers to youth mental health care as they not only affect help-seeking behavior, but also predict actual service utilization rates and treatment outcomes (Corrigan, 2004; Gonzalez, Alegria, and Prihoda, 2005). Studies suggest that many minority groups hold negative attitudes toward individuals with mental health problems, viewing them as dangerous or as outcasts of society (Whaley, 1997; Pescosolido, Monahan, Link, Stueve, and Kikuzawa, 1999). Evidence shows that minorities are less likely to seek help even when a mental health problem is distressing and unlikely to resolve on its own due to negative attitudes and stigma toward mental health problems and toward seeking help for problems (for mental health concerns as well as problems in general). Current literature suggests that many minority groups hold extremely negative attitudes towards individuals with mental health problems; one study found that Asian Americans, Hispanic Americans, and African Americans viewed mentally ill individuals as dangerous (Whaley, 1997). For many Asian groups, mental illness is highly stigmatizing and reflects poorly on one's family lineage, and can influence the community's beliefs about how suitable someone is for marriage and economic/career pursuits (Sue and Morishima, 1982; Ng, 1997). Many Asians with mental health problems become so ashamed of their illness and so fearful of the impact it could have on their societal status that they often conceal their symptoms around others (Wahl, 1999), leading to a decision not to seek help. It is hypothesized that similar stigmatizing attitudes exist in many Latino cultures (USDHHS, 2001), although studies that examine these attitudes specifically for Latino youths are currently lacking.

In many minority cultures, seeking help for any problems (not just mental health related) is viewed negatively and considered undesirable. In many East Asian cultures, requiring help from sources outside one's family for any problems is regarded as shameful and a "loss of face" (Zane and Yeh, 2002; Cheung and Snowden, 1990; Liao, Rounds, and Klein, 2005). Therefore, Asian American families make every attempt to deal with the child's emotional/behavioral problems within the family before going to outside sources (Lin, Inui, Kleinman, and Womack, 1992). This is supported by the finding that among Asians, only 12% mentioned their mental health problems to friends/relatives, and only 7% consulted a mental health professional or a physician, rates that are much lower than those for non-Hispanic Whites (Zhang, Snowden, and Sue, 1998). This is also supported by the finding that APIs are the most severe in their symptom presentation at initial service use compared to other racial/ethnic groups (Brown et al., 1973; Bui and Takeuchi, 1992; Durvasula and Sue, 1996; Sue and Sue, 1974).

Latino families value stoicism and, similar to Asians, prefer to handle all problems within the family (Alvidrez, 1999; Martinez, 1993; Rosello and Bernal, 1996). African Americans are more inclined than Whites to handle distress on their own without others' help (Sussman, Robins, and Earls, 1987) and strive to overcome mental health problems through self-reliance and determination (Snowden, 1998); African American youths are encouraged by adults to use willpower to overcome adversity or to "tough out" certain difficult situations (Poulin et al., 1997). These cultural values and beliefs encourage many minority individuals to deal with problems on their own or within the immediate family, and lead to a lesser likelihood of seeking help in any setting, mental health or otherwise, formal or informal.

There is some evidence that cultural values related to help-seeking may vary by acculturation level. Findings with Asian adolescents and young adults show that those more aligned with values of their indigenous culture were least likely to recognize a need for professional help, least tolerant of stigma associated with deciding to seek help, and least open to discussing problems with a professional (Atkinson and Gim, 1989). Results of this study suggest that acculturation or the degree to which one is affiliated with mainstream American culture and one's indigenous culture is important to consider when examining the level of impact cultural values may have in help-seeking for a particular family.

Service Selection

Once a problem is recognized and the decision to seek help of some type is made, cultural factors may act as barriers for minority families to seek help in the mental health sector. Minority families are more likely to hold stigma attached specifically to mental health service use and negative attitudes toward mental health care professionals (USDHHS, 2001), and thus are less inclined than Whites to seek services in the mental health sector (Gallo, Marino, Ford, and Anthony, 1995; Chun et al., 1996). For example, studies show that minorities are wary of unfair treatment or discrimination due to their cultural background. Minority parents tend to be fearful of professional mental health services because they were afraid that family members will be in appropriately labeled, medicated, or hospitalized

(Staggers, 1987). African Americans are more suspicious and fearful of mental health treatment and hospitalization compared to Whites (Sussman et al., 1987; Uba, 1994), and Latinos felt that health care providers have treated them badly because of their race/ethnicity (LaVeist et al., 2002). These fears of being mistreated may deter minority families from selecting services in the specialty mental health sector. Once in services, minority families are more likely to continue to hold these negative attitudes toward mental health care and tend to endorse negative expectations of treatment outcomes (Richardson, 2001). Negative expectations may act as an important barrier to staying in services, as studies show that these attitudes predict subsequent barriers to participation in services, premature dropout, and poor outcomes (USDHHS, 2001; Nock and Kazdin, 2001). These results reiterate the importance of parental attitudes in youth mental health care, and suggest that attitudes may not only influence parents' decisions to seek services in the mental health sector but also influences their interest in ongoing involvement with mental health treatment for their child (McKay et al., 2004).

Many minority families prefer other sources of care that are more consistent with their cultural practices, norms, and/or beliefs, and often favor informal sources of care such as family, friends, clergy, and traditional healers over formal sources of care such as general health care in the medical setting or specialty mental health care (Harrison et al., 2004; Snowden, 2001; Peifer, Hu, and Vega, 2000). African American, Mexican American, and American Indian youth and adults often turn to their friends, relatives, or immediate family members for assistance with mental health concerns (Bee-Gates, Howard-Pitney, LaFromboise, and Rowe, 1996). African Americans also tend to rely more on spirituality to help them cope with adversity and symptoms of mental illness than other cultural groups (Broman, 1996; Neighbors et al., 1998), and prayer and seeking guidance from ministers are among some of their most common coping responses (Taylor and Chatters, 1991; USDHHS, 2001; Levin, 1986). African Americans often utilize alternative treatments for mental health problems (USDHHS, 2001). Latinos and American Indian adolescents and adults often use folk remedies or indigenous healers for their psychiatric concerns (Novins et al., 2004; Keegan, 1996), and Asian/Pacific Islanders often used complementary therapies such as Chinese medicine (USDHHS, 2001). While use of alternative services in itself a barrier to mental health service use (as it does not necessarily preclude concurrent use of specialty mental health services), there is evidence that minority groups utilize informal networks or traditional healing options in lieu of services in the mental health sector, and that specialty mental health services were not preferred. For over two-thirds of parents of minority youth, seeking help from professionals was not their first choice (McMiller and Weisz, 1996), and they often exhibit a reluctance to utilize and participate in mental health services (Tolan and McKay, 1996). Minority parents were about one-third as likely as non-Hispanic White parents to contact professionals during the initial stages of help-seeking and service selection, and much more likely to make initial contact for assistance with family and community members (McMiller and Weisz, 1996). African Americans often utilize alternative treatments for mental health problems instead of seeking mainstream health care (USDHHS, 2001), and Asian Americans are likely to see formal treatment as a last resort and will only utilize professional services after exhausting all other resources (Lin et al., 1992; Okazaki, 2000).

When minority groups do decide to seek any type of mainstream professional help, they are twice as likely to seek treatment in general health care settings as opposed to specialty mental health settings (Cooper-Patrick et al., 1999). This service choice is related to unfamiliarity with psychotherapy and mental health service options, which is common among minority families. Different cultural groups may be less knowledgeable and less informed about mental health treatment options (USDHHS, 2001; McCabe, 2002), which may be due in part to other factors such as an unfamiliarity with American culture and Westernized mental health care, especially for recent immigrants or the less acculturated (Yeh et al., 2003; Keefe and Casas, 1980; USDHHS, 2001), negative attitudes towards mental health care (e.g., minority individuals may be less willing or less motivated to learn about mental health treatment due to stigma associated with using services), or socioeconomic status (e.g., poorer families may not have the resources to access information about available services). This lack of knowledge, which may be related to some of these other cultural or contextual factors, may act as a barrier to service use in the mental health sector simply because families are unaware of service availability.

Beyond unfamiliarity, minority families also seem to have important differences when compared to non-Hispanic White families regarding expressions of illness and views on what types of treatment may be appropriate for their symptoms. Specifically, minority individuals seem to have different symptom experiences and idioms of distress from White individuals (USDHHS, 2001) and are more likely to view mental disorders as physiological problems that should be treated by primary care physicians (Acosta et al., 1983, Vega et al., 1999). However, there is concern that primary care providers may not be adequately trained to recognize mental disorders and may not be equipped to provide the specific services patients need for their mental health problems, especially if they have co-existing physical disorders (Rost et al, 2000). In fact, minorities are at greater risk than non-minorities for missed and/or incorrect diagnoses in primary health care, resulting in inappropriate treatments in the general medical setting (Borowsky et al., 2000). Specialty mental health services may offer more appropriate assessments and specific treatments for individuals with mental health problems, but these services in the mental health sector are usually not preferred or selected by minorities due to a number of cultural factors, some of which were highlighted here.

Provider Barriers

Provider barriers in this discussion include factors that are present on the service delivery side of mental health treatment for minority youths. These provider barriers can be presented in two broad classifications: agency barriers and clinician characteristics.

Agency Barriers

System Barriers

Among the most often mentioned barriers to service use for low income minority families were factors at the agency level such as inconvenient agency hours, scheduling problems, waiting lists, and unresponsive service providers (Staudt, 1999; McKay, Pennington, Lynn, and McCadam, 2001). These barriers seem to be ones that may be more readily reduced by providers to effect greater service use and improve quality of care for youths of all cultural groups (including non-Hispanic Whites); nevertheless, attrition is largely associated with these factors, especially for low-income families (McKay et al., 2001). On a larger agency level, fragmented community mental health care that lacks adequate communication between agencies, inadequacy of community-based services to deliver appropriate care for minority families with mental health concerns, and an overreliance on institutional care for minority youth (often resulting in unnecessary hospitalizations) are other barriers that impede service utilization and improved mental health care for minority children and their families (Collins and Collins, 1994; USDHHS, 2001). These barriers may be more difficult to address as they involve the larger systems of care of the mentally ill youth (nonminority and minority) in the U. S.

Lack of Availability of Same-language Therapist

There is a limited availability of mental health professionals that speak a language other than English fluently (USDHHS, 2001). The effects of language barriers are heightened during the treatment process, when it is crucial for clinicians and families to communicate effectively in order to facilitate change. Lack of availability of same-language therapists for minority youths (especially recent immigrants or those less acculturated to mainstream American society) can be a deterrent to utilizing services and reduce quality of care and treatment retention. One study found that language match between therapist and youth significantly predicted dropout and total number of sessions attended for Mexican American adolescents ages 12-17 (Yeh, Eastman, and Cheung; 1994), which suggests that language match is an important factor to consider in the treatment process for minority families and warrants further investigation in future studies.

Lack of Availability of Same-culture Clinicians

The current U. S. population mainly consists of White practitioners, and there is evidence that ethnic mismatch between clients and therapists leads to higher rates of dropout before service completion for minority families (USDHHS, 2001). Evidence suggests that ethnic match is a significant predictor of dropout for African American, Mexican American, and Asian American adolescents, and number of sessions attended for Mexican American and Asian American adolescents (Yeh et al., 1994). These findings suggests that ethnic match is an important factor to consider in the treatment process for minority families, perhaps due to a sense of comfortability in relating personal issues to a professional that appears to be familiar with the family's culture of origin.

Clinician Characteristics

Clinicians bring their own personal cultures, beliefs, and experiences to the therapy setting (Hunt, 1995; Porter, 1997), and as such, can be said to have a "culture" of their own (USDHHS, 2001). The "culture" of the clinician is reflected in the jargon members use, and in their mindset and worldviews, which may be very different from the culture of their patients. Specifically, clinicians and patients may have different beliefs about the causes of mental health problems, different ideas about each individual's roles in treatment, and find certain symptoms to be more or less important to address in therapy than youth and parents (USDHHS, 2001). The barriers discussed in this section involve characteristics of the client that may significantly impact client-therapist interactions in treatment.

Miscommunication and Inadequate Communication

With the current limited availability of therapists who are themselves cultural minorities, the most commonly occurring pairings of therapist-client relationships will involve the intersection of more than one ethnic culture. When the clinician and the patient are from different cultural backgrounds, misalliance and miscommunication is more likely to occur (USDHHS, 2001). Miscommunication between therapists can obviously occur when the language preferred by the therapist is different from language preferred by the parent or youth; however, it can also occur when the clinician and patient speak the same language but are from different cultural backgrounds (USDHHS, 2001).

Misdiagnosis largely originates from ineffective communication regarding symptomatology and difficulties that clinicians have in addressing cultural differences (Pumariega, Rogers, and Rothe 2005), resulting in a higher likelihood for inaccurate diagnoses or missed diagnoses for minorities. Studies have shown that assessment results are affected by whether Latino adult patients were interviewed in Spanish or in English (Price and Cuellar, 1981; Malgady and Constantino, 1998). Specifically, more psychopathology was communicated when patients reported their problems in Spanish than when they reported problems in English, resulting in more diagnoses when interviews were conducted in Spanish. Other literature for minority adults show that Asian Americans were more likely to receive an inaccurate diagnosis than non-Hispanic Whites (Strakowski et al., 1997), Latinos with mood disorders were more likely to have been diagnosed with a psychotic disorder than non-Hispanic Whites (Mukherjee, Shukla, Woodle, Rosen, and Olarte, 1983), and Asian Americans were likely to not be diagnosed with any mental health illness even when they present with mental health concerns (USDHHS, 2001).

Although evidence for misdiagnoses is less clear for youths, there is mounting evidence that diagnoses disparities exist for minority youths compared to their non-Hispanic White counterparts. African American youth in mental health services were less likely to be diagnosed with ADHD or a mood disorder compared to non-Hispanic White youth (Yeh et al., 2002), Latino youth were more likely than non-Hispanic White youth to be diagnosed with adjustment disorders, anxiety disorders, and psychotic disorders, and less likely to be diagnosed with ADHD than non-Hispanic White youth (Yeh et al., 2002). Asian American youth were more likely to receive diagnoses of anxiety and adjustment disorder, and less likely to receive diagnoses of ADHD and depression than non-Hispanic Whites (Nguyen et al., 2004; Yeh et al., 2002). American Indian youth were less likely to be diagnosed with anxiety disorders and more likely to be diagnosed with ADHD and substance use disorders than non-Hispanic White youth (Schaffer et al., 1996). These results may reflect real differences in prevalence rates of disorders in different cultural groups, differential use of mental health services, or could be evidence of misdiagnoses for minority youth largely due to miscommunication or inadequate communication by therapists. Other clinician characteristics, such as clinician biases and stereotypes about different groups or lack of knowledge of possible differences in symptom presentation by minorities compared to non-Hispanic Whites may also result in inaccurate or missed diagnoses (Smedley et al., 2003). Epidemiological studies that examine the rates of mental illness among different cultural groups and studies comparing the diagnoses minority youth receive from different providers are needed to elucidate the implications of these findings of differential diagnoses in minority youth in mental health services.

The responsibility rests on the therapist, as the service provider, to communicate assessment results and elements of the treatment process as clearly as possible to patients. Inadequate communication or miscommunication by the therapist post-assessment may act as a significant barrier to treatment retention and eventual outcomes, and may lead to incongruent ideas and expectations for treatment by both parties (therapist and client). Findings suggest that a mismatch between client and therapist expectations for the treatment process leads to greater dropout (Acosta, et al., 1983). Parents are likely to dropout prematurely when they have different expectations from the therapist in terms of how long treatment will last, how quickly their child will begin to improve, and how much parents will be expected to participate in the process (Kupst and Shulman, 1979; Morrissey-Kane and Prinz, 1999). In addition, parents who expected their child to recover quickly were more likely to drop out of treatment after attending only one session (McCabe et al., 1999).

Clinician's Personal Biases and Inadequate Consideration of Cultural Factors

While results suggest that lack of availability of same-language and same-ethnicity therapists may be important barriers to minority youth mental health care, the bigger and more relevant issue may be a lack of culturally sensitive therapists who are able to understand the patient's culture and identify culturally-related needs in the therapeutic process. Taken one step further, there may be a lack of cultural competence in current service delivery, a concept that goes beyond awareness and sensitivity to include the possession of cultural knowledge and respect for different cultural perspectives, and having the ability to use these skills effectively in cross-cultural situations (Cross, Bazron, Dennis, and Issacs, 1989; Orlandi, 1995; Tirado, 1996; Brach, 2000).

Therapists' personal biases regarding minorities and/or lack of consideration of the client's cultural values may serve as barriers that deter minority families from continuing services once enrolled (USDHHS, 2001). Lack of availability of clinicians trained in cultural issues can lead to failure to form effective therapeutic alliances (Cooper et al., 2003) and lower satisfaction with treatment (USDHHS, 2001). In one study, adult participants endorsed a lower satisfaction with cultural sensitivity of therapists compared to general satisfaction ratings for services received (Leveille, 2004). Client's ratings of the cultural competence of therapist appear to be closely related to client's overall competence ratings of the therapist (Constantine, 2002), suggesting that consideration of client's cultural values and needs may improve the experience of services for minority families.

Clinician's Inadequate Involvement of Families in Treatment

Inadequate involvement of families in therapy by the treatment staff may also be a significant barrier to minority youth mental health service use. Because parents are the gatekeepers to youth mental health care (McMiller and Weisz, 1996), parents are often viewed as essential components to youth's treatment success (Henggeler, 1994); thus, engaging the family in the treatment process is integral to service retention. The issue of engagement is prevalent across all cultural groups in youth mental health care (including non-Hispanic Whites) and inadequate attention to engagement can act as a barrier for both minority and nonminority families. However, there is evidence that minority families in youth mental health services may experience even higher dropout rates than non-Hispanic Whites (Kazdin, Stolar, and Marciano, 1995), suggesting that family involvement in services may be both a challenge with minority families as well as even more critical for treatment retention and success as compared to non-Hispanic Whites. For example, studies show that the degree to which families are involved in service planning and family perception of aspects of the therapeutic relationship are predictive of premature dropout (Garcia and Weisz, 2002). In one study, client/family reported therapeutic relationship problems was the greatest predictor of premature termination (Garcia and Weisz, 2002), and matching parental preference for type of service offered to children and what the child actually receives was significantly associated with higher number of sessions attended (Bannon and McKay, 2005). Poor family involvement and therapeutic alliance may act as barriers to service use and have a significant negative impact on treatment retention, and eventual outcomes in therapy.

Summary of Barriers

As illustrated in the above examples, there are a number of barriers that minority families experience in service utilization, retention, and treatment outcomes in mental health care. The context in which the family experiences the youth's emotional/behavioral problem and its associated burdens can act as a severe impediment to receiving and staying in needed services. Barriers perceived by the family and how these are created and maintained by cultural variables also contribute to the disparities evident for minority families in the youth mental health literature. Finally, provider characteristics, including both those present at the agency level as well as at the individual level, may serve to affect not only the utilization process but also the client-therapist relationship in treatment. Please see Appendix 1 for a summary of barriers discussed in this section.

A CONCEPTUAL MODEL

Researchers have consistently demonstrated that disrupted care continues to occur for minority clients after barriers to initial access have been surmounted (Snowden and Yamada, 2005). To better understand why disparities in mental health care occur beyond access, more attention should be paid to the development of the provider-client relationship and the role of cultural factors in its formation (Snowden and Yamada, 2005, Martin et al., 2000). The factors that act as barriers to service utilization as outlined previously may also impact the treatment relationship. At the level of the therapeutic relationship, the impact of these various barriers intersect (contextual, client, provider) and can seriously jeopardize the quality of care (actual or perceived), the investment in the treatment process by all parties involved (e.g., youth, parent, therapist), and treatment outcomes. Limited evidence supports a relationship between the quality of the therapeutic relationship and treatment outcomes for children and adolescents (Shirk and Karver, 2003). Therefore, bringing the therapeutic relationship to the forefront when examining disparities in mental health care may be helpful to increase understanding of how and at which junctures various factors interact in the treatment process, and identify mechanisms to target for disparity reduction.

We present a diagram here that highlights how the influence of sociopolitical, contextual, and cultural factors culminate in the client-clinician interaction. In this diagram, we also show the possible interaction of client and clinician characteristics that lead to various cultural outcomes, such as cultural congruence/incongruence (the degree of agreement and/or consensus in cultural values, beliefs, behaviors, and treatment goals between the client and therapist), cultural alliance/misalliance (the degree to which there is a mutual understanding of cultural values and beliefs of the client and therapist and a sense of teamwork or camaraderie in the treatment process), and cultural competence/incompetence (the degree to which there is respect for different cultural perspectives between the client and therapist, and whether the therapists possesses the skills to use this knowledge effectively in the therapeutic milieu).

The larger sociopolitical and cultural environment represents the daily practices, social norms and group worldviews and ideologies in which an individual is immersed on a continual basis. In addition, the historical context of a cultural group, along with specific cultural beliefs, values, and attitudes also shape an individual's experience and affect daily interactions with others. Within this larger sociopolitical/cultural environment, contextual factors and agency factors (described in detail in the above section) may act as barriers or facilitators for using services and for the development of the client-therapist relationship. At the level of the client and clinician characteristics, individual experiences stemming from the larger sociopolitical/cultural, contextual, and agency environments, along with specific beliefs and attitudes toward mental health illness, mental health treatment, and expectancies of the therapeutic process directly influence the client-clinician relationship, and subsequently, outcomes from therapy. In summary, we believe that racially disparate problem recognition and decision making primarily takes place within the larger sociopolitical, contextual, and cultural environments, and that racially disparate outcomes primarily result as a product of the client-clinician interaction, which is a culmination of the influences of these larger environments (i.e., sociopolitical, contextual, cultural).

Table 1. A diagram illustrating the contribution of various factors to the client-clinician interaction

This diagram specifies the mechanisms that may be influential to the client-clinician relationship, and takes multi-level influences into account. We hope that this further illustrates the complexities of mental health care for minority youth, elucidates the various interrelationships between factors that can act as barriers, and helps to identify potential mechanisms to reduce barriers and improve mental health care for these populations.

Recommendations

The evidence provided in this review supports the conclusion that there are disparities for minority youth and families in mental health care. In addition, we have reviewed barriers that may impede effective mental health care for these populations, ranging from contextual factors to characteristics of the client and provider. In addition, we have discussed the therapeutic relationship as a key vehicle to effect improvement in the delivery of mental health services for minority youth, and we described a diagram that highlights how various sociopolitical, contextual, and agency factors may play a role in the development of this relationship in the mental health treatment process. We now discuss the results from this review for current mental health care and suggest recommendations that may help to reduce barriers, promote access, and improve outcomes for minority youths in mental health services.

Include Racial/Ethnic Minorities in Services and Outcomes Research
In this review, we have summarized existing data regarding the disparities in care that ethnic minority families currently face in the youth mental health care system. However, it is difficult to draw finite, generalizable conclusions based on the paucity of studies that include minorities in their samples and the limited number of studies that have examined relationships between variables in the mental health treatment process. The existing body of knowledge is often inconsistent, and although we continue to observe disparities in mental health care for minority families, we cannot adequately explain these findings. In recent years, national agencies have recognized ethnic minorities as a priority population in research. In March 1994, the policies of the National Institutes of Health (NIH) regarding inclusion of racial/ethnic minorities in research populations were significantly strengthened (NIH Guidelines, 1994), requiring inclusion of ethnic minorities in all NIH-funded research. In 2002, NIH reiterated the importance of not excluding minority populations unless it is scientifically justifiable (NIH, 2002).

Other national agencies such as Agency for Healthcare Research and Quality (AHRQ) and Substances and Mental Health Services Association (SAMHSA) have also prioritized minority mental health access and outcome issues into special funding initiatives (AHRQ, 2002). Inclusion of minority participants in mental health research is the first step to increasing the knowledge base for racial/ethnic youth.

Including enough minority participants in samples to be able to examine racial/ethnic differences between groups on a number of mental health treatment variables is also a priority. Data is especially lacking for minorities in clinical trials research that examines the efficacy of mental health treatment, although much of community-based effectiveness research also fails to include an adequate number of minorities in their samples. Many existing studies rely on small samples of minority groups which limits generalizability of findings and likely produces inconsistencies in results; as such, oversampling minorities (e.g., using block designs and random sampling by strata) for research samples may be appropriate in order to facilitate statistical comparisons (Miranda, Nakamura, and Bernal, 2003). Inclusion of cultural groups that have been largely neglected in research such as American Indian and Alaskan Native youth is needed to examine variables impacting mental health care for these groups more systematically. Care must also be taken to ensure that samples of minority participants reflect the demographics (e.g., income, parental education, immigration status) of the increasingly diverse nation so that results are applicable and generalizable. Researchers should be cautious with inclusionary/exclusionary criteria for their participants so that certain subpopulations of minority families (e.g., non-English speakers, low income families) are not systematically excluded from participation (Walsh and Ross, 2003; Kataoka et al., 2002; USDHHS, 2001). Whenever possible, broad categorizations of race/ethnicity should be broken down to examine cultural differences for specific minority groups. For example, APIs are usually categorized into one ethnic group for research purposes, but this grouping is broad and heterogeneous, as there are many notable cultural differences between specific cultural groups (e.g., Filipino American, Cambodian American, Chinese Americans, Japanese Americans) that may uniquely contribute to disparities in mental health care. The relationships between cultural factors and variables in mental health care need to be more clearly elucidated for different ethnic groups.

Inclusion of ethnic minority families in youth mental health research is important to address current gaps in research, to increase our understanding of access, utilization, treatment, and outcomes for different cultural groups, and to guide outreach programming and program design efforts that are culturally appropriate (USDHHS, 2001; Snowden and Yamada, 2005). Ensuring that minorities are included in research will help us to obtain invaluable information to advise and improve current mental health care for minority youth.

Develop and Utilize Culturally Valid Assessment in Research and Practice

Both as a deterrent and a consequence of the inadequate inclusion of minorities in mental health research, there is a paucity of appropriate and valid measures for different cultural groups in research and practice. Researchers and practitioners often utilize measures and assessment instruments that are not culturally valid and lack cultural sensitivity. To address this problem, it is pertinent to evaluate existing measures used in research and in practice for cultural appropriateness with minorities. For example, English measures are often used with individuals who have limited English proficiency because an appropriate translation was not readily available, a practice that may result in misunderstandings due to linguistic barriers. Researchers and clinicians should be responsive to these language-related issues that may inhibit performance on tests and ensure that the content of measures used is suitable for age, educational, and proficiency levels. Mental health professionals should also ascertain whether the subjects/clients have some familiarity with completing these measures, and make sure that subjects/clients do not have strong negative psychological reactions to instruments used (Olmedo, 1981; Padilla and Medina; 1996). If measures have established reliability and validity, but are only available in English, appropriate translations of these measures may alleviate some of these linguistic barriers. However, most translations of measures are not conducted using methodologically sound procedures. In addition to the translation-back translation process involved in most translations, recommendations have drawn attention to the importance of establishing equivalence of measures (Allen and Walsh, 2000; Okazaki and Sue, 1995), specifically, semantic, content, and conceptual equivalence (Bravo, 2003; Padilla and Medina, 1996).

In certain circumstances, there may be no existing reliable and valid assessment tool to measure a construct or psychological syndrome, and the development of new measures are needed. In such circumstances, care should be taken to construct culturally appropriate measures that are sensitive to cultural variations (e.g., differential symptom expression). To develop reliable and valid measures, using focus groups that are representative of the cultural group that the measure is intended for in the development phase, and conducting multiple assessments of its validity and reliability on larger samples is necessary (Geisenger, 1994).

Regarding selection of assessment instruments and interpretation of results, whenever possible, researchers and practitioners should ensure measures of symptomatology are valid and reliable for minorities, particularly given possible differences in idioms of distress and symptom experience, and note whether norms are based on samples that include an adequate proportion of minorities (Okazaki and Sue, 1995). Using multiple measures and methods of assessment (e.g., structured, self-report, qualitative) may be especially informative, and may provide information about the convergent and incremental validity of the measures (Okazaki and Sue, 1995).

It is important to note that clinician bias and other clinician factors often act as barriers to appropriate diagnosis and assessment, and disparities in diagnoses of minority clients has been demonstrated in several studies (USDHHS, 2001). Research needs to examine how culture influences the expression and identification of problems in order to improve diagnostic accuracy (Yeh et al., 2002). For clinicians, developing a knowledge base of these potential differences between specific cultural definitions of mental health problems utilized by different ethnic groups and those used within the formal mental health system may help to create better understanding between mainstream treatment providers and minority youth. In addition, clinicians should be more aware of how their own biases and assumptions affect their assessment (Porter, Garcia, Jackson, and Valdez, 1997), and agencies should provide training in anti-racist/anti-discriminatory practices (Walker, 2005).

Examine Underlying Cultural Variables and How they Relate to Mental Health and Mental Health Care

Most existing research relies on examining mental health care across racial/ethnic groups to identify barriers, cultural factors impacting mental health care, and to explain differential access, utilization, and outcomes. Although reporting differences between racial/ethnic groups is an informative starting point and has helped us to advance the knowledge base regarding minority mental health care, future studies should also include examinations of the underlying cultural variables that are hypothesized to produce racial/ethnic group differences (Clark, 1987; Betancourt and Lopez, 1993; Okazaki and Sue 1995; Miranda, Nakamura, and Bernal, 2005). For example, some current investigations have examined specific cultural variables such as acculturation (Berry, 1997), ethnic identity (Helms, 1986; Phinney, 1996), years in the U.S., immigrant status, and beliefs about causes of mental health illness (Yeh, Forness et al., 2004) to identify relationships to variables relevant to mental health care. Results that suggest the existence of relationships between underlying cultural variables and variables relevant to mental health care may be applicable to people from various cultures, provide information on possible intervention points, and aid in designing interventions to reduce disparities.

Improve Access to Treatment and Increase Availability of Services

Conduct Research to Identify Access Barriers

There is consistent evidence that racial and ethnic minority youth, especially those who are poor, have less access than white Americans to mental health services (Snowden and Yamada, 2005). Despite the attention given to disparities in access to mental health care, a relative low percentage of funding is given toward improving access to youth mental health services (Snowden and Yamada, 2005). Race/ethnicity, culture, language, and other social factors affect the perception, availability, use, and outcomes of mental health services (USDHHS, 2001), and attention must be focused on reducing barriers to service use for individuals with high unmet need. Yeh and colleagues (2003) found that caregivers of Asian/Pacific Islander and Latino youth were significantly more likely to endorse language barriers, and that caregivers of minority youth were less likely than non-Hispanic Whites to endorse economic (African American and Asian/Pacific Islanders) and accessibility (African American, Asian/Pacific Islanders, and Latinos) barriers. These results are somewhat unexpected given that financial problems and access issues have been found to impede youth entry to mental health services, and may indicate the importance of taking cultural factors (e.g., values, beliefs, and attitudes) into account when measuring barrier endorsement with minority families. Future research should continue to examine and identify specific access barriers for different cultural groups, to guide outreach, to develop incentive strategies for potential clients, and to increase provider awareness of access barriers for minority families.

Utilizing Episode-oriented Approaches to Studying Access

Existing research usually presents help seeking and access to services as an event that did or did not occur over a certain specified interval. Although useful, this type of approach (event-oriented) fails to capture the complexities of the service utilization process. A more dynamic approach is episode-oriented, which examines access and utilization using analytic units that are defined by clinically meaningful segments of time (Snowden and Yamada, 2004). The use of this approach in research with minority youth populations has not yet been published, but may potentially yield important findings. Another extension of the episode-oriented approach, the "network-episode" model (Pescosolido, 1992), may also be very useful in giving a more comprehensive account of cultural influences in help-seeking. This approach takes into account the influence of sociocultural factors on various help-seeking sources (e.g., mental health, alternative therapies, general medical setting) concurrently and sequentially (e.g., unidirectional, bi-directional, feedback loops), and represents an attempt to incorporate "process" into the understanding of mental health care. This model has been adapted for children and adolescents to take into account the development from childhood to young adulthood, and highlights the important role of families and schools for youth mental health service use (Costello, Pescosolido, Angold, and Burns, 1998). Both of these latter approaches may be better able to capture the cultural influences and explanations for barriers for minority mental health care than the currently predominating event-oriented approach (Snowden and Yamada, 2005).

Address Financial and Language Barriers to Access

Minorities are more likely to be poor and uninsured, and many live in areas where specialty mental health care is limited in availability (USDHHS, 2001). Strategies for training providers on the impact of sociocultural factors on mental health care and creating incentives for providers to service underserved areas may provide greater geographic access to mental health services for youths in need. A major barrier to effective mental health treatment occurs when provider and patient do not speak the same language. For persons with limited English proficiency, the "language barrier" is also an important deterrent to receiving needed services (Sue, Fujino, Hu, and Takeuchi, 1991). Efforts to reduce this barrier go beyond the clinician-client level. Existing federal law states that providers have an obligation under the 1964 Civil Rights Act to ensure that persons with limited English proficiency have meaningful and equal access to benefits and services (DHHS, 2000). Providers should identify and document the language needs of the client population, provide a range of translation options and ensure their quality, and provide written materials in languages other than English wherever a significant percentage of the target population has limited English proficiency free of charge. Following guidelines such as this will help to improve access for a significant proportion of racial/ethnic minorities, especially recent immigrants and those less acculturated to mainstream American society.

Provide Services in Socially Acceptable Settings

To further reduce the impact of barriers, it is important to provide needed services in community settings where diverse populations feel comfortable (Pumariega, Rogers, and Rothe, 2005; Mirand et al., 2003). Ethnic-specific services in the community that address language concerns and cultural sensitivity in treatment may be more effective than mainstream mental health care that does not specifically cater to cultural groups Sue et al., 1991). Yeh, Takeuchi, and Sue (1994) found that the use of parallel centers, established to specifically provide mental health services to the Asian community, was associated with lower dropout rates, greater number of sessions, and higher functioning scores compared to use of mainstream centers for Asian American youth. In addition, associating services with institutions that are viewed favorably in the community or are aligned with cultural values (e.g., religious institutions, primary care settings, schools) are usually viewed as less threatening and provide easier access than specialty mental health clinics (Pumariega et al., 2005). Strengthening the identification and referral process in schools by providing training to school personnel may help to reduce current disparities in school-based services utilization. Adopting important components of evidence-based Multisystemic Therapy (MST) can increase access by bringing the service to the family's sociocultural milieu (e.g., providing therapy in youths' homes, in culture specific multifamily therapy groups).

Examine and Integrate Mental Health Services with General Medical Care and Alternative Treatments

Given the higher occurrence of service-seeking by minority families in traditional care and primary care settings compared to specialty mental health settings (Cooper=Patrick et al., 1999; Peifer et al., 2000), research examining the integration of these services may be helpful in improving access to those in need. Many minority families prefer to enter services through the primary care setting as it is more easily accessed and there is a lower level of stigma associated with receiving care through physicians. The Federal Government, in collaboration with the private sector, is working to bring quality mental health care to the primary health care system (USDHHS, 2001). Efforts to strengthen the capacity of primary care providers to meet the demand for mental health services and to encourage the delivery of integrated care in primary care and specialty mental health care settings will help to meet the needs and preferences of diverse populations in services. Furthermore, developing relationships between primary care and community mental health systems will encourage continuity of care when intensive mental health services are warranted in the specialty sector.

Many racial/ethnic minority families also prefer to utilize traditional care in lieu of mental health services, or sometimes use these complementary treatments in conjunction with mental health services (Neighbors and Jackson, 1984; Peifer et al., 2000, USDHHS, 2001). Researchers have not directly evaluated complementarity-substitution of these alternative treatments for mental health care in ethnic youth and families, and it is important to examine patterns of use in order to rule this out as an explanation/barrier to minority Western-based mental health care (Snowden and Yamada, 2005). In addition, investigations of indigenous healing practices, including its therapeutic components, and the beliefs behind seeking care in this sector may facilitate a better understanding of the help seeking process and rationale for different cultural groups. Integrating consultation and intervention by traditional healers is an important component of culturally competent care (Pumariega et al., 2005), and working with consultants and indigenous healers (Porter, Garcia, Jackson, and Valdez, 1997) in the development of a holistic treatment plan may increase treatment retention and eventual outcomes for minority youths. It is also important to research the process and outcomes for complementary therapies and identify any possible interactions (positive or negative) with western mental health treatment, and apply these findings to the development of treatment options for families in the mental health sector.

Increase Availability of Types of Services

A variety of services current exist in the U. S. youth mental health care system to address the emotional/behavioral needs of children (please see Appendix 2 for a list of these services organized by categories), however, they are disproportionately accessed and used by minority families, and may not be available to certain populations (e.g., poor or uninsured). It is important to increase the availability of treatment options whenever possible (e.g., school-based therapy, outpatient group therapy, outpatient individual therapy) to encourage use of community-based alternatives to hospitalization or more restrictive services. It is possible these disproportionate numbers in restrictive services reflect an unavailability of more desirable or less restrictive services, and efforts to increase treatment options for high need youths and utilize innovative methods in treatment delivery are needed (e.g., delivery of services in client's home). To understand their potential role in reducing mental health care disparities, more research is needed on the impact of ethnically-focused programs on youth services utilization. Identifying specific organizational variables (e.g., structural characteristics, organizational culture) and linking these to utilization, retention, and outcomes for minority youth would be especially helpful (Snowden and Yamada, 2005).

Improve Quality of Care to Minorities

Provide State-of-the-art, Evidence-based Care

Evidence in this review suggests racial/ethnic disparities in the quality of mental health services, and the Nation's mental health service system needs to ensure that all Americans receive state-of-the-art care (USDHHS, 2001). Racial/ethnic minorities are less likely than whites to receive evidence-based care, and there are only a handful of studies documenting minority outcomes for evidence-based treatments (Miranda et al., 2005), although initial results appear promising. Evidence-based care for depression improves outcomes for African American and Latino youths at rates equal to or greater than for non-Hispanic White youths, and established psychosocial care for Asians may be effective, and while research on effectiveness for American Indian and Alaskan Natives are lacking, available literature on prevention strategies appear helpful (Miranda et al., 2005). Given these limited but promising results, there is a great need to examine outcomes for minority youth in evidence-based care in larger, more representative studies. Strategies for increasing training of therapists to provide evidence-based care to minority youths is also necessary, as the level of therapists' engagement skills is critical to retention (McKay, Stoewe, McCadam, and Gonzales, 1998).

Provide Culturally-adapted Treatments when Appropriate

Culture and language may significantly affect the perception, utilization, retention, and eventual outcomes of mental health services (USDHHS, 2001). Clear evidence exists for the development of tailored interventions in order to increase acceptability and accessibility of services to minorities (Miranda, Nakamura, and Bernal, 2003), and the provision of culturally and linguistically appropriate mental health services is key to meet the needs of diverse populations. Efficacy studies with youth suggest that culturally-adapted treatments are effective for African American and Latino youths, and more work is currently underway to adapt existing efficacious treatments for minority populations (e.g., McCabe, Yeh, Garland, Lau, and Chavez, 2005). To continue the advancement of appropriate efficacious and effective care for minority youth, we need theory and evidence to inform when interventions need to be culturally adapted. Conducting theory driven research examining the extent to which evidence-based treatments are effective across different cultural groups and how they are affected by cultural constructs (e.g., collectivism) would be useful (Miranda et al., 2003). In addition, developing systematic methodologies to tailor evidence-based interventions for specific populations would also be extremely helpful (Miranda et al., 2005). Much more research is needed on culturally adapted interventions not only to evaluate effectiveness, but also to compare adapted care to standard interventions (Miranda et al, 2005).

Utilize Cultural Competence in Treatment

As suggested in our literature review and highlighted in our diagram, the client-therapist relationship may be key in effecting change and improving care for minority youth in mental health services. It is clear that a one-size-fits all health care system cannot meet the needs of an increasingly diverse American population, and embracing and utilizing cultural competence in the delivery of services should be a priority among all service providers. Cultural competence goes beyond cultural awareness and sensitivity to include the possession of cultural knowledge and respect for different cultural perspectives and having the ability to use these skills effectively in cross-cultural situations (Cross et al., 1989; Orlandi, 1995; Tirado, 1996; Brach, 2000). These three general areas of cultural competency defined by Sue, Ivey, and Pederson (1996) (i.e., cultural awareness and beliefs, cultural knowledge, and cultural skills) have been adopted by APA's Multicultural Guidelines (APA, 2003) to urge the Nation to improve quality of care for minority groups. Careful and appropriate implementation of sound cultural competency techniques in delivering health services can reduce disparities (Brach, 2000); but there have been difficulties in the translation of cultural competency as a philosophical concept to a practice/research-oriented construct (Sue, 2006). As such, future research needs to establish a definition of cultural competence that is readily operationalized and standard instruments to measure cultural competence across samples (Beach et al., 2005). Research thus far has mainly focused on the examination of techniques to reduce language barriers within the cultural competency framework for minority adults, and studies are needed to evaluate the impact of other specific cultural competency techniques on treatment for children. Specifically, the hypothesis that cultural competent practices improves patient adherence to therapy, process of service delivery, and mental health outcomes have yet to be empirically tested (Beach et al., 2005). Research is also needed to compare culturally competent interventions with those uninformed by patient's culture and language. This type of research is critical to rule out confounders such as education and socioeconomic status as causes of treatment disparities. Accumulating evidence is essential if cultural competency is to be widely adopted by mental health systems in the U. S. (Brach, 2000).

In practice, going from a philosophical definition of cultural competence to a practice-oriented definition has also presented many challenges. Sue (2006) suggested concrete steps in treatment that present opportunities for providers to adopt and utilize cultural competent techniques in treatment: self-awareness and stimulus value, assessment of client, pretherapy intervention, hypothesizing and testing hypotheses, attending to credibility and giving, understanding the nature of discomfort and resistance, understanding client's perspectives, strategy or plan for intervention, assessment of treatment session, and willingness to consult. In addition, learning (through research or clinical practice) which cultural competence techniques are most useful for facilitating greater engagement and enhancing outcomes for minority families, and identifying effective methods of teaching cultural competence to service providers are integral to an ongoing commitment of appropriate practice and policies for diverse populations and improving quality of care for minority families.

Enhance Engagement and Involvement of Families in Services

Evidence suggests that consideration of families' input in treatment planning and engaging them in services improves service retention and may affect eventual outcomes, and although literature is inconsistent, some evidence shows that minority families may be particularly difficult to engage. As such, research focusing on identifying specific strategies to engaging minorities is extremely important (Miranda et al., 2005). Without more intensive treatment efforts, 56% of clients can be lost between the call to request services and the first intake appointment (McKay, McCadam, Gonzales, 1998). Engaging families in treatment, especially highly resistant minority families, is best addressed with an ecological multilevel approach that integrates interventions at the child, parent, social network, school, agency, and community level. This includes involving ethnic minorities in planning and reviewing services (Walker, 2005). Successful engagement strategies that have been attempted in the past include letter writing (Lown and Britton, 1991), intensive telephone contact (McKay, Stoewe et al., 1998), parent orientation meetings (Wenning and King, 1995), modifying treatment to address parents' expressed needs (Prinz and Miller, 1994), influencing the client's social networks (Carr, 1990; Pescosolido, 1996), and more comprenhensive engagement strategies based on Strategic Structural Systems Engagement (Santisteban et al., 1996) and Multidimensional Family Therapy (Liddle, 1995). To encourage parents' commitment to bringing youth to treatment (Morrissey-Kane and Prinz, 1999), adapting strategies in motivational interviewing can help parents be more motivated (Miller and Rollnick, 1991). The effectiveness of engagement strategies largely rests on the therapist's competence in administering these techniques, and providing engagement training to clinicians in order to facilitate engagement and retention for their clients is crucial (McKay, Stoewe et al., 1998).

An illustrative example of a treatment that may move the field toward increasing family involvement more systematically is evidence-based MST. MST originates from the theory that an adolescent's social ecology, which includes parental factors, affects their psychosocial adjustment and are related to their likelihood of developing and maintaining emotional and behavioral problems (Henggeler and Borduin, 1990). Understanding ways in which to best engage parents in treatment is important for the success of MST and similar types interventions (Coffey, 2004). MST has demonstrated both efficacy and effectiveness (Huey et al., 2004; Curtis, Ronan, and Borduin, 2004; Rowland et al., 2005), and outcome studies documenting the success of MST provide support for the importance of collaborating with parents in the treatment process. These findings also provide support for the importance of considering others' perspectives in establishing a strong therapeutic relationship and the application of the model described above.

CONCLUSION

This review presents compelling evidence that racial and ethnic minorities experience a high level of burden from unmet mental health needs and encounter a number of barriers that influence help-seeking, service selection, service utilization, process in treatment, and outcomes. Despite the progress made in recent research efforts, the knowledge base concerning mental health and mental health care for minority youth is limited and inconsistent.

The goal of eliminating racial and ethnic disparities in mental health is extremely challenging but not unrealistic. As the country continues to increasingly diversify and as the number of minority individuals increases in proportion the U. S. population, improving the care of minority youths will enhance the care of all youths in the U.S. as a whole. As studies have repeatedly found disparities in utilization and access, now is the time to move beyond identification and awareness of these problems to generating possible solutions. It is necessary to expand and improve programs to deliver culturally, linguistically, and geographically accessible mental health services for minority families that have identified a need and have made the decision to seek help (USDHHS, 2001), but it is equally important to begin outreach with at-risk populations even before this juncture; it is essential to develop programs that aim to increase public awareness of mental illness and effective treatments, and prioritize using education to overcome shame, stigma, discrimination, and mistrust (USDHHS, 2001). Once in services, delivering state-of-the-art, evidence-based interventions and applying cultural competence in all clinical interactions will be integral to treatment success for these families. Rigorous research is still needed to evaluate evidence-based treatments and culturally adapted interventions for minority youth, and to identify key ingredients in culturally sensitive practices that significantly enhance the therapeutic relationship and increase productivity in achieving desired outcomes. While significant strides have been made in the evidence base for minority youth mental health and mental health care, gaps still exist in the documentation of prevalence, perception, course, detection, and treatment of racial/ethnic minorities (USDHHS, 2001). Training individuals to carry out programs of research to examine the mental health and mental health care process for these groups is needed, and researchers should take advantage of national agendas that support such research by providing special funding initiatives for the study of minority mental health care. Finally, considering the voices of racial and ethnic minority families and their opinions regarding their experiences of mental illness and preferences for care is critical. For clinicians, being open to other cultural views regarding mental health treatment and embracing these differences will serve to empower clients and facilitate a more positive therapeutic relationship, a component of the treatment process we have highlighted as essential to creating change for families in need. Beyond understanding the existence of disparities and barriers to mental health care for ethnic youths, being able to appreciate other worldviews will make all of us better educators, researchers, and clinicians who are able to effect progress in the youth mental health care system.

APPENDIX 1. A SUMMARY OF CONTEXTUAL BARRIERS, CLIENT BARRIERS, AND PROVIDER BARRIERS

Contextual Barriers

- Concrete Barriers
  - Inaccessible locations
  - Financial difficulties
  - Lack of insurance
  - Transportation problems
  - Lack of time
  - Lack of child care
- Stressor Barriers
  - Lack of social support
  - Stress associated with poverty
  - Family dysfunction
  - Negative life events
  - Caregiver burden
- Referral Barriers
  - Gatekeepers
  - Differential referral to systems of care
  - Misidentification

Client Barriers

- Perceived Barriers
- Cultural Barriers
  - Problem Recognition and Definition: Failure to recognize problem as mental health related
  - Decision to Seek Help: Failure to seek help in any setting
  - Service Selection: Failure to seek help in mental health sector

Provider Barriers

- Agency Barriers
  - System Barriers: inconvenient hours, scheduling problems, waiting lists, unresponsive service providers, fragmented community mental health care that lack adequate communication between agencies, inadequacy of community-based services to deliver appropriate care for minority families with mental health concerns, and an overreliance on institutional care for minority youth
  - Lack of availability of same-language therapists
  - Lack of availability of same-culture therapists
- Clinician Characteristics
  - Miscommunication and inadequate communication
  - Clinician's personal biases and inadequate consideration of cultural factors
  - Clinician's inadequate involvement of families in treatment

APPENDIX 2. SERVICE TYPES

A variety of services currently exist in the U. S. youth mental health care system to address the emotional/behavioral needs of children, and can be generally categorized into the following treatment types: inpatient mental health services, outpatient mental health services, school-based mental health services, and mental health clinical trials. Note that this categorization may not be used by all researchers, and others may have different ways of grouping youth mental health services.

We have modeled three of the four service type groupings (inpatient mental health services, outpatient mental health services, school-based mental health services) after the organization scheme used in the Service Assessment for Children and Adolescents (SACA; Horowitz et al., 2001). The SACA is a valid and reliable measure (Hoagwood et al., 2000; Horwitz et al., 2001; Stiffman et al., 2000) used to assess the types of mental health services children use, the rationale for service use, the specific treatments (e.g., behavioral management, parent training) received within three broad service types, the rationale for service use, and the quality of services. We have added an additional service type to this organizational scheme that warrants consideration and discussion: mental health clinical trials for youth with emotional/behavioral problems. Clinical trials are similar to the other three service types named in the SACA, specifically, that there is an intervention/treatment application, but differ in important areas such as client enrollment, treatment protocol application, and measurement of outcomes. We briefly describe each of these four service types below.

Inpatient Mental Health Services

This service type includes youth mental health care that required one or more overnight stays in a number of settings (e.g., psychiatric hospital, psychiatric unit within a hospital, residential treatment center, and inpatient alcohol and drug-abuse treatment).

Outpatient Mental Health Services

Includes services received from a mental health care professional (e.g., psychiatrist, psychologist, social worker, or family counselor) in specialty outpatient care such as community mental heath clinics or private providers. Nonspecialty outpatient care (e.g., visit to a pediatrician for emotional/behavioral issues) and outpatient alcohol and drug abuse treatment are also classified in this category.

School-based Mental Health Services

Includes services received from a mental health care professional in the school setting for emotional, behavioral, or drug/alcohol problems. This may consist of counseling received in a special school or special classroom in a regular school, special help in a regular classroom, or counseling/therapy with a school psychologist or counselor.

Mental Health Clinical Trials

Clinical trials are well-controlled research studies specially designed to evaluate or compare specific novel or established treatments. Clinical trials differ from the above three service types in that they typically have specific inclusionary and exclusionary criteria for client enrollment in treatment/services, rigid treatment administration procedures (e.g., protocol application, number of sessions for treatment completion), and systematic measurement to assess outcomes across clients. Although the high specificity of enrollment in this service type may limit the generalizability of these studies to the community population at large, we have included this service type in our discussion because it is similar to the previous three service types in that one or more intervention(s) was(were) administered by mental health professionals to help youth with emotional, behavioral, and/or alcohol/drug problems, and therefore can be regarded as an option for mental health care (especially for families who might not otherwise have the financial access to services for their youth).

REFERENCES

Abe-Kim, J., Takeuchi, D., and Hwang, W-C. (2002). Predictors of help seeking for emotional distress among Chinese Americans: Family matters. *Journal of Consulting and Clinical Psychology*, 70, 1186-90.

Acosta, F. X., Yamamoto, J., Evans, L. A., and Skilbeck, W. M. (1983). Preparing low-income Hispanic, Black, and White patients for psychotherapy: Evaluation of a new orientation program. *Journal of Clinical Psychology, 39*, 872-877.

Agency for Healthcare Research and Quality (2002). *Testimony on AHRQ's Role in Eliminating Racial and Ethnic Disparities in Health.* Agency for Healthcare Research and Quality, Rockville, MD, Retrieved March 1, 2006 from *http://www.ahrq.gov/news/test52102.htm.*

Akustu, P. D., Tsuru, G. K., and Chu, J. P. (2004). Predictors of nonattendance of intake appointments among five Asian American groups. *Journal of Consulting and Clinical Psychology*, 72, 891-896.

Allen, J. and Walsh, J. A. (2000). A construct-based approach to equivalence: Methodologies for cross-cultural/multicultural personality assessment research. In R. H. Dana (Ed)., *Handbook of cross-cultural and multicultural personality assessment. Personality and clinical psychology series.* (pp.63-85). Mahwah, NJ: Lawrence Erlbaum Associates.

Alonso, M., Val, E., and Rapaport, M.M. (1997). An open-label study of SSRI treatment in depressed Hispanic and non-Hispanic women. *Journal of Clinical Psychiatry, 58,* 31.

Alvidrez, J. (1999). Ethnic variations in mental health attitudes and service use among low-income African American, Latina, and European American young women. *Community Mental Health Journal, 35*(6), 515-530.

American Psychological Association (2003). Guidelines on multicultural education, training, research, practice, and organizational change for psychologists. *American Psychologist, 58,* 377-402.

appointments among five Asian American client groups. *Journal of Consulting and Clinical Psychology, 72,* 891-896.

Arcia, E. and Fernandez, M. C. (2003). From awareness to acknowledgement: The development of concern among Latina mothers of children with disruptive behaviors. *J Atten Disord.* 2003 Jun; 6(4):163-75

Atkinson, D. R. and Gim, R. H. (1989). Asian-American cultural identity and attitudes toward mental health services. *Journal of Counseling Psychology, 36,* 209-212.

Atkinson, D. R., Poterotto, J. G., and Sanchez, A. R. (1984). Attitudes of Vietnamese and Anglo-American students toward counseling. *Journal of College Student Personnel, 25,* 448-452. *Attention Disorders, 6,* 163-175.

Baekeland, F., and Lundwall, L. (1975). Dropping out of treatment: A critical review. *Psychological Bulletin, 82,* 738–783.

Bannon, W. M., and McKay, M. M. (2005). Are barriers to service and parental preference match for service related to urban child mental health service use? *Families in Society: The Journal of Contemporary Social Services, 86,* 30-34.

Barker, L. A. and Adelman, H. S. (1994). Mental health and help-seeking among ethnic minority adolescents. *Journal of Adolescence, 17,* 251-263.

Beach, M. C., Price, E. G., Gary, T. L., Robinson, K. A., Gozu, A., Palacio, A., Smarth, C., Jenckes, M. W., Feuerstein, C., Bass, E. B., Powe, N. R., and Cooper, L. A. (2005). Cultural competence: A systematic review of health care provider educational interventions. *Medical Care, 43,* 356-373.

Beals, J., Piasecki, J., Nelson, S., Jones, M., Keane, E., Sauphinais, P., Red Shirt, R., Sack, W., and Manson, S. M. (1997). Psychiatric disorder among American Indian adolescents: Prevalence in Northern Plains youth. *Journal of the American Academy of Child and Adolescent Psychiatry, 36,* 1252-1259.

Bee-Gates, D., Howard-Pitney, B., LaFromboise, T., and Rowe, W. (1996). Help-seeking behavior of Native American Indian high school students. *Professional Psychology: Research and Practice, 27,* 495-499.

Berry, J. W. (1997). Immigration, acculturation and adaptation (Lead article). *Applied Psychology: An International Review, 46,* 5 - 68.

Betancourt, H. and Lopez, S.R. (1993). The study of culture, ethnicity, and race in American psychology. *American Psychologist, 48,* 629-637.

Bond, C. F., DiCandia, C. G., MacKinnon, J. R. (1988). Responses to violence in a psychiatric setting: The role of patient's race. *Personality and Social Psychology Bulletin, 14,* 448–458.

Borduin, C.M., Mann, B.J., Cone L.T., Henggeler, S.W., Fucci, BR, et al. (1995). Multisystemic treatment of serious juvenile offenders: Longterm prevention of criminology and violence. *Journal of Consulting and Clinical Psychology, 63,* 569–578.

Borowsky, S. J., Rubenstein, L. V. Meredith, L. S., Camp, P., Jackson-Triche, M., and Wells, K. B. (2000). Who is at risk of nondetection of mental health. Problems in primary care? *Journal of General Internal Medicine, 15,* 381-388.

Borduin, C. M., and Henggeler, S. W. (1990). A multisystemic approach to the treatment of serious delinquent behavior. In R. J. McMahon and R. DeV. Peters (Eds.), *Behavior disorders of adolescence: Research, intervention, and policy in clinical and school settings* (pp. 62-80). New York: Plenum.

Boyd-Franklin, N. (1993). Black families. In F. Walsh (Ed.), *Normal family process* (pp. 361-376). New York: Guilford Press.

Brach, C. (2000). Can cultural competency reduce racial and ethnic health disparities? A review and conceptual model. *Medical Care Research and Review, 57,* 181-217.

Brannan, A. M., Heflinger, C. A., and Bickman, L. (1997). The Caregiver Strain Questionnaire: Measuring the impact on the family of living with a child with serious emotional disturbance. *Journal of Emotional and Behavioral Disorders, 5,* 212-222.

Brannan, A. M., Heflinger, C. A., and Foster, E. M. (2003). The role of caregiver strain and other family variables in determining children's use of mental health services. *Journal of Emotional and Behavioral Disorders, 11,* 78-92.

Bravo, M. (2003). Instrument development: Cultural adaptations for ethnic minority research. In G. Bernal, J. E. Trimble, A. K. Burlew, and F. T. L. Leong (Eds.), *Handbook of Racial and Ethnic Minority Psychology* (pp. 220-236). Thousand Oaks, CA: Sage.

Breaux, C, and Ryujin, D. (1999). Use of mental health services by ethnically diverse groups within the United States. *The Clinical Psychologist, 52,* 4-15.

Browman, C. L. (1996). Coping with personal problems. In H. W. Neighbors and J. S. Jackson (Eds.), *Mental health in black America* (pp. 117-129). Thousand Oaks, CA: Sage.

Brown, J., Cohen, P., Johnson, J. G., and Smailes, E. M. (1999). Childhood abuse and neglect: Specificity of effects on adolescent and young adult depression and suicidality. *Journal of the American Academy of Child and Adolescent Psychiatry, 38,* 1490–1496.

Brown, R. T., and Sexson, S. B. (1988). A controlled trial of methylphenidate in black adolescents. *Clinical Pediatrics, 27, 74–81.*

Brown, T. R., Huang, K., Harris, D. E., and Stein, K. M. (1973). Mental illness and the role of ·mental health facilities in Chinatown. In S. Sue and N. Wgner (Eds.), Asian American: Psychological perspectives (p. 212-231). Palo Alto, CA: Science and Behavior Books.

Bui, K. V. T. and Takeuchi, D. T. (1992). Ethnic minority adolescents and the use of community mental health care services. *American Journal of Community Psychology, 20,* 403-417.

Burns, B. J., Costello, E. J., Angold, A., Tweed, D., Stangl, D., Farmer, E. M. Z., and Erkanli, A. (1995). Children's mental health service use across service sectors. *Health Affairs, 14,* 147-159.

Bussing, R., Schoenberg, N. E., Rogers, K. M., Zima, B. T., and Angus, S. (1998). Explanatory models of ADHD: Do they differ by ethnicity, child gender, or treatment status? *Journal of Emotional and Behavioral Disorders, 6*(4), 233-242.

Carr, A. (1990). Failure in family therapy: A catalogue of engagement mistakes. *Journal of Family Therapy, 12,* 371-386.

Cauce, A. M., Paradise, M., Domenech-Rodriguez, M., Cochran, B. N., Shea, J. M., Srebnik, D., and Baydar, N. (2002). Cultural and contextual influences in mental health help-seeking: a focus on ethnic minority youth. *Journal of Consulting and Clinical Psychology, 70*, 44-55.

Centers for Disease Control and Prevention (2000). Youth Risk Behavior Surveillance-United States, 1999. Morbidity Mortality Weekly Representation, 49, 1-96.

Chabra, A., Chavez, G. F., Harris, E. S., and Shah, R. (1999). Hospitalization for mental illness in adolescents: risk groups and impact on the health care system. *Journal of Adolescent Health, 24,* 349-356.

Cheung, F. L., and Snowden, L. R. (1990). Community mental health and ethnic minority populations. *Community Mental Health Journal, 26,* 277-291.

Chun, C., Enomoto, K., and Sue, S. (1996). Health-care issues among Asian Americans: Implications of somatization. In P. M. Kata and T. Mann (Eds.), *Handbook of diversity issues in health psychology* (p. 347-366). New York: Plenum.

Clark, L. A. (1987). Mutual relevance of mainstream and cross-cultural psychology. *Journal of Consulting and Clinical Psychology , 55,* 461-70.

Coffey, E. P. (2004). The heart of the matter 2: Integration of ecosystemic family therapy practices with systems of care mental health services for children and families. *Family Process, 43,* 161-173.

Collins, B. G., and Collins, T. M. (1994). Child and adolescent mental health: Building a system of care. *Journal of Counseling and Development, 72,* 239-243.

Comas-Diaz, L. (1981). Effects of cognitive and behavioral group treatment on the depressive symptoms of Puerto Rican women. *Journal of Consulting and Clinical Psychology, 49,* 627–632.

Constantine, M.G. (2002). Predictors of satisfaction with counseling: Racial and ethnic minority clients' attitudes toward counseling and ratings of their counselors' general and multicultural counseling competence. *Journal of Counseling Psychology, 49*, 255-263.

Cooper, L., Roter, D., Johnson, R., Ford, D. Steinwachs, D., and Powe, N. (2003). Patient-centered communication, ratings of care, and concordance of patient and physician race. *Annals of International Medicine, 139*, 907-916.

Corrigan, P. (2004). How stigma interferes with mental health care. *American Psychologist, 59*, 614-625.

Costello, E. J., Farmer, E. M., Angold, A., Burns, B. J., and Erkanli, A. (1997). Psychiatric disorders among American Indian and white youth in Appalachia: The Great Smoky Mountains Study. *American Journal of Public Health, 87*, 827-832.

Costello, E. J., and Janiszewski, S. (1990). Who gets treated? Factors associated with referral in children with psychiatric disorders. *Acta Psychiatric Scandinavia, 81*, 523-529.

Costello, E. J., Pescosolido, B. A., Angold, A., and Burns, B. J. (1998). A family network-based model of access to child mental health services. *Research in Community and Mental Health, 9*. 165-190.

Cross, T. L., Bazron, B. J., Dennis, K. W., and Issacs, M. R. (1989). *Towards a culturally competent system of care*. Washington, DC: CAASP Technical Assistance Center.

Curtis, N. M., Ronan, K. R. and Bordouin, C. M. (2004). Multisystemic treatment: a meta-analysis of outcome studies. *Journal of family psychology*, 18, 411-419.

D'Amico, E. J. (2005). Factors that impact adolescents' intentions to utilize alcohol-related prevention services. *Journal of Behavioral Health Services and Research, 32*, 332-340.

Dubow, E.F., Huesmann, L.R., and Eron, L.D. (1987). Childhood correlates of adult ego development. *Child Development*, 58, 859–869.

Duncan, B. B., Forness, S. R., and Hartsough, C. (1995). Students identified as seriously emotionally disturbed in school-based day treatment: cognitive, psychiatric, and special educational characteristics. *Behavioral Disorders, 20*, 238-252.

Durvasula, R. S., and Sue, S. (1996). Severity of disturbance among Asian American outpatients. *Cultural Diversity and Mental Health, 2*, 43-52.

Edgerton, R., and Karno, M. (1971). Mexican-American bilingualism and perception of mental illness. *Archives of General Psychiatry, 24*, 236-290.

Fabrega, H., Jr., Ulrich, R., Mezzich, J. E. (1993). Do Caucasian and black adolescents differ at psychiatric intake? *Journal of American Academy Child Adolescent Psychiatry 32*(2), 407-413.

Flaskerud, J. H. and Lui, P. Y. (1991). Effects of an Asian client-therapist language, ethnicity, and gender match on utilization and outcome of therapy. *Community Mental Health Journal, 27*, 1991.

Flisher, A. J., Kramer, R. A., Grosser , R. C., Alegria, M., Bird, H. R., Bourdon, K. H. et al. (1997). Correlates of unmet need for mental health services by children and adolescents. *Psychological Mewdicine*, 27, 1145-1154.

Forness, S. R. (2003). Barriers to evidence-based treatment: developmental psychopathology and the interdisciplinary disconnect in school mental health practice. *Journal of School Psychology, 41*, 61-67.

Gallo, J. J., Marino, S., Ford, D., and Anthony, J. C. (1995). Filters on the pathway to mental health care, II. Sociodeomographic factors. *Psychological Medicine*, 25, 1149-1160.

Garcia, J. A., and Weisz, J. R. (2002). When youth mental health care stops: Therapeutic relationship problems and other reasons for ending youth outpatient treatment. *Journal of Consulting and Clinical Psychology, 70*, 439-443.

Garland, A. F., Hough, R. L., McCabe, K., Yeh, M., Wood, P., and Aarons, G. (2001). Prevalence of psychiatric disorders for youth in public sectors of care. *Journal of the American Academy of Child and Adolescent Psychiatry, 40*, 409-418.

Garland, A. F., Kruse, M., and Aarons, G. A. (2003). Clinicians and outcome measurement: What's the use? *Journal of Behavioral Health Services and Research, 30*, 393-405.

Garland, A. F., Lau, A. S., Yeh, M., McCabe, K. M., Hough, R. L., and Landsverk, J. A. (2005). Racial and ethnic differences in utilization of mental health services among high-risk youths. *The American Journal of Psychiatry, 162,* 1336-1343.

Garland, A. F., Saltzman, M. D., and Aarons, G. A. (2000). Adolescent satisfaction with mental health services: Development of a multidimensional scale. *Evaluation and Program Planning, 23*, 165-175.

Geisenger, K. F. (1994). Cross-cultural normative assessment: Translation and adaptation issues influencing the normative interpretation of assessment instruments. *Psychological Assessment, 6,* 304-312.

Gibbs, J. T., and Huang, L. N. (1989). *Children of color: Psychological interventions with minority youth*. San Francisco: Jossey-Bass.

Ginsburg, G.S., and Drake, K.L. (2002). School-based treatment for anxious African-American adolescents: A controlled pilot study. *Journal of the American Academy of Child and Adolescent Psychiatry, 41*, 768–775.

Gonzalez, J. M., Alegria, M., and Prihoda, T. J. (2005). How do attitudes toward mental health treatment vary by age, gender, and ethnicity/race in young adults? *Journal of Community Psychology, 33,* 611-629.

Hahn, E. J. (1995). Predicting Head Start parent involvement in an alcohol and other drug prevention program. *Nursing Research, 44*, 45-51.

Halfon, N., Berkowitz, G. and Klee, L. (1992). Mental health service utilization by children in foster care in California. *Pediatrics, 89,* 1238–1244.

Harrison, M. E., McKay, M. M., and Bannon, W. M. (2004). Inner-city child mental health service use: The real question is why youth and families do not use services. *Community Mental Health Journal, 40,* 119-131.

Helms, J. E. (1986). Expanding racial identity theory to cover counseling process. *Journal of Counseling Psychology, 33*, 62-64.

Henggeler, S. (1994). A consensus: Conclusionss of the APA task force report on innovative models of mental health services for children, adolescents, and their families. *Journal of Clinical Child Psychology, 23*, 3-6.

Henggeler, S. W., and Borduin, C. M. (1990). *Family therapy and beyond: A multisystemic approach to treating the behavior problems of children and adolescents*. Pacific Grove, CA: Brooks/Cole Publishing Company.

Hill, N. E. and Herman-Stahl, M. A. (2002). Neighborhood safety and social involvement: Associations with parenting behaviors and depressive symptoms among African American and Euro-American mothers. *Journal of Family Psychology, 16*, 209-219.

Hoagwood, K., Horwitz, S., Stiffman, A., Weisz, J., Bean, D., Rae, D., Compton, W., Cottler, L., Bickman, L., and Leaf, P. (2000). Concordance between parent reports of children's mental health services and service records: The Services Assessment for Children and Adolescents (SACA). *Journal of Child and Family Studies, 9*, 315-331.

Hoagwood, K., and Johnson, J. (2003). School psychology: a public health framework. I. From evidence-based practices to evidence-based policies. *Journal of School Psychology, 41*, 3-21.

Hohmann, A. A., and Parron, D. L. (1996). How the new NIH Guidelines on Inclusion of Women and Minorities apply: efficacy trials, effectiveness trials, and validity. *Journal of Consulting and Clinical Psychology, 64*, 851-855.

Horwitz, S. M., Hoagwood, K., Stiffman, A. R., Summerfeld, T., Weisz, J. R., Costello, E. J., Rost, K., Bean, D. L., Cottler, L., Leaf, P. J., Roper, M., and Norquist, G. (2001). Reliability of the services assessment for children and adolescents. *Psychiatric Services, 52*, 1088-1094.

Hough, R. L., Hazen, A. L., Soriano, F. I., Wood, P. A., McCabe, K., and Yeh, M. (2002). Mental health services for Latino adolescents with psychiatric disorders. *Psychiatric Services, 53*, 1556-1562.

Hu, T. W., Snowden, L. R., Jerrell, J. M., and Nguyen, T. D. (1991). Ethnic populations in public mental health: Services choice and level of use. *American Journal of Public Health, 81*, 1429–1434.

Hudley, C., and Graham, S. (1993). An attributional intervention to reduce peer-directed aggression among African-American boys. *Child Development, 64*, 124–138.

Huey, S. J., Henggeler, S. W., Rowland, M. D., Halliday-Boykins, C. A., and Cunningham, P. B. et al. (2004). Multisystemic therapy effects on attempted suicide by youths presenting psychiatric emergencies. *Journal of American Academic Child And Adolescent Psychiatry, 43*, 183-90.

Hunt, G. J. (1995). Social and cultural aspects of health, illness, and treatment. In H. H. Goldman (Ed.), *Review of general psychiatry*. Norwalk, CT: Appleton and Lange.

Karno, M., and Edgerton, R. (1969). Perception of mental illness in a Mexican American community. *Archives of General Psychiatry, 20*, 233-238.

Kataoka, S. H., Zhang, L., and Wells, K. B. (2002). Unmet need for mental health care among U.S. children: variation by ethnicity and insurance status. *American Journal of Psychiatry, 159*, 1548-1555.

Kazdin, A. (1993). Premature termination from treatment among children referred for antisocial behavior. *Journal of Clinical Child Psychology, 31*, 415-425.

Kazdin, A. E., Holland, L., and Crowley. (1997). Family experience of barriers to treatment and premature termination from child therapy. *Journal of Consulting and Clinical Psychology, 65,* 453-463.

Kazdin, A.E., Mazurick, J. L., and Siegal, T. C. (1994). Treatment outcome among children with externalizing disorder who terminate prematurely versus those who complete health services for ethnic minority groups: A test of the cultural responsiveness hypothesis. *Journal of Consulting and Clinical Psychology, 59*, 533-54.

Kazdin, A. E., Stolar, M. J., and Marciano, P. L. (1995). Risk factors for dropping out of treatment among White and Black families. *Journal of Family Psychology, 9,* 402-417.

Keefe, S.E. and Casas, M.J. (1980). Mexican Americans and mental health: A selected review and recommendations for mental health service delivery. *American Journal of Community Psychology, 303,* 319-320.

Keegan, L. (1996). Use of alternative therapies among Mexican Americans in the Texas Rio Grande Valley. *Journal of Holistic Nursing, 14*, 277-294.

Kleinbaum, D. G., Kupper, L. L., Muller, K.E., and Nizam, A. (1998). *Applied regression analysis and other multivariate methods, 3rd edition.* Pacific Grove, CA: Brooks/Cole Publishing Co.

Koroloff, N. M., Elliot, D. J., Koren, P. E., and Friesen, B. J. (1994). Connecting low-income families to mental health services: The role of the family associate. *Journal of Emotional and Behavioral Disorders, 4,* 2-11.

Kupst, M. J., and Shulman, J. L., (1979). Comparing professional and lay expectations of psychotherapy. *Psychotherapy,: Theory, Research and Practice, 16,* 237-243.

LaFromboise, T. D., and Low, K. G. (1989). American Indian children and adolescents. In: Gibbs, J. T., and Huang, L. N. (Eds.). *Children of color: Psychological Interventions with Minority Youth.* San Francisco: Jossey-Bass.

Larsen, D. L., Nguyen, T. D., Green, R. S., and Attkisson, C. C. (1983). *Enhancing the utilization of outpatient mental health services.* New York: Human Sciences Press.

LaVeist, T. A., Diala, C., and Jarrett, N. C. (2000). Social status and perceived discrimination: Who experiences discrimination in the health care system, how, and why? In C. Hogue, M. Hargraves, and K. Scott-Collins (Eds.), *Minority health in America* (p. 194-208). Baltimore, MD: Johns Hopkins University Press.

Leong, F. T. L. (1994). Asian Americans' differential patterns of utilization of inpatient and outpatient public mental health services in Hawaii. *Journal of Community Psychology, 22,* 82-89.

Leong, F. T. L., Wagner, N. S., and Tata, S. P. (1995). Racial and ethnic variations in help seeking attitudes. In J. G. Ponterotto, J. M. Casas, L. A. Suzuki, and C. M. Alexander (Eds.), *Handbook of multicultural counseling* (pp. 415^438). Thousand Oaks, CA: Sage.

Leveille, C.C. (2004). Satisfaction with psychotherapy at a college counseling center: A comparison between ethnic minority and ethnic majority clients. *Dissertation Abstracts International: Section B: The Sciences and Engineering, 65,* 444.

Levin, J. (1986). Roles for the black pastor in preventive medicine. *Pastoral Psychology, 35,* 94–103.

Liao, H., Rounds, J., and Klein, A. G. (2005). A test of Cramer's (1999) help-seeking model and acculturation effects with Asian and Asian American college students. *Journal of Counseling Psychology, 52,* 400-411.

Liddle, H.A. Conceptual and clinical dimensions of a multidimensional, multisystems engagement strategy in family-based adolescent treatment. *Psychotherapy: Theory, Research, Practice, Training. Special Issue: Adolescent Treatment: New Frontiers and New Dimensions, 32,* 39-58.

Lin, J. C. H. (1994). How long do Chinese-Americans stay in psychotherapy? *Journal of Counseling Psychology, 41,* 288-291.

Lin, K., Inui, T. S., Kleinman, A. M., and Womack, W. M. (1992). Socio-cultural determinants of the help-seeking behavior of patients with mental illness. *Journal of Nervous and Mental Disease, 170,* 78-85.

Lochman, J.E., Coie, J.D., Underwood M.K., and Terry R. (1993). Effectiveness of a social relations intervention program for aggressive and nonaggressive rejected children. *Journal of Consulting and Clinical Psychology, 61,* 1053–1058.

Lopez, M., Forness, S. R., MacMillan, D. L., Bocian, K., and Gresham, F. M. (1996). Children with attention deficit hyperactivity disorder and emotional or behavioral disorders in the primary grades: inappropriate placement in the learning disability category. *Education and Treatment of Children, 19*, 286-299.

Lown, N. and Britton, B. (1991). Engaging families through the letter writing technique. *Journal of Strategic and Systemic Therapies, 10*, 43–48.

MacNaughton, K. (2001). Predicting adherence to recommendations by parents of clinic-referred children. *Journal of Consulting and Clinical Psychology, 69*, 262-270.

Malgady, R. G., and Costantino, G. (1998). Symptom severity in bilingual Hispanics as a function of clinician ethnicity and language of interview. *Psychological Assessment, 10*, 120-127.

Martin, D. J., Garske, J. P., and Davis, M. K. (2000). Relation of the therapeutic alliance with outcome and other variables: A meta-analytic review. *Journal of Consulting and Clinical Psychology, 68*(3), 438-450.

Martinez, C. (1993). Psychiatric care of Mexican Americans. In A. C. Gaw (Ed.), *Culture, ethnicity, and mental illness* (pp. 431-466). Washingotn, DC: American Psychiatric Press.

McCabe, K. M. (2002). Factors that predict premature termination among Mexican-American children in outpatient psychotherapy. *Journal of Child and Family Studies, 11*, 347-359.

McCabe, K., Yeh, M., Hough, R. L., Landsverk, J., Hurlburt, M. S., Culver, S. W., and Reynolds, B. (1999). Racial/ethnic representation across five public sectors of care for youth. *Journal of Emotional and Behavioral Disorders, 7*, 72-82.

McCabe, K., Yeh, M., Garland, A., Lau, A., and Chavez, G. (2005). The GANA Program: A Tailoring Approach to Adapting Parent-Child Interaction Therapy for Mexican Americans. *Education and Treatment of Children, 28*, 111-129.

McKay, M. M., Hibbert, R., Hoagwood, K., Rodriguez, J., Murray, L., Legerski, J., and Fernandez, D. (2004). Integrating evidence-based engagement interventions into "real world" child mental health settings. *Brief Treatment and Crisis Intervention, 4*, 177-186.

McKay, M. M., McCadam, K., and Gonzales, J. J. (1996). Addressing the barriers to mental health services for inner city children and their caretakers. *Community Mental Health Journal, 32*, 353-361.

McKay, M. M., Pennington, J., Lynn, C. J., and McCadam, K. (2001). Understanding urban child mental health service use: Two studies of child, family, and environmental correlates. *The Journal of Behavioral Health Services and Research, 28*, 475-483.

McKay, M. M., Stoewe, J., McCadam, K., and Gonzales, J. (1998). Increasing access to child mental health services for urban children and their caregivers. *Health and Social Work, 23*, 9-15.

McMiller, W. P., Weisz, J. R. (1996). Help-seeking preceding mental health clinic intake among African-American, Latino, and Caucasian youths. *Journal of American Academy of Child and Adolescent Psychiatry, 35*, 1086-1094.

McNeil, J. S., and Kennedy, R. (1997). Mental health services to minority groups of color. In T. R.Watkins and J. W. Callicutt. (Eds). *Mental Health Policy and Practice Today* (pp. 235-257). Thousand Oaks, CA: Sage Publications.

Melfi, C., Croghan, T., Hanna, M., and Robinson, R. (2000). Racial variation in antidepressant treatment in a Medicaid population. *Journal of Clinical Psychiatry, 61*, 16–21.

Miller, W. R. and Rollnick, S. (1991). Motivational Interviewing: Preparing People to Change Addictive Behavior. New York, NY: Guilford Press.

Miranda, J., Bernal, G., Lau, A., Kohn, L., Hwang, W., and LaFromboise, T. (2005). State of the science on psychosocial interventions for ethnic minorities. *Annual Review of Clinical Psychology, 1*, 113-142.

Miranda, J., Nakamura, R., and Bernal, G. (2003). Including ethnic minorities in mental health intervention research: A practical approach to a long-standing problem. *Culture, Medicine, and Psychiatry, 27*, 467-486.

Mohammed, S. (2001). Toward an understanding of cognitive consensus in a group decision-making context. *Journal of Applied Behavioral Science, 37*, 408-425.

Mohammed, S., and Dumville, B. C. (2001). Team mental models in a team knowledge framework: Expanding theory and measurement across disciplinary boundaries. *Journal of Organizational Behavior, 22*(2), 89-106.

Mohammed, S., and Ringeis, E. (2001). Cognitive diversity and consensus in group decision making: The role of inputs, processes, and outcomes. *Organizational Behavior and Human Decision Processes, 85*, 310-335.

Morrissey-Kane, E., and Prinz, R. J. (1999). Engagement in Child and Adolescent Treatment: The Role of Parental Cognitions and Attributions. *Clinical Child and Family Psychology Review, 2*, 183-198.

MTA Cooperative Group. (1999). A 14-month randomized clinical trial of treatment strategies for attention-deficit/hyperactivity disorder. *Archives of General Psychiatry, 56*, 1073–1086.

Mukherjee, S., Shukla, S. Woodle, J., Rosen, A. M., and Olarte, S. (1983). Misdiagnosis of schizophrenia in bipolar patients: a multiethnic comparison. *American Journal of Psychiatry, 140,* 1571-1574.

National Center for the Dissemination of Disability Research. (2002). *Disability, Diversity, and Dissemination - The Scope of Concern.* Retrieved May 14, 2003, from http://www.ncddr.org/du/products/dddreview/scope.html.

National Institute of Mental Health (2002). Retrieved online from *www.nimental health.gov on April 15, 2003.*

National Institute of Health (2002). NIH Policy and guidelines on the inclusion of women and minorities as subjects in clinical research – Amended, October, 2001. Retrieved April 5, 2006 from *http://grants.nih.gov/grants/funding/women_min/guidelines_amended_10_ 2001.htm*

National Institutes of Health (1994). NIH guidelines on the inclusion of women and minorities as subjects in clinical research. Retrieved March 9, 2006, from http://grants.nih.gov/grants/policy/emprograms/overview/women-and-mi.htm.

Neighbors, H. W., Jackson, J. S., Campbell, L., and Williams, D. R. (1989). The influence of racial factors on psychiatric diagnosis: a review and suggestions for research. *Community Mental Health Journal, 24,* 301-311.

Neighbors, H. W., Musick, M. A., and Williams, D. R. (1998). The African American minister as a source of help for serious personal crises: Bridge or barrier to mental health care? *Health Education and Behavior, 25*, 759-777.

Ng, C. H. (1997). The stigma of mental illness in Asian cultures. *Australian and New Zealand Journal of Psychiatry, 31*, 382-390.

Nguyen, L., Arganza, G. F., Huang, L. N., Liao, Q., Nguyen, H. T., Santiago, R. (2004). Psychiatric diagnoses and clinical characteristics of Asian American youth in children's services. *Journal of Child and Family Studies, 13*, 483-495.

Nock, M. K., and Kazdin, A. E. (2001). Parent expectancies for child therapy: Assessment and relation to participation in treatment. *Journal of Child and Family Studies, 10*, 155-180.

Novins, D. K., Beals, J., Moore, L. A., Spicer, P., Manson, S. M., and the AI-SUPERPFP Team. (2004). Use of biomedical services and traditional healing options among American Indians: Sociodemographic correlates, spirituality, and ethnic identity. *Medical Care, 42,* 670-679.

Novins, D. K., Feming, C. M., Beals, J., and Manson, S. M. (2000). Quality of alcohol, drug, and mental health services for American Indian children and adolescents. *American Journal of Medical Quality, 15,* 148-156.

Office of Technology Assessment (1986). *Children's mental health: Problems and services – A background paper.* Washington, D. C.: U. S. Government Printing Office.

Okazaki, S. and Sue, S. (1995). Methodological issues in assessment research with ethnic minorities. *Psychological Assessment, 7,* 367-375.

Okazaki, S. (2000). Treatment delay among Asian-American patients with severe mental illness. *American Journal of Orthopsychiatry, 70,* 58-64

Olmedo, E. L. (1981). Testing linguistic minorities. *American Psychologist, 36,* 1078-1085.

Orlandi, M. A. (1995). *Cultural Competence for Evaluators: A Guide for Alcohol and Other Drug Abuse Prevention Practitioners Working with Ethnic/Racial Commun*ities. (2nd ed.). Rockville, MD: U. S. Department of Health and Human Services.

O'Sullivan, M. J., Peterson, P. D., Cox, G. B., and Kirkeby, J (1989). Ethnic populations: Community mental health services ten years later. *American Journal of Community Psychology, 17,* 17-30.

Padilla, A. M. (1980). Acculturation: Theory, Models and Some New Findings. Boulder, CO: Westview Press.

Padilla, A. M. and Medina, A. (1996). Cross-cultural sensitivity in assessment: Using tests in culturally appropriate ways. In L. A. Suzuki, P. J. Meller, and J. G. Ponterotto (Eds.), *Handbook of Multicultural Assessment: Clinical, Psychological, and Educational Applications* (pp. 3-28). San Francisco, CA: Jossey-Bass Publishers.

Pantin, H., Coatsworth, J.D., Feaster, D.J., Newman, F.L., Briones, E., et al. (2003). Familias unidas: the efficacy of an intervention to increase parental investment in Hispanic immigrant families. *Prevention Science, 4,* 189–201.

Paris, M. Jr., Anez, L. M., Bedregal, L. E., Andres-Hyman, R. C., and Davidson, L. (2005). *Journal of Community Psychology, 33,* 299-312.

Peifer, K. L., Hu, T. W., and Vega, W. (2000). Help seeking by persons of Mexican origin with functional impairments. *Psychiatric Services, 51,* 1293-1298.

Pescosolido, B. A. (1992). Beyond rational choice: the social dynamics of how people seek help. *American Journal of Sociology, 97,* 1096-1138.

Pescosolido, B.A. (2001). The role of social networks in the lives of persons with disabilities. In G L. Albrecht, K. D., Seelman and M. Bury (Eds.) *Handbook of Disability Studies* (pp. 468-489). Thousand Oaks, CA: Sage Publications .

Pescosolido, B. A., Monahan, J., Link, B. G.; Stueve, A., and Kikuzawa, S. (1999). The public's view of the competence, dangerousness, and need for legal coercion of persons with mental health problems. *American Journal of Public Health, 89,* 1339-1345.

Phinney, J. S. (1996). Understanding ethnic diversity: The role of ethnic identity. A*merican Behavioral Scientist, 40,* 143-152.

Pickrel, S. G., and Edwars, J. (2004). Multisystemic therapy effects on attempted suicide by youths presenting psychiatric emergencies. *Journal of the American Academy of Child and Adolescent Psychiatry, 43,* 183 –190.

Pinderhughes, E. E., Nix, R., Foster, E. M., Jones, D., and The Conduct Problems Prevention Research Group. (2001). Parenting in context: Impact of neighborhood poverty, residential stability, public services, social networks, and danger on parental behaviors. *Journal of Marriage and the Family, 63,* 941-953.

Pingitore, D., Snowden, L. R., Sansome, R., and Klinkman, M. (2001). Persons with depression and the treatments they receive: A comparison of primary care physicians and psychiatrists. *International Journal of Psychiatry in Medicine, 31,* 41-60.

Porter, N., Garcia, M., Jackson, H., and Valdez, D. (1997). The rights of children in adolescents of color in mental health systems. *Women and Therapy, 20,* 57-74.

Porter, R. (1997). *The greatest benefit to mankind: A medical history of humanity.* New York: Norton.

Poulin, F., Cillessen, A. H. N., Hubbard, J. A., Coie, J. D., Dodge, K. A., and Schwartz, D. (1997). Children's friends and behavioral similarity in two social contexts. *Social Development, 6,* 225-237.

President's New Freedom Commission on Mental Health (2003). *Achieving the Promise: Transforming Mental Health Care in America.* Rockville, MD: President's New Freedom Commission on Mental Health.

Price, C. S. A. and Cuellar, I. (1981). Effects of language and related variables on the expression of psychopathology in Mexican American psychiatric patients. *Hispanic Journal of Behavioral Sciences, 3,* 145-160.

Prinz, R. J. and Miller, G. E. (1994). Family-based treatment for childhood antisocial behavior: Experimental influences on dropout and engagement. *Journal of Consulting and Clinical Psychology, 62,* 645-650.

Pumariega, A. J., Glover, S., Holzer III, C. E., and Nguyen, H. (1998). Utilization of mental health services in a tri-ethnic sample of adolescents. *Community Mental Health Journal, 34,* 145-156.

Pumariega, A. J., Holzer, C. A., and Nguyen, H. (1993). Utilization of mental health services in a tri-ethnic sample of adolescents. In C. Liberton, K. Kutash, and R. Friedman (Eds.), *The Eighth Annual Research Conference Proceedings, A system of* care *for children's mental health: Expanding the research base* (pp. 359364). Tampa: University of South Florida.

Pumariega, A. J., Rogers, K. and Rothe, E. (2005). Culturally competent systems of care for children's mental health: advances and challenges. *Community Mental Health Journal, 41,* 539-555.

Ramos-Sanchez, L. (2001). The relationship between acculturation, specific cultural values, gender, and Mexican American's help-seeking intentions. *Dissertation Abstracts International: Section B: the Sciences and Engineering, 62,* 1595.

Redden, S. C., Forness, S. R., Ramey, S. L., Ramey, C. T., Zima, B. T., Brezausek, C. M., and Kavale, K. A. (1999). Head Start Children at third grade: preliminary special education identification and placement of children with emotional, learning, or related disabilities. *Journal of Child and Family Studies, 8,* 285-303.

Regier, D. A., Narrow, W. E., Rae, D. S., Manderscheid, R. W., Locke, B., and Goodwin, F. K. (1993). The de facto US mental and addictive disorders service system: Epidemiologic catchment area prospective 1-year prevalence rates of disorders and services. *Archives of General Psychiatry, 50,* 85-94.

Reid, M.J., Webster-Stratton, C., and Beauchaine, T.P. (2001). Parent training in Head Start: A comparison of program response among African American, Asian American, Caucasian, and Hispanic mothers. *Prevention Science, 2,* 209–227.

Richardson, L. A. (2001). Seeking and obtaining mental health services: What do parents expect? Archives of Psychiatric Nursing, 15, 233-241.

Roberts, R. E., and Chen, Y. (1995). Depressive symptoms and suicidal ideation among Mexican-origin and Anglo adolescents. *Journal of the American Academy of Child and Adolescent Psychiatry, 34,* 81-90.

Roberts, R. E., and Sobhan, M. (1992). Symptoms of depression in adolescence: a comparison of Anglo, African, and Hispanic Americans. *Journal of Youth and Adolescence, 21,* 639-651.

Ross, L. F., and Walsh, C. (2003). Minority children in pediatric research. *American Journal of Law and Medicine, 29,* 319-336.

Rossello J., and Bernal, G. (1999). The efficacy of cognitive-behavioral and interpersonal treatments for depression in Puerto Rican adolescents. *Journal of Consuling and Clinical Psychology,* 67, 734–45.

Rost, K., Nutting, P., Smith, J., Coyne, J. C., Cooper-Patrick, L., and Rubenstein, L. (2000). The role of competing demands in the treatment provided primary care patients with major depression. *Archives of Family Medicine, 9,* 150-154.

Rowland, M. D., Halliday-Boykins, C. A., Henggeler, S. W., Cunningham, P. B, Lee, T. G., Kruesi, M. J. P., and Shapiro, S. B. (2005). A randomized trial of multisystemic therapy with Hawaii's Felix class youths. *Journal of Emotional and Behavioral Disorders, 13,* 13-23.

Santisteban, D. A., Szapocznik, J., Perez-Videl, A., Kurtines, W. M., Murray, E. J., and LaPerrier, A. (1996). Efficacy of intervention for engaging youth and families into treatment and some variables that may contribute to differential effectiveness. *Journal of Family Psychology,* 10, 35-44.

Scheffler, R. M., and Miller, A. B. (1991). Differences in mental health service utilization among ethnic subpopulations. *International Journal of Law and Psychiatry, 14,* 363-376.

Sclar, D. A., Robison, L. M., Skaer, T. L., and Galin, R. S. (1999). Ethnicity and the prescribing of antidepressant pharmacotherapy: 1992-1995. *Harvard Review of Psychiatry, 7,* 29-36.

Sen, B. (2004). Adolescent propensity for depressed mood and help seeking: Race and gender differences. *Journal of Mental Health Policy and Economics, 7,* 133-145.

Shaffer, D., Fisher, P., Dulcan, M. K., Davies, M., Piacentini, J., Schwab-Stone, M. E., Lahey, B. B., Bourdon, K., Jensen, P. S., Bird, H. R., Canino, G., and Regier, D. A. (1996). The NIMH Diagnostic Interview Schedule for Children Version 2.3 (DISC–2.3): Description, acceptability, prevalence rates, and performance in the MECA study. *Journal of American Academy of Child Adolescent Psychiatry, 35,* 865–877.

Shaffer, D., Fisher, P., Duncan, M. K., Davies, M., Piacentini, J., Schwab-Stone, M. E., Lahey, B. B., Bourdon, K., Jensen, P. S., Bird, H. R., Canino, G., and Regier, D. A. (1996). The Mental Health Diagnostic Interview Schedule for Children Version 2.3 (DISC-2.3): Description, acceptability, prevalence rates, and performance in the MECA study. *Journal of American Academy of Child Adolescent Psychiatry, 35,* 865-877.

Shirk, S. R., and Karver, M. (2003). Prediction of treatment outcomes from relationship variables in child and adolescent therapy: A meta-analytic review. *Journal of Consulting and Clinical Psychology, 71*, 452-464.

Silverman, W.K., Kurtines, W.M., Ginsburg, G.S., Weems, C.F., Lumpkin, P.W., Carmichael D.H., et al. (1999). Treating anxiety disorders in children with group cognitive-behavioral therapy: A randomized clinical trial. *Journal of Consulting and Clinical Psychology, 67*, 995–1003.

Smedley, B.D., Stith, A.Y., Nelson, A.R., (Eds.). (2003) Unequal treatment: Confrontingracial and ethnic disparities in health care. Washington DC: Institute of Medicine, The National Academy Press, 160-179.

Snowden, L. R. (1998). Managed care and ethnic minority populations. *Administrative Policy and Mental Health, 25*, 581-593.

Snowden, L. R. (2001). Barriers to effective mental health services for African Americans. *Mental Health Services Research, 3*, 181-187.

Snowden, L. R., and Cheung, F. K. (1990). Use of inpatient mental health services by members of ethnic minority groups. *American Psychologist, 45,* 347–355.

Snowden, L. R., and Yamada, A. (2005). Cultural differences in access to care. *Annual Review of Clinical Psychology, 1*, 143-166.

Staudt, M. (1999). Barriers and facilitators to use of services following intensive family preservation services. *The Journal of Behavioral Health Services and Research, 26*, 39-49.

Staudt, M. (2003). Helping children access and use services: a review. *Journal of Child and Family Studies, 12*, 49-60.

Stehno, S. M. (1982). Differential treatment of minority children in service systems. *Social Work, 27*, 39-45.

Stiffman, A. R., Horwitz, S. M., Hoagwood, K., Compton, W. I., Cottler, L., Bean, D. L. et al. (2000). The Service Assessment for Children and Adolescents (SACA): Adult and child reports. *Journal of the American Academy of Child and Adolescent Psychiatry, 39*, 1032-1039.

Strakowski, S. M., Hawkins, J. M., Keck, P. E., McElroy, S. L., West, S. A., Bourne, M. L., Sax, K. W., and Tugrul, K. C. (1997). The effects of race and information variance on disagreement between psychiatric emergency service and research diagnoses in first-episode psychosis. *Journal of Clinical Psychiatry, 58,* 457-463.

Sue, S. (1977). Community mental health services to minority groups: Some optimism, some pessimism. *American Psychologist, 32,* 616-624.

Sue, S. (1998). In search of cultural competence in psychotherapy and counseling. *American Psychologist, 53,* 440-448.

Sue, S. (2006). Cultural competency: From philosophy to research and practice. *Journal of Community Psychology, 34*, 237-245.

Sue, S., Fujino, D. C., Hu, L. T., and Takeuchi, D. T., et al. (1991). Community mental health services for ethnic minority groups: A test of the cultural responsiveness hypothesis. *Journal of Consulting and Clinical Psychology, 59,* 533-540.

Sue, D. W., Ivey, A. E., and Pedersen, P. B. (1996). *A theory of multicultural counseling and therapy*. San Francisco: Brooks/Cole Publishing.

Sue, S. and McKinney, H.(1975). Asian Americans in the community mental health care system. *American Journal of Orthopsychiatry, 45,* 111-118.

Sue, S., McKinney, H. L., and Allen, D. B. (1976). Predictors of the duration of therapy for clients in the community mental health system. *Community Mental Health Journal, 12,* 365-375.

Sue, S., and Morishima, J. K. (1982). *The mental health of Asian Americans.* San Francisco: Jossey-Bass.

Sue, S., and Sue, D. W. (1974). MMPI comparisons between Asian- and non-Asian-American students utilizing a university psychiatric clinic. *Journal of Counseling Psychology, 21,* 423-427.

Sussman, L., Robins, L., and Earls, F. (1987). Treatment seeking for depression by black and white Americans. *Social Science and Medicine, 24,* 187-196.

Swartz, M. S., Wagner, H. R., Swanson, J. W., Burns, B. J., George, L. K., and Padgett, D. K. (1998). Comparing use of public and private mental health services: The enduring barriers of race and age. *Community Mental Health Journal, 34,* 133–144.

Szapocznik, J., Santisteban, D., Rio, A., Perez-Vidal, A., Santisteban, D., and Kurtines,W.M. (1989). Family effectiveness training: An intervention to prevent drug abuse and problem behaviors in Hispanic adolescents. *Hispanic Journal of Behavioral Sciences, 11,* 4–27.

Takayama, J. I., Bergman, A. B., and Connell, F. A. (1994). Children in foster care in the State of Washington: Health care utilization and expenditures. *Journal of the American Medical Association, 271,* 1850–1855.

Takeuchi, D. T., Bui, K. V.T., and Kim, L. (1993). The referral of minority adolescents to community mental health centers. *Journal of Health and Social Behavior, 34,* 153-164.

Takeuchi, D. T., Leaf, P. J., and Kuo, H-S. (1988). Ethnic differences in the perception of barriers to help-seeking. *Social Psychiatry and Psychiatric Epidemiology, 23,* 273-280.

Takeuchi, D. T., Mokuau, N., and Chun, C-A. (1992). Mental health services for Asian Americans and Pacific Islanders. *The Journal of Mental Health Administration, 19,* 237-245.

Takeuchi, D. T., and Uehara, E. S. (1996) Ethnic minority mental health services: Current research and future conceptual directions. In. B. L. Levin and J. Petrila (Eds.), *Mental health services: A public health perspective* (pp. 63–80). New York: Oxford University Press.

Tata, S. P. and Leong, F. T. L. (1994). Individualism-collectivism, social-network orientation, and acculturation as predictors of attitudes toward seeking professional psychological help among Chinese Americans. *Journal of Counseling Psychology, 41,* 280-287.

Taylor, R. J., and Chatters, L. M. (1991). Religious life. In J. S. Jackson (Ed.), *Life in black America.* Newbury Park, CA: Sage.

Telles, C., Karno, M., Mintz, J., Paz, G., Arias, M., Tucker, D., and Lopez, S. (1995). Immigrant families coping with schizophrenia: Behavioural family intervention v. case management with a low-income Spanish-speaking population. *British Journal of Psychiatry, 167,* 473-479.

Tirado, M. D. (1996). *Tools for Monitoring Cultural Competence in Health Care.* San Francisco: Latino Coalition for a Healthy California.

Tolan, P. H. and McKay, M. M. (1996). Preventing serious antisocial behavior in inner-city children: An empirically based family intervention program. *Family Relations: Journal of Applied Family and Child Studies, 45,* 148-155.

U. S. Department of Commerce (1999). *Minority Population Growth: 1995-2050.* Washington, D. C.: U. S. Department of Commerce.

U. S. Department of Education (1990). *Elementary and secondary school civil rights survey.* Washington D.C.: author.

U.S. Department of Health and Human Services. (1999). *Mental health: A report of the Surgeon General.* Rockville, MD: U.S. Department of Health and Human Services, Substance Abuse and Mental Health Services Administration, Center for Mental Health Services, National Institutes of Health, National Institute of Mental Health.

U. S. Department of Health and Human Services. (2000). Healthy People 2010 (2nd ed.). With *Understanding and improving health and Objectives for improving health* (2 vols.). Washington, DC: Author.

U.S. Department of Health and Human Services. (2001). *Mental health: Culture, race, and ethnicity - A supplement to mental health: A report of the Surgeon General.* Rockville, MD: U.S. Department of Health and Human Services, Office of the Surgeon General.

U.S. Public Health Service. (2000). *Report of the Surgeon General's conference on children's mental health: A national action agenda.* Washington, D.C.: Department of Health and Human Services.

Uba, L. (1994). *Asian Americans: Personality patterns, identity, and mental health.* New York: Guilford.

Vanderbleek, L. M. (2004). Engaging families in school-based mental health treatment. *Journal of Mental Health Counseling, 26,* 211-224.

Vega, W. A., Kolody, B., Aguilar-Gaxiola, S., and Catalano, R. (1999). Gaps in service utilization by Mexican Americans with mental health problems. *American Journal of Psychiatry, 156,* 928-934.

Vetter, H. M. (2004). Effects of ethnicity and consumer-provider ethnic match on adult client satisfaction with a community mental health center. *Dissertation Abstracts International: Section B: The Sciences and Engineering, 64,* 4069.

Walker, S. (2005). Towards culturally competent practice in child and adolescent mental health. *International Social Work, 48,* 49-62.

Walsh, C., and Ross, L. F. (2003). Are minority children under- or overrepresented in pediatric research? *Pediatrics, 112,* 890-895.

Wang, P. S., Berglund, P., and Kessler, R. C. (2000). Recent care of common mental disorders in the United States. *Journal of General Internal Medicine, 15,* 284–292.

Weisz, J. R., and Weiss, B. (1991). Studying the "referability of child clinical problems. *Journal of Consulting and Clinical Psychology, 59,* 266-273.

Weisz, J. R., Weiss, B., Walter, B. R., Suwanlert, S., Chaiyasit, W., Anderson, W. W. (1988). Thai and American Perspectives on Over- and Undercontrolled Child Behavior Problems: Exploring the Threshold Model Among Parents, Teachers, and Psychologists. *Journal of Consulting and Clinical Psychology, 4,* 601-609.

Wells, K. B., Golding, J. M., Hough, R. L., Burnam, M. A., and Karno, M. (1989). Factors affecting the probability of use of general and medical health and social/community services for Mexican-Americans and non-Hispanic Whites. *Medical Care, 26,* 441-452.

Wenning, K. and King, S. (1995). Parent orientation meetings to improve attendance and access at a child psychiatric clinic. *Psychiatric Services, 46,* 831-833.

Whaley, A. (1997). Ethnic and racial differences in perceptions of dangerousness of persons with mental illness. *Psychiatric Services, 48,* 1328-1330.

Wintersteen, M. B., Mensinger, J. L., and Diamond, G. S. (2005). Do gender and racial differences between patient and therapist affect therapeutic alliance and treatment retention in adolescents? *Professional Psychology: Research and Practice, 36,* 400-408.

Yeh, C. (2002). Taiwanese students' gender, age, interdependent and independent self-construal, and collective self-esteem as predictors of professional psychological help-seeking attitudes. *Cultural Diversity and Ethnic Minority Psychology, 8,* 19-29.

Yeh, M., Eastman, K., and Cheung, M. G. (1994). Children and adolescents in community health centers: Does the ethnicity or the language of the therapist matter? *Journal of Community Psychology, 22,* 153-163.

Yeh, M., Forness, S. R., Ho, J., McCabe, K., and Hough, R. L. (2004). Parental etiological explanations and disproportionate racial/ethnic representation in special education services for youths with emotional disturbance. *Behavioral Disorders, 29,* 348-358.

Yeh, M., Hough, R. L., McCabe, K., Lau, A., and Garland, A. (2004). Parental beliefs about the causes of child problems: Exploring racial/ethnic patterns. *American Academy of Child and Adolescent Psychiatry, 43,* 605-612.

Yeh, M., McCabe, K., Hough, R., Dupuis, D. and Hazen A. (2003). Racial/ethnic differences in parental endorsement of barriers to mental health services for youth. *Mental Health Services Research, 5,* 65-77.

Yeh, M., McCabe, K., Hough, R. L., Lau, A., Fakhry, F., and Garland, A. (2005). Why bother with beliefs? Examining relationships between race/ethnicity, parental beliefs about causes of child problems, and mental health service use. *Journal of Consulting and Clinical Psychology, 73,* 800-807.

Yeh, M., McCabe, K., Hurlburt, M., Hough, R. L., Hazen, A., Culver, S., Garland, A., and Landsverk, J. (2002). Referral sources, diagnoses, and service types of youth in public outpatient mental health care: a focus on ethnic minorities. *Journal of Behavioral Health Services and Research, 29(1),* 45-60.

Yeh, M. and Weisz, J. R. (2001). Why are we here at the clinic? Parent-child (dis)agreement on referral problems at outpatient treatment entry. *Journal of Consulting and Clinical Psychology, 69,* 1018–1025.

Ying, Y. and Miller, L. S. (1992). Help-seeking behavior and attitude of Chinese Americans regarding psychological problems. American Journal of Community Psychology, 20, 549-556.

Young, A. S., Klap, R., Shebourne, C. D., Wells, K.B. (2001). The quality of care for depressive and anxiety disorders in the United States. *Archives of General Psychiatry, 58,* 55–61.

Zane, N., Enomoto, K., and Chun, C.-A. (1994). Treatment outcomes of Asian- and White-American clients in outpatient therapy. *Journal of Community Psychology, 22(2),* 177-191.

Zane, N. and Yeh, M. (2002). The use of culturally-based variables in assessment: Studies on loss of face. K. Kurasaki, S. Okazaki, and S. Sue (Eds.), *Asian American mental health: Assessment theories and methods. International and cultural psychology series.* (pp. 123-138). New York, NY, US: Kluwer Academic/Plenum Publishers.

Zhang, N., and Dixon, D. N. (2003). Acculturation and attitudes of Asian international students toward seeking psychological help. *Multicultural Counseling and Development, 31,* 205-222.

Zhang, A. Y., Snowden, L. R., and Sue, S. (1998). Differences between Asian and White Americans' help seeking and utilization patterns in the Los Angeles area. *Journal of Community Psychology, 26,* 317-326.

Zwaanswijk, M., Verhaak, P. F. M., Bensing, J. M., van der Ende, J., and Verhulst, F. C. (2003). Help seeking for emotional and behavioural problems in children and adolescents: A review of recent literature. *European Child and Adolescent Psychiatry, 12,* 153-61.

In: Racial and Ethnic Disparities in Health and Health Care
Editor: Elene V. Metrosa, pp. 205-217
ISBN 1-60021-268-9
© 2006 Nova Science Publishers, Inc.

Chapter 8

THE IMPACT OF DRUG ABUSE ON POOR AND MINORITY FAMILIES AND CHILDREN

Patrick B. Johnson[*,1]
Department of Human Development and Learning, Dowling College, New York, USA
Micheline Malow-Iroff
Department of Special Education, Manhattanville College, New York, USA

ABSTRACT

This paper provides a brief overview of the devastating impact of drug abuse on many poor and/or minority American families. While all groups experience drug abuse and its negative consequences, research has classified individuals into broad groups that include Native Americans (which include American Indians and Alaska Natives), Hispanics, and African Americans. Within each broad minority grouping, fall many distinct ethnic populations; however for research purposes these groups are placed into these broad categories. Research has found that the adverse health consequences related to drug abuse and the associated violence are experienced disproportionately by members of minority groups. In this paper, drug abuse among the poor and specific minority groups will be examined with the following statements in mind:

- The relatively greater threat of drug use and its consequences for poor and minority adults and youth
- The reduced likelihood of drug abuse treatment and the inferior medical treatment of the poor and minority populations
- The greater risk of drug-related HIV/AIDS infection in these populations
- The developmental complexities observed among children residing in poor and/or minority families and their connections to drug abuse

[*] Correspondence should be with first author at School of Education, Dowling College, Oakdale, New York 11769 or johnsonp@dowling.edu
[1] Preparation of this chapter was supported in part by funds from the Annie Casey Foundation.

INTRODUCTION

This paper provides a brief overview of the devastating impact of drug abuse on many poor and/or minority American families. While all groups experience drug abuse and its negative consequences, research has classified individuals into broad groups that include Native Americans (which include American Indians and Alaska Natives), Hispanics, and African Americans. Within each broad minority grouping, fall many distinct ethnic populations; however for research purposes these groups are organized into broad categories. With this in mind, research has found that adverse health consequences related to drug abuse and its associated violence are experienced disproportionately by members of minority groups including Native Americans (Beauvais, 1998), Hispanics (Caetano, Clark and Tam, 1998; Helzer and Canino, 1992; Sorlie, Backlund, Johnson and Rogot, 1993) and African Americans (Caetano and Kaskutas, 1995; Jones-Webb, 1998; National Institute on Alcohol Abuse and Alcoholism, 2001). Drug abuse among the poor and the three identified minority groups will be examined with the following statements in mind:

- The relatively greater threat of drug use and its consequences for poor and minority adults and youth.
- The reduced likelihood of drug abuse treatment and the inferior medical treatment of the poor and minority populations.
- The greater risk of drug-related HIV/AIDS infection in these populations.
- The developmental complexities observed among children residing in poor and/or minority families and their connections to drug abuse.

DRUG ABUSE AND POOR AND/OR MINORITIES AND ITS CONSEQUENCES

Results from the 2002 National Survey of Drug Use and Health (Substance Abuse and Mental Health Services Administration, 2003) revealed that the rate of current illicit drug use—use within the previous month—among respondents 12 and older was highest among American Indian/Alaska natives (10.1%) and lowest among Asian Americans (3.5%). African-Americans had the second highest rate (9.7%), followed by whites (8.5%), and Hispanics (7.2%). Rates of substance use dependence – defined by the need or desire for the substance, and abuse – improper and/or excessive use, follow a similar pattern. American Indian/Alaska natives possessed the highest rates of dependence and abuse (14.1%), followed in order by African Americans (9.5%), whites (9.3%), and Asians (4.2%). Hispanics were an exception to the pattern of similarity. Although this group was ranked the lowest in current illicit drug use, the Hispanic group was ranked second in overall substance use dependence and abuse following the American Indian/Alaska Native minority grouping with a rate of 10.4%.

The picture with respect to racial/ethnic differences in youth drug use is somewhat more complicated. The National Survey of Drug Use and Health Survey results (Office of Applied Studies, 2004) conducted on individuals 12 years of age and older revealed that American

Indians (12.1%) and biracial Americans (12%) were most involved with drugs while Hispanics (8%) and Asian Americans (3.8%) were least involved. In contrast, Monitoring the Future school-based survey results (Johnston, O'Malley, Bachman, and Schulenberg, 2004), which examined youth in eighth through twelfth grades, revealed African Americans were far less likely than Whites to be involved with drugs while Hispanics generally fell between these two groups. However, in the Monitoring the Future survey, eighth grade Hispanic students reported greater use of almost all categories of drugs while among the twelfth grade students, Hispanics only reported greater crack use and heroin use with a needle. The relatively high dropout rates of Hispanics (Spring, 2004) may account in large measure for their different eighth and twelfth grade patterns of Hispanic students' drug use. In any event, it is clear that illicit drug use certainly is found in relatively high rates among members of each minority group.

Recently research has highlighted the sharp increases in adolescents' nonmedical use of prescription drugs including oxycontin and vicodin (Sung, Richter, Vaughan, Johnson, and Thom, 2005). More specifically, a secondary analyses of National Household Survey data (Office of Applied Studies, 2004) revealed sharper increases among African American youth and youth from lower socioeconomic backgrounds in this category of drug use.

With respect to alcohol use and abuse, results from nationwide surveys have found that rates of current drinking and heavy drinking among adults are most prevalent in the Native American population (Kim, Coletti, Crutchfield, Williams, and Hepler, 1995; Office of Applied Studies, 2004). In addition, interviews with admissions to alcohol treatment centers has revealed that while American Indian respondents reported initiating alcohol use at the earliest mean age (15.1) and Hispanic respondents reported initiating at the latest mean age (19.7). Between these extremes were White respondents (16.6), African American respondents 17.2) and Asian Americans (17.9) (Drug and Alcohol Services Information System, 2002).

Alcohol-related death rates appear to be highest among African-American adults, and alcohol-related mortality rates among Hispanic males are twice as high as non-Hispanic white mortality rates (National Institute on Alcohol Abuse and Alcoholism, 2001). Additionally, Native Americans die from alcohol-related liver disease and cirrhosis more frequently than the rest of the general population in the United States combined (Beauvais, 1998).

Not surprisingly, Hispanic and African-American men also succumb to drug-related death in disproportionate numbers (Harlow, 1990; Schai, 1992). A study of polydrug abuse and mortality rates in New York City, for example, found disproportionately high rates among African-American and Hispanic males (Tardiff, et al., 1996).

Because the Hispanic racial/ethnic category includes many subgroups, studies have also been conducted to determine the extent of subgroup differences in substance use/abuse. Results from the 1999 National Household Survey of Drug Abuse revealed relatively high rates of alcohol use/abuse among both Puerto Rican and Mexican-American respondents, while low rates of alcohol use/abuse were found among Cuban respondents. The survey also revealed relatively high rates of cigarette use in the two largest Hispanic subgroups, Puerto Ricans and Mexican Americans (Substance Abuse and Mental Health Services Administration, 2002). An earlier report on racial/ethnic differences produced by the Office of Applied Studies (1998) revealed similar patterns as Mexican Americans and Puerto Ricans possessed relatively elevated rates of drug use while Cubans and Central Americans possessed relatively attenuated rates compared with the general population.

For Hispanics, one might assume that increasing acculturation would be associated with reduced drug use and related problems. Unfortunately, the opposite pattern has emerged in the literature. Among Hispanics increasing acculturation has been linked to increases in youth and adult smoking (Crespo, Smit, Carter-Pokras and Anderson, 2001; Landrine, Richardson, Klonoff, and Flay, 1994), drug use (Black and Markides, 1993; Epstein, Botvin, and Diaz, 2001; Farabee, Wallisch, and Maxwell, 1995; Rogler, Cortes, and Malgady, 1991), and AIDS risk (Epstein, Dusenbury, Botvin and Diaz, 1994). Thus, even when Hispanics adopt mainstream customs and practices, their drug use and related behaviors do not moderate, nor do they become more comfortable with mainstream health-related structures and services in ways that generate more effective utilization and health benefits (Opler, Ramirez, Dominguez, Fox, and Johnson, 2003).

Interestingly, while African American adults are at relatively high risk of alcohol and drug use, the opposite is generally true of African American youth (Johnston, et al., 2004). The reason(s) for this unfortunate transition remain largely speculative and some researchers suggest that it may be an artifact of the samples employed in different national surveys (Office of Applied Studies, 1998). At the same time, a recent investigation (Johnson, Richter, Kleber, McLellan, and Carise, 2005) suggested that these age shifts may represent a cohort phenomenon with younger generations of African American youth not differing substantially in age of alcohol use onset from other racial/ethnic groups.

The picture with respect to substance abuse and socioeconomic status generally suggests an inverse relation. For example, results from the 2002 National Survey on Drug Use and Health (NSDUH) revealed that while 17.4% of unemployed respondents indicated using an illicit drug in the past month, only 8.2% of full-time employed respondents indicated such use (Substance Abuse and Mental Health Services Administration, 2003). Moreover, while 19.7% of unemployed respondents met criteria for substance dependence/abuse or both, only 10.6% of full-time employed respondents met the same criteria. At the same time, a recent study observed an inverse relation between hospitalization for alcohol-related disorders and socioeconomic status (Hwang, Agha, Creatore, and Glazier, 2005) as individuals hospitalized for such disorders came disproportionately from lower socioeconomic strata.

It is important to bear in mind that considerable overlap has been observed between minority group membership and socioeconomic status (Comer, 1980; Blau, 1981; Substance Abuse and Mental Health Services Administration, 1998). A study examining the links between socioeconomic status, drug use, and depression found that, although there was generally an inverse SES-drug use linkage, the precise nature of the relation depended upon the individual's racial/ethnic background (Goodman, and Huang, 2002). While some researchers have postulated that this relationship and its link to drug abuse is part of an intergenerational selection drift of less adaptable individuals into lower socioeconomic strata, a recent study by Miech and Chilcoat (2005) found evidence that supported a social causation perspective. The position put forth by the social causation perspective is that social conditions give rise to poor functioning and maladaptive behaviors which include drug abuse.

DRUG ABUSE TREATMENT AMONG
POOR AND/OR MINORITY POPULATIONS

According to the Institute on Medicine (IOM) report, *Unequal Treatment: Understanding Racial and Ethnic Disparities in Health Care* (IOM, 2002), "Disparities in health care are among this nation's most serious health care problems. Research has extensively documented the pervasiveness of racial and ethnic disparities." In recent years, attention has shifted in the health research field from documenting minority health disparities to identifying and overcoming disparities in their health treatment access and quality.

Research findings suggest that minority group members are less likely to enter mental health and substance abuse treatment (Cervantes, and Pena, 1998; Woll, 1995), and generally arrive only when their symptoms have reached critical levels (Baker, and Bell, 1999). Minorities are also far more likely to terminate treatment prematurely—before they have had the opportunity to benefit fully from it (Baekeland, and Lundwall, 1975; Pekarik, 1992).

With regard to Hispanic mental health treatment, the Surgeon General's Report suggested that standard mental health treatment may be ineffective or, in some cases, may even exacerbate their presenting symptoms (US Department of Health and Human Services, 1999). A clinical patient study supports this by revealing that the use of standard medical assessment and treatment procedures with Dominican adults initially led to culturally insensitive treatment and increased treatment noncompliance and client dropout (Opler, et al., 2003).

Another way of exploring the relationship between disadvantaged status and drug abuse treatment is to examine the links between insurance status and substance abuse treatment. To the extent that poor Americans and American minority group members are unable to access treatment, they are disproportionately disadvantaged. Researchers (Wu, Kouzis, and Schlenger, 2003) have found that only 9% of uninsured substance-dependent individuals received any treatment in previous years. Non-Hispanic Whites who were uninsured, however, were three times more likely than uninsured African Americans to have received some form of treatment for their substance abuse. Although the uninsured are more likely to possess a drug abuse problem, they are less likely than the insured to receive treatment for it especially if they are African American.

Research once again indicates that minorities are least likely to address the negative health consequences of drug abuse with effective treatment or to overcome these consequences with timely and appropriate medical care (McKay, Rutherford, Cacciola, Kabasakalian-McKay and Alterman, 1996; National Institute on Alcohol Abuse and Alcoholism, 2001). A report by Wells and colleagues (2001) indicated that compared to non-Hispanic Whites, African Americans were much less likely to have access to alcoholism services and that Hispanics received less care and experienced longer delays in obtaining treatment.

The link between drug abuse treatment and the disadvantaged members of society can also be observed in relation to relapse following treatment (Drug and Alcohol Services Information System-DASIS, 2002). For example, 80% of those patients that had received treatment five or more times in the past were currently unemployed. In addition, while 17% of those who had received treatment five or more times were on public assistance, only 8% of new admissions were on public assistance.

HIV/AIDS AND ITS TREATMENT

Minority group members experience a disproportionate burden with respect to HIV/AIDS. Intravenous drug use is one of the two primary routes of contracting HIV/AIDS, the other being sexual contact with infected partners. The chance of contracting AIDS from intravenous drug use is not shared equally by members of all racial/ethnic groups. In 2001, Alan Leshner (2001), then Director of National Institute on Drug Abuse (NIDA), cited research findings indicating that twice as many African American injection drug users developed AIDS as White injection drug users. This occurred despite the fact that there were far more White injection drug users.

While Hispanics and African Americans together constituted only 25% of the country's population in 1999, these two minority groups accounted for approximately 55% of adult AIDS cases. More disturbingly, they also accounted for 82% of pediatric AIDS cases (Center for Disease Control, 2003). Although African Americans make up but 12% of the nation's population, they accounted for 54% of new HIV/AIDS diagnoses in 2002. Of the estimated 385,000 Americans currently living with AIDS, 42% are African American (Villarosa, 2004).

In 2002 almost twice as many African American as White AIDS patients died from the disease (Villarosa, 2004). Among men ages 25-44 African Americans were six times more likely than Whites to die from HIV/AIDS; among women in the same age category, African Americans were 13 times more likely to die from the disease. Researchers speculate that these differences result from later diagnoses, inferior health care treatment, and co-occurring medical complications including heart disease and diabetes.

Again, many of the deaths associated with late diagnosis AIDS are African Americans. Drug abuse may be one reason for the failure to diagnose the disease in a timely fashion. As one African American AIDS patient stated recently, "I had so much heroin and cocaine in my body that I couldn't feel anything, so I had no idea I was sick or not." (Villarosa, 2004). In addition, lack of insurance or inability to pay for treatment may also be involved in the late diagnoses of AIDS among African Americans.

Minority group members are also disadvantaged when it comes to HIV/AIDS treatment. A report by the Institute of Medicine (2002) emphasizes that even in the absence of economic differences between African American and White AIDS patients, African American patients obtain less sophisticated treatment. Highly active, antiretroviral therapy or HAART has been associated with decreased HIV load blood levels, increased CD4+ cell counts, and longer lives (Macalino, et al.,2004). However, a hospital-based study revealed that the homeless, women, substance abusers, and African Americans were less likely to be included in HAART regimen programs in Cook County Hospital in Chicago (Pulvirenti, et al., 2003).

Research findings also reveal that members of "distressed" groups are at increased risk of dropping out of HIV group counseling (Beadnell, et al., 2003). Included among the characteristics of those in such groups were heavy substance abusers and those residing in unstable living arrangements.

DEVELOPMENTAL COMPLEXITIES
AND POOR AND/OR MINORITY CHILDREN

Developmentally children move toward increasing autonomy and self-direction at the same time that their understanding of the world becomes more structured and differentiated. All this occurs within the context of the child's care giving environment, which provides the raw material or data that the child uses to construct a view of self and a view of the world that seem to predict experience (Sameroff, Seifer, Barocas, Zax, and Greenspoon, 1987).

For infants born into poverty, the course of these basic developmental processes may be skewed by pressures on the care-giving environment (Johnson, Nusbaum, Bejarano, and Rosen, 1998). When the resources available to families are limited, both directly and by virtue of support networks that are themselves impoverished and attenuated, an increased amount of energy must be directed toward basic survival issues such as procurement of food and shelter (Okongwu, 1995). Uncertainty about fulfillment of these basic needs, diminished personal control over daily living, and increased vulnerability to victimization combine to restrict the emotional resources available for parenting. At the same time, these forces frequently induce feelings of powerlessness and depression in mothers who must confront them which, in turn, lead in some instances to substance abuse.

At the same time, infants born into these impoverished conditions are also subjected to multiple pressures or stresses that can combine to negatively impact their developmental trajectories. For example, poor children are more likely to experience combinations of the following stressors: parental drug use, divorce, interpersonal conflict, maternal depression, parental health problems, and parent-child conflict. According to Rutter's theory of cumulative stress (1979), as the number of family stressors increases, child maladjustment increases. Drug use represents, but one manifestation of such maladjustment.

Support for the cumulative stress theory comes from a variety of research studies (Forehand, Biggar, and Kotchick, 1998; Luster, and McAdoo, 1994; Sameroff, Seifer, Barocas, Zax, and Greenspan, 1987). These studies support Rutter's empirical finding that increasing the number of family stressors is associated with increasing maladjustment in at-risk children. In fact, Rutter found that increasing the number of family stressors from three to four increased child maladjustment almost four times.

Werner's (1989) intensive longitudinal study indicated that exposure to adverse social conditions is ten times more likely than perinatal complications to result in restricted developmental outcomes. St. Pierre and Layzer (1999) concluded, "...the effects of poverty on homes and communities represent indirect threats to a child's development" (p. 4). These conditions and threats are frequently heightened in the households of drug-abusing mothers. It should be obvious that the cumulative stress theory is also applicable to single mothers who are likely to be exposed to multiple stresses for extended periods of time. It is likely that some of these women use licit or illicit drugs to cope with the pressurized circumstances in which they find themselves (Johnson, Dunlap, and Maher, 1998).

It has been suggested elsewhere that developmental outcomes, including drug use, result from repeated and ongoing transactions between caretakers and children (Sameroff, et al., 1987). Chess and Thomas (1987) demonstrated that it is not the particular characteristics of the child that determine developmental outcomes including the use of illicit drugs, so much as the goodness of fit between the child's endowments and the environment, that is the fit between the child and key individuals in the child's environment including parents, siblings, and teachers. There are many reasons to assume that the fit is often not particularly good between drug-abusing mothers and their drug-exposed infants. Profiles of addicted mothers indicate higher levels of depression and stress and lower levels of self-esteem than in matched non-drug-abusing controls (Fiks, Johnson, and Rosen, 1985; Luthar, D'Avanzo, and Hites, 2003). Furthermore, cocaine-abusing mothers have been found to be less attentive and responsive to their infants (Mayes, Bornstein, Chawarska, Haynes, and Granger, 1996); while addicted mothers hold more negative perceptions of their children (Bernstein, and Hans, 1994).

At the same time, research suggests that the drug-exposed infant is more likely to be characterized as a "difficult baby" using the classic description of Chess and Thomas (1987). The infant often presents a distinctly intense cry, and is irritable and difficult to comfort and console (Lester, et al., 2001). Some of the characteristics may actually represent symptoms of neonatal narcotics abstinence syndrome (Finnegan, 1976). In any event, these characteristics make the task of providing love and responsive care particularly demanding.

Together, these two groups of characteristics, those of the substance-abusing mother and those of the drug-exposed infant, produce a potentially destructive mismatch between the drug-addicted mother's limited emotional resources and the infant's intense care giving needs and demands (Johnson et al., 1998). The tension within the dyad created by this lack of fit or mismatch is likely to limit the mother's emotional responsiveness to her infant.

Drug-exposed children are sometimes characterized as "damaged goods" and abnormal in their interactions with the environment (Johnson et al., 1999). To a great extent, however, many of the characteristics of these children make sense as reactions or adaptations to their experience. Thus, a child whose caregiver is erratic or abusive, as would be the case with many drug-addicted mothers, may well learn not to engage in extended social interactions-there are no models for these interactions in the child's experience, and the interaction carries with it the possibility of negative consequences (Johnson, Bejarano, Nusbaum, and Rosen, 1996). For many drug-exposed children, remaining unengaged and non-communicative is adaptive. So here, normal adaptive processes can result in deviant outcomes (Sameroff, et al.,1987), and the disorders reported in drug-exposed children may in fact reflect the operation of normal developmental processes in response to atypical infant-mother transactions.

At the same time, it is important to understand that the same parenting style may have widely different impacts depending on the circumstances surrounding its use. For example, while authoritarian parenting, characterized by harsh discipline, has frequently been associated with alcohol abuse and anti-social behaviors in Anglo youth (Kandel, 1990), the same parental behavior may exert a positive influence on the substance use of non-Anglo children living in primarily non-Anglo sociocultural environments (Baumrind, 1972; Johnson, and Johnson, 1999).

Importantly, Werner's research (1989) on the impact of poverty and family stressors on at-risk children found that many of these children "...were able to rebound in their twenties and thirties" (p. 110). While this finding is hopeful, other researchers (Forehand, and Wierson, 1993) have suggested that such early stressors often set in motion a destructive set of dynamic circumstances that result in long-term negative consequences for the child's later adjustment. Unfortunately, this is all too often the case with maltreated children who show little resilience possibly because of the cumulative deficits so often characterizing their environments including poverty, discrimination, parental conflict, and psychopathology (Bolger, 2002).

CONCLUSION

The relationship between socioeconomic status and minority group membership has been frequently highlighted in the social sciences. In the present review, we have sought to highlight the specific connections between socioeconomic status, minority group membership, drug abuse and the pernicious effects of this abuse. Drug abuse is disproportionately found among these groups and such abuse can be found relatively early in life, at least among some of these groups including Native Americans and Hispanic males. At the same time, drug abuse exacts devastating health and social costs on poor and minority communities through its relationship to various chronic and ultimately fatal diseases including HIV/AIDS, Hepatitis C and chronic liver disease.

While it is important for researchers and policy makers to be aware of these disproportionate and inequitable linkages, it is probably more important that we redouble our efforts to ameliorate them using a variety of strategies, some focused on drug use prevention and treatment, and others focused on addressing poor living conditions and social discrimination. We fear, however, that less rather than more will be done to enhance the effectiveness of our drug prevention and drug treatment programs especially those aimed specifically at poor and minority children and their families. Some support for this fear can be found in welfare-reform legislation and the reduced funding for social safety network programs such as Women, Infants, and Children or WIC. Let us hope that we are wrong in this regard.

REFERENCES

Baekeland, F., and Lundwall, L. (1975). Dropping out of treatment: A critical review. *Psychological Bulletin, 82*, 738-783.

Baker, F. M., and Bell, C. C. (1999). Issues in the psychiatric treatment of African Americans. *Psychiatric Services, 50*, 362-368.

Baumrind, D. (1972). An exploratory study of socialization effects on black children: Some black-white comparisons. *Child Development, 42*, 261-267.

Beadnell, B., Baker, S., Knox, K., Stielstra, S., Morrison, D.M., Degooyer, E., et al. (2003). The influence of psychosocial difficulties on women's attrition in an HIV-STD prevention program. *AIDS Care, 15*, 807-820.

Beavais, F. (1998). American Indians and alcohol. *Alcohol Health Research World, 22*, 253-259.

Bernstein, V. J., and Hans, S. L., (1994). Predicting the developmental outcome of two-year old children born exposed to methadone: The impact of social-environmental risk factors. *Journal of Clinical Child Psychology, 23*, 349-359.

Black, S.A., and Markides, K.S. (1993). Acculturation and alcohol consumption in Puerto Rican, Cuban American and Mexican American females in the United States. *American Journal of Public Health, 83*, 890-893.

Blau, Z.S. (1981). *Black children/white children: Competence, socialization, and social structure*. New York: Free Press.

Bolger, K.E., and Patterson, C.J. (2003). Sequelae of child maltreatment : Vulnerability and resilience. In S.S. Luthar (Ed.). *Resilience and Vulnerability: Adaptation in the Context of Childhood Adversity*. (pps. 156-181). Cambridge, UK: Cambridge University Press.

Caetano, R., Clark, C. L., and Tam, T. (1998). Alcohol consumption among racial/ethnic minorities: Theory and research. *National Institute on Alcohol Abuse and Alcoholism (NIAAA) Publications, 22*, 233-241.

Caetano, R., and Kaskutas, L. A. (1995). Changes in drinking patterns among Whites, Blacks, and Hispanics, 1984-1992. *Journal of Studies on Alcohol, 56*, 558-565.

Center for Disease Control (2003). Fact Sheet: Racial and Ethnic Disparities in Health Status. http://cdc.gov/od/media/pressrel

Cervantes, R. C., and Pena, C. (1998). Evaluating Hispanic/Latino programs ensuring cultural competence. *Alcoholism Treatment Quarterly, 16*, 109-131.

Chess, S., and Thomas, A. (1987). *Origins and evolution of behavior disorders: From infancy to early adult life*. Cambridge, MA: Harvard University Press.

Comer, J.P. (1988). Educating poor minority children. *Scientific American, 259,* 42-48.

Crespo, C.J., Smit, E., Carter-Pkras, O., and Anderson, R. (2001). Acculturation and leisure-time physical inactivity in Mexican-American adults: Results from the NHANES III, 1988-1994. *American Journal of Public Health, 91*, 1254-1257.

Drug and Alcohol Services Information System (2002). Characteristics of Repeat Admissions to Substance Abuse Treatment. *The DASIS Report* (June).

Drug and Alcohol Services Information System (2002). Characteristics of Primary Alcohol Admissions by Age of First use of Alcohol: 2002, (September).

Epstein, J.A., Botvin, G.J., and Diaz, T. (2001). Alcohol use among Dominican and Puerto Rican adolescents residing in New York City: Role of Hispanic group and gender. *Developmental and Behavioral Pediatrics, 22*, 113-118.

Epstein, J.A., Dusenbury, L., Botvin, G.J., and Diaz, T. (1994). Acculturation, beliefs about AIDS and AIDS education among New York City Hispanic parents. *Hispanic Journal of Behavioral Science, 16*, 342-354.

Farabee, D., Wallisch, L., and Maxwell, J.C. (1995). Substance use among Texas Hispanics. *Hispanic Journal of Behavioral Sciences, 17*, 523-536.

Fiks, K., Johnson, H., and Rosen, T. (1985). Methadone maintained mothers: Three-year follow-up of parental functioning. *International Journal of Addictions, 20*, 651-660.

Finnegan, L. P. (1976). Clinical effects of pharmacological agents on pregnancy and the fetus and the neonate. *Annals of the New York Academy of Science, 281*, 74-89.

Forehand, R., Biggar, H., and Kotchick, B. A. (1998). Cumulative risk across family stressors: Short- and long-term effects for adolescents. *Journal of Abnormal Child Psychology, 26*, 119-128.

Forehand, R., and Wierson, M. (1993). The role of developmental factors in planning behavioral intervention for children: Disruptive behavior as an example. *Behavior Therapy, 24*, 117-141.

Goodman, E. and Huang, B. (2002). Socioeconomic status, depressive symptoms, and adolescent substance use. *Archives of Pediatric and Adolescent Medicine, 156*, 448-453.

Harlow, K.C. (1990). Patterns of rates of mortality from narcotics and cocaine overdose in Texas, 1976-1987. *Public Health Reports, 105*, 455-462.

Helzer, J.E. and Canino, G.J. (1992). Comparative analysis of alcoholism in ten cultural regions. In J.E. Helzer and G.J. Canino (Eds.). *Alcoholism in North America, Europe, and Asia.* (pp.289-308). New York: Oxford University Press.

Hwang, S.W., Agha, M.M., Creatore, M.I. and Glazier, R.H. (2005). Age- and sex-specific income gradients in alcohol-related hospitalization rates in an urban area. *Annals of Epidemiology, 15*, 56-63.

Institute of Medicine (2002). *Unequal Treatment: Understanding Racial and Ethnic Disparities in Health Care.* Washington, D.C.: National Academy Press.

Johnson, B. D., Dunlap, E., and Maher, L. (1998). Nurturing for careers in drug use and crime: Conduct norms for children and juveniles in crack-using households. *Substance Use and Misuse, 33*, 1511-1546.

Johnson, H. L., Nusbaum, B. J., Bejarano, A., and Rosen, T. S. (1999). An ecological approach to development in children with prenatal drug exposure. *American Journal of Orthopsychiatry, 69*, 448-455.

Johnson, P. B., and Johnson, H. L. (1999). Cultural and familial influences that maintain the negative meaning of alcohol. *Journal of Studies on Alcohol, Supplement, 13,* 79-83.

Johnson, P.B., Richter, L., Kleber, H.D., McLellan, A.T., and Carise, D. (2005). Telescoping of gender related behaviors: Gender, racial/ethnic, and age comparisons. *Substance Use and Misuse, 40,* 1139-1151.

Johnston, L. D., O'Malley, P. M., Bachman, J. G., and Schulenberg, J. E. (2004). *Monitoring the Future: National results on adolescent drug use: Overview of key findings, 2003.* (NIH Publication No. 04-5506). Bethesda, MD: U.S. Department of Health and Human Services, Public Health Service, National Institute on Drug Abuse.

Jones-Webb, R. (1998). Drinking patterns and problems among African-Americans: recent findings. *Alcohol Health Research World, 22*, 260-264.

Kandel, D. B. (1990). Parenting styles, drug use, and children's adjustment in families of young adults. *Journal of Marriage and the Family, 52*, 183-196.

Kim, S., Coletti, S.D., Crutchfield, CC., Williams, C. and Hepler, N. (1995). Benefit-cost analysis of drug abuse prevention programs: a macroscopic approach. *Journal of Drug Education, 25*, 111-127.

Landrine, H., Richardson, J.L., Klonoff, E.A., and Flay, B. (1994). Cultural diversity in the predictors of adolescent cigarette smoking: The relative influence of peers. *Journal of Behavioral Medicine, 17*, 331-346.

Leshner, A.I. (2001). Addressing the medical consequences of drug abuse. *NIDA Notes, Director's Column, 15*.

Lester, B., ElSohy, M., Wright, L. L., Smeriglio, V., Verter, J., and Bauer, C. R., et al. (2001). The Maternal Lifestyle Study: Drug use by meconium toxicology and maternal self report. *Pediatrics, 107*, 309-317.

Luster, T., and McAdoo, H. P. (1994). Factors related to the achievement and adjustment of young African American children. *Child Development, 65*, 1080-1094.

Luthar, S.S., D'Avanzo, K., and Hites, S. (2003). Maternal drug abuse versus other psychological disturbances: Risks and resilience among children. In S.S. Luthar (Ed.).

Resilience and Vulnerability: Adaptation in the Context of Childhood Adversity. (pps. 104-129). Cambridge, UK: Cambridge University Press.

Macalino, G. E., Mitty, J. A., Bazerman, L. B., Singh, K., McKenzie, M., and Flanigan, T. (2004). Modified directly observed therapy for the treatment of HIV-seropositive substance users: Lessons learned from a pilot study. *Clinical Infectious Diseases, 38* (Supplement 5), S393-S397.

Mayes, L. C., Bornstein, M. H., Chawarska, K., Haynes, O. M., and Granger, R. H. (1996). Impaired regulation of arousal in 3-month-old infants exposed prenatally to cocaine and other drugs. *Development and Psychopathology, 8,* 29-42.

McKay, J. R., Rutherford, M. J., Cacciola, J. S., Kabasakalian-McKay, R., and Alterman, A. I. (1996). Gender differences in the relapse experiences of cocaine patients. *Journal of Nervous and Mental Disease, 184,* 616-22.

Miech, R., and Chilcoat, H. (2005). Maternal education and adolescent drug use: A longitudinal analysis of causation and selection over a generation. *Social Science and Medicine, 60,* 725-735.

National Institute on Alcohol Abuse and Alcoholism (2001). *Prevention of Alcohol-Related Problems among Adolescents. RFA: AA-01-001.* Alexandria, VA: National Institutes of Health.

Office of Applied Studies. (1998). *Prevalence of substance use among racial and ethnic subgroups in the U.S.* DHHS Publication. Contract # 283-95-0002. Rockville, MD. Web:http//www:samhsa.gov/oas.

Office of Applied Studies. (2004). *Overview of Findings from the 2003 National Survey on Drug Use and Health.* NSDUH Series H-24, DHHS Publication No. SMA 04-3963. Rockville, MD. Web:http//www:samhsa.gov/oas.

Okongwu, A.F. (1995). Looking for the bottom of the ceiling of the basement floor: Single-parent, female-headed families surviving on $22,000 or less. *Urban Anthropology, 24,* 3-4.

Opler, L.A., Ramirez, P., Dominguez, L., Fox, R., and Johnson, P.B. (2003). Rethinking medication prescribing practices in an inner-city Hispanic mental health clinic. *Journal of Psychiatric Practice, 10,* 134-140.

Pekarik, G. (1992). Relationship of clients' reasons for dropping out of treatment to outcome and satisfaction. *Journal of Clinical Psychology, 48,* 91-98.

Pulvirenti, J. J., Glowacki, R., Muppiddi, U., Surapaneni, N., Gail, C., Kohl, B., et al. (2003). Hospitalized HIV-infected patients in the HAART era: A view from the inner city. *AIDS Patient Care and Standards, 17,* 565-573.

Rogler, L. H., Cortes, D.E., and Malgady, R.G. (1991). Acculturation and mental health status among Hispanics. *American Psychologist, 46,* 585-597.

Rutter, M. (1979). Protective factors in children's responses to stress and disadvantage. In W. M. Kent and J. E. Roll (Eds.), *Primary Prevention of Psychopathology: Vol. 3* (pp. 49-74). Hanover, NH: University Press of New England.

Sameroff, A. J., Seifer, R., Barocas, R., Zax, M., and Greenspan, S. (1987). Intelligence quotient scores of 4-year-old children: Social-environmental risk factors. *Pediatrics, 79,* 343-350.

Schai, D. (1992). Mortality associated with drug misuse among blacks in New York City, 1979-1981. *International Journal of Addictions, 27,* 1433-1443.

Sorlie, P. D., Backlund, E., Johnson, N. J., and Rogot, E. (1993). Mortality by Hispanic status in the United States. *Journal of the American Medical Association, 270*, 2464-2468.

Spring, J. (2004). *American Education*. New York: McGraw-Hill Publishing.

St. Pierre, R.G., and Layzer, J.I. (1999). Using home visits for multiple purposes: The Comprehensive Child Development Program. *Future Child, 9*, 134-151.

Substance Abuse and Mental Health Services Administration. (2003). *Results from the 2002 National Survey on Drug Use and Health: National findings.* (Office of Applied Studies, NHSDA Series H022, DHHS Publication No. SMA 03-3836). Rockville, MD.

Sung, H., Richter, L., Vaughan, R.D., Johnson, P.B., and Thom, B. (2005). Nonmedical use of prescription opiods among teenagers in the United States: Trends and correlates. *Journal of Adolescent Health, 37*, 44-51.

Tardiff, K., Marzuk, P.M., and Leon, A.C. (1996). Accidental fatal overdoses in New York City, 1990-1992. *Journal of Drug and Alcohol Abuse, 22*, 135-146.

US Department of Health and Human Services, Center for Mental Health Services. (1999). *Mental Health: A Report of the Surgeon General.* Rockville, MD, National Institute of Mental Health.

Villarosa, L. (2004, August 7). Patients with H.I.V. seen as separated by a racial divide. *New York Times*.

Wells, K., Klap, R., Koike, A., and Sherbourne, C. (2001). Ethnic disparities in unmet need for alcoholism, drug abuse, and mental health care. *American Journal of Psychiatry, 158*, 2027-2032.

Werner, E. E. (1989, April). Children of the Garden Island. *Scientific American, 260*, 106-111.

Woll, C. (1995). *Cultural competence in women's alcohol and drug programs: Addressing cultural diversity in recovery* (Women's Alcohol and Drug Program Services Technical Assistance Training Series). Van Nuys, CA: California Women's Commission on Alcohol and Drug Dependencies.

Wu, L. T., Kouzis, A. C., and Schlenger, W. E. (2003). Substance use, dependence, and service utilization among the US uninsured nonelderly population. *American Journal of Public Health, 93*, 2079-85.

INDEX

J

K

L

M

N

S

T

U

V

W

Y